Anaesthesia:
Review 5

Edited by

Leon Kaufman

MD, FFARCS

Consultant Anaesthetist,
University College Hospital and St Mark's Hospital, London;
Honorary Senior Lecturer, Faculty of Clinical Sciences,
University College, London;
Examiner in Physiology Primary FRCS (Edin);
Formerly Examiner Primary (Pharmacology),
Final FFARCS and MB ChB, London

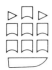

CHURCHILL LIVINGSTONE
EDINBURGH LONDON MELBOURNE AND NEW YORK 1988

CHURCHILL LIVINGSTONE
Medical Division of Longman Group UK Limited

Distributed in the United States of America by
Churchill Livingstone Inc., 1560 Broadway, New
York, N.Y. 10036, and by associated companies,
branches and representatives throughout the world.

First published 1988
  Reprinted 1989

ISBN 0-443-03774-4

British Library Cataloguing in Publication Data

Anaesthesia. — Review 5.
  1. Anaesthesia — Periodicals
  617'.96'05   RD78.3

Produced by Longman Singapore Publishers (Pte) Limited
Printed in Singapore

Preface

The purpose of this Review series has been to select literature which may be relevant to anaesthesia and anaesthetic practice. Readers will have noticed that the presentation may vary from a formal essay to a chapter which contains recent information collated under a wide variety of headings. For a complete review of a particular subject, previous volumes may have to be consulted.

Repetition is unfortunately unavoidable but reflection on material from more than one approach may be beneficial. Thus fluid balance has been considered in the endocrine response to surgery, the colloid-crystalloid controversy and in the influence of hyperglycaemia on ischaemic brain damage, the pathophysiology and treatment of which are also discussed. There are sections on spinal anaesthesia, pain relief which may be influenced by the absorption of analgesic drugs and the place of the computer in anaesthesia. Helpful critics have drawn my attention to omissions of subject material worthy of consideration. The present volume includes problems in cardiac surgery and advances in the pathophysiology and treatment of the adult respiratory distress syndrome, as well as anaesthesia for ENT, ophthalmology, dentistry and obstetrics.

As in previous volumes there is a distinct emphasis on medicine which might be related to anaesthesia, and there is also a chapter on the psychological aspects of surgical operations. A miscellany of subjects from the recent literature is considered in the update chapters.

The relative merits of the Harvard and Vancouver systems of references have been discussed with the publishers, colleagues and many readers and after due consideration it has been decided to continue with the Harvard system.

The success of this series is in no small measure due to the contributors for their enthusiastic participation and for readily accepting editorial comment without resentment. The brunt of the secretarial assistance was shared by Miss S. Wiggins, Miss S. D'Cruz and Mrs M. Pitts, with assistance from Wordstar.

London, 1987   L.K.

Contributors

Bernard Adams MSc FRCP FRCPsych DPM
Consultant Psychiatrist, University College Hospital, London

Nayef R F Al-Rodhan MD
Laboratory of Neurosurgical Research, Mayo Clinic, Rochester, Minnesota, USA

Michael P Barrowcliffe MA FFARCS
Senior Registrar in Anaesthesia, Southampton General Hospital and Royal Hampshire
County Hospital, Winchester

James M Borthwick BSc MB ChB FFARCS
Senior Registrar, Department of Anaesthesia, Royal Hallamshire Hospital, Sheffield

P E R De Silva MB BS FFARCS
Consultant Anaesthetist, Moorfields Eye Hospital, London

William Fitch BSc MB ChB PhD FFARCS MRCP
Reader, University Department of Anaesthesia, Royal Infirmary, Glasgow

R A Harrison MS FRCS
Lecturer, Department of Surgery, University College, London

J Gareth Jones MD FRCP FFARCS
Professor of Anaesthesia, University of Leeds; Honorary Consultant in Anaesthesia, Leeds
General Infirmary

Michael J Jordan MA MB BChir FFARCS
Consultant Anaesthetist, St Bartholomew's Hospital, London

Leon Kaufman MD FFARCS
Consultant Anaesthetist, University College Hospital and St Mark's Hospital, London;
Honorary Senior Lecturer, Faculty of Clinical Sciences, University College, London

J H McClure BSc MB ChB FFARCS
Consultant Anaesthetist, Royal Infirmary, Edinburgh; Honorary Senior Lecturer, University
of Edinburgh

R K Mirakhur MD PhD FFARCS FFARCSI
Consultant Anaesthetist, Royal Victoria Hospital, Belfast

Erling Mjanger MD
Laboratory of Neurosurgical Research, Mayo Clinic, Rochester, Minnesota, USA

Walter S Nimmo BSc MD FRCP FFARCS
Professor of Anaesthesia, University of Sheffield

Adrian Padfield MB BS FFARCS DA
Consultant Anaesthetist, Royal Hallamshire Hospital and Charles Clifford Dental Hospital, Sheffield; Honorary Clinical Lecturer, University of Sheffield

J R Pepper MChir MA MB FRCS
Consultant Cardiothoracic Surgeon, St George's Hospital, London and St Helier Hospital, Carshalton, Surrey

A J Rampton BSc MB BS FFARCS
Lecturer, Anaesthetics Unit, The London Hospital Medical College, London

P J Simpson MD FFARCS
Consultant Anaesthetist, Frenchay Hospital, Bristol

Krystyna Tusiewicz BSc MD FRCP(C) FFARCS
Consultant Anaesthetist, University College Hospital, Shaftesbury Hospital and St Paul's Hospital, London

Duncan Weir BSc MB ChB FFARCS
Senior Registrar in Anaesthetics, Royal Infirmary, Glasgow

J A W Wildsmith MD FFARCS
Consultant Anaesthetist, Royal Infirmary, Edinburgh; Part-time Senior Lecturer, University of Edinburgh

Tony L Yaksh PhD
Laboratory of Neurosurgical Research, Mayo Clinic, Rochester, Minnesota, USA

Contents

Medicine relevant to anaesthesia (1)

CARDIOVASCULAR SYSTEM

Myocardial infarction

Muller et al (1985) deduced from a study of a large number of patients that there was a marked circadian rhythm in the frequency of onset of acute myocardial infarction. The onset of myocardial infarction was assessed objectively by measuring plasma creatine kinase MB(CK-MB). The peak frequency of onset was at 9 a.m. compared with the reduced incidence at 11 p.m. The circadian rhythm was not present in patients receiving beta-adrenergic blocking agents. The use of intravenous beta-blocking agents on selected patients during the early stage of infarction is reasonably safe and may be beneficial (Leading Article Lancet 1986a).

There have been reports that although morphine relieves the pain of myocardial infarction it did have a vagal effect which might produce hypotension. Semenkovich & Jaffe (1985) studied the records of 244 patients with suspected acute myocardial infarction and found only four patients who had temporary hypotension associated with morphine administration. They found no evidence of narcotic-induced conduction defects.

The cardiovascular effects of coffee are due to the caffeine content. Ordinary coffee led to a rise in blood pressure, a fall in heart rate and an increase in plasma catecholamines, whereas decaffeinated coffee induced a smaller increase in diastolic pressure without affecting the other parameters (Smits et al 1985). There was a definite link between the incidence of coronary artery disease and heavy coffee drinkers (La Croix et al 1986).

Smoking as a risk factor has been investigated in survivors of cardiac arrest following resuscitation. It was found that there was a reduced incidence of recurrent cardiac arrest in those patients who had given up smoking. Smoking may also increase the long term atheromatous damage to the coronary vessels (Hallstrom et al 1986).

Congestive cardiac failure

The biochemical basis of myocardial contraction has recently been reviewed by Colucci et al (1986) with an explanation for the rational use of drugs in the management of congestive cardiac failure. Dopamine has actions at alpha, beta and dopaminergic receptor sites as well as releasing endogenous noradrenaline. The main cardiac-stimulating action of dopamine is on the cardiac beta receptors. Dopexamine, a dopamine analogue, stimulates dopamine and beta receptors but not alpha receptors. In contrast to dopamine dopexamine causes an increase in renal blood flow.

Dobutamine is a racemic mixture the l isomer having marked alpha$_1$-adrenergic agonist actions whereas the d isomer is a potent beta$_1$ and beta$_2$ agonist. Dobutamine results in less tachycardia and gives rise to fewer arrhythmias than other sympathomimetic amines. Loss of beta-adrenergic responsiveness is also discussed and it is recommended that treatment should consist of full rather than partial agonists and that administration of the drug should be continuous rather than intermittent.

Pure alpha-adrenergic stimulation results in intense vasoconstriction and is unlikely to be of benefit in the treatment of congestive cardiac failure. In contrast vasodilator drugs, such as hydralazine and isosorbide, when added to existing therapy which includes digoxin and diuretics, lead to an improvement in left ventricular function and decrease mortality (Cohn et al 1986).

The value of drugs such as glucagon and the possibility of H$_2$ agonists appears to be negligible. Drugs which release the endogenous supply of noradrenaline such as metaraminol have also limited value in chronic heart failure. Beta-adrenergic drugs may act by releasing or mimicking the action of cAMP. Phosphodiesterase inhibitors increase cAMP and therefore cardiac contractility. This may explain the action of theophylline and the methylxanthines but these agents do not appear to have achieved much clinical importance. However, Colucci et al (1986) commented that the action of many of the agents outlined above in the treatment of cardiac failure is complex.

Hypertension

The pharmacology of a new alpha$_1$ adrenoceptor antagonist, doxazosin, has been described by Alabaster & Davey (1986). It is long acting and is well tolerated in a daily dose of 1–16 mg. Doxazosin is recommended either as the sole treatment of hypertension or as an adjunct to thiazide diuretics or beta-blockers (Cox et al 1986).

The benefits of treatment with adrenergic blocking agents have mostly been ascribed to their effects on the systemic circulation. It is possible to speculate on their effect on the pulmonary circulation as Guazzi et al (1986) have shown that in systemic hypertension adrenaline and noradrenaline have also vasoconstrictor effects on the pulmonary circulation. The treatment of primary hypertension appears more encouraging with more accurate diagnosis and treatment with vasodilators such as epoprostenol, anticoagulant therapy or possibly even heart-lung transplantation (Leading Article Lancet 1986b).

Angiotensin-converting enzyme (ACE) inhibitors

Captopril

An advantage of angiotensin-converting enzyme inhibitors such as captopril is that they reduce blood pressure without reflex tachycardia. Ajayi et al (1985) suggest that the parasympathetic effect of captopril is a direct consequence of the removal of angiotensin II.

Enalapril

There have been reports of hypotension, renal failure and angioneurotic oedema in association with enalapril. The allergic responses included oedema of the tongue, glottis and larynx leading to respiratory difficulties and have occurred after the first dose of the drug. The manufacturers recommend that enalapril should only be used as a second line of treatment in treatment of hypertension when standard therapy has been ineffective. When used for cardiac failure the patient should be in hospital under close supervision, the recommended dose being reduced for patients over 65. When a diuretic is given in association with the ACE inhibitor the dose should be reduced and renal function closely monitored (Committee on Safety of Medicines 1986).

Pulmonary oedema

Acute pulmonary oedema following myocardial infarction carries a high mortality and may be caused by transient ischaemia rather than acute mycardial infarction or fluid overloading. Treatment of the first group would involve nitrates, beta-blockers and calcium antagonists while the latter groups would require digoxin, diuretics or vasodilators. Kunis et al (1985) reported four patients with recurrent acute pulmonary oedema due to ischaemia and which was refractory to therapy. Coronary bypass surgery was performed successfully resulting in prolonged relief of symptoms.

Postural hypotension

The paraphysiology and management have been reviewed by Bradshaw & Edwards (1986). On standing there is pooling of between 300 ml and 800 ml of blood in the legs and trunk leading to an immediate fall in cardiac output and blood pressure. The baroreceptors in the aortic arch and carotid bodies sense the fall in pressure and impulses are passed to the vasomotor centre via the vagus initiating sympathetic activity resulting in reflex vaso-constriction and an increase in cardiac output. There is an increase in muscle tone on standing which promotes an increase in venous return. There are also hormonal changes with increased release of noradrenaline, antidiuretic hormone and production of aldosterone.

Postural hypotension occurs when the systolic blood pressure falls by 20 mmHg or the diastolic by 100 mmHg on standing. It occurs particularly in the elderly and is thought to be a failure in the composite mechanisms which support blood pressure while standing.

Bradshaw & Edwards (1986) have classified the causes of postural hypotension as follows.

1. The elderly
   Slow or diminished responsiveness of baroreceptors
   'Inefficient' vasomotor centre
   Increased arterial and arteriolar rigidity
   Autonomic dysfunction
   Postprandial hypotension
2. Neurological causes of postural hypotension
   Central lesions
   > Parkinson's disease
   > Shy-Drager syndrome
   > Parasellar and posterior fossa tumours
   > Multiple cerebral infarcts
   > Olivopontocerebellar degeneration
   > Wernicke's encephalopathy
   > Cerebral hypoxia
   > Ageing
   > Drugs
   Peripheral lesions
   a. Cord lesions
   > Tabes dorsalis
   > Syringomyelia
   > Traumatic/inflammatory myelopathy (above T_6)
   > Transverse myelitis
   b. Associated peripheral neuropathy
   > Diabetes mellitus
   > Guillain-Barré syndrome
   > Alcohol
   > Thiamine deficiency
   > Toxic neuropathies
   > Rheumatoid arthritis
   > Idiopathic orthostatic hypotension
   > Porphyria
   > Carcinomatous neuropathy
   > Amyloidosis
   > Dialysis

Extensive sympathectomy
Chagas' disease
Riley-Day syndrome
Pandysautonomia

The cardiovascular causes of postural hypotension are as follows.

1. Low cardiac output
   Arrhythmias
   Cardiac failure
2. Restricted cardiac output
   Aortic stenosis
   Atrial myxoma
   Cardiomyopathy
   Pericardial effusion
   Constrictive pericarditis
3. Hypovolaemia
   a. Absolute hypovolaemia
      Shock
      Blood loss
      Dehydration, diuretic treatment
      Hypoproteinaemia
      Diabetes insipidus
      Salt wasting
   b. Relative hypovolaemia
      (i) Varicose veins
          Hyperlordosis
          Pregnancy
          Hemiplegia
          Parkinsonism
      (ii) Vasodilatation
           Heat
           Hypoxia
           Alcohol
           Paget's disease
           ? Prostaglandins
           Hyperbradykininism

Drugs likely to produce postural hypotension are as follows.

1. Centrally acting
   Levodopa
   Methyldopa
   Clonidine
   Mono-amine oxidase inhibitors
   Tranquillisers
   Sedatives

Hypnotics
Antidepressants
2. Peripherally acting
   Guanethidine
   Bethanidine
   Phentolamine
   Chlorpromazine
3. Vasodilators
   Nitrates
   Prazosin
   Alcohol
4. Diuretics
   Frusemide
   Thiazide diuretics
   Combination of diuretics
5. Others
   Insulin
   Calcium-channel inhibitors

There are also a variety of other miscellaneous disorders including the following.
1. Endocrine disorders
   Addison's disease
   Hypopituitarism
   Myxoedema
   Carcinoid syndrome
2. Hypokalaemia
3. Prolonged bed rest
4. Anaemia
5. Gastrectomy
6. Starvation

Treatment of postural hypotension depends on the cause which may involve extensive investigation. Mechanical methods may be required to decrease pooling for surprisingly raising the head of the bed promotes sodium retention and stimulated renin-angiotensin. Bradshaw & Edwards (1986) also refer to the use of drugs such as 9-alpha-fludrocortisone which acts by increasing the sensitivity of blood vessels to noradrenaline and dihydroergotamine which has powerful alpha-adrenergic receptor activity.

The beta-receptor antagonists such as propranolol are of value in postural hypotension associated with tachycardia whereas other drugs with intrinsic sympathomimetic activity such as pindolol are of value in patients with postural hypotension and supine hypotension. Indomethacin is of value by inhibiting prostaglandin synthesis and also acts as a peripheral vasoconstrictor. Other drugs of value include noradrenaline, phenylephrine, midodrine, prealterol and even metoclopramide.

Anti-arrhythmic drugs

Group 1 — membrane stabilising drugs
Group 2 — beta-blocking agents
Group 3 — drugs prolonging repolarisation (increased duration of action potential)
Group 4 — calcium-channel blocking agents

Group 1. Membrane stabilising drugs

Tocainide is an analogue of lignocaine which makes it more suitable for long term therapy. It decreases the duration of the action potential and the effective refractory period: there is a slight shortening of QT but the QRS is unchanged. It is very effective in the management of ventricular ectopic arrhythmias. No drug interactions have been reported but adverse effects include nausea, vomiting, dizziness, tremors and paraesthesia. A more serious side effect reported has been agranulocytosis and its use is now restricted for life saving ventricular arrhythmias which do not respond to other forms of therapy (Roden & Woosley 1986a).

Flecainide, which has a formula not unlike that of procainamide, prolongs the effective refractory period, has no effect on the action potential duration but increases the PR and QRs intervals. It is effective in the treatment of non-sustained ventricular arrhythmias and its use in patients with sustained ventricular tachycardia may lead to ventricular fibrillation and difficulty in resuscitation. Cimetidine reduces its clearance and there may be interactions with digoxin and propranolol (Roden & Woosley 1986b).

Encainide undergoes extensive first-pass metabolism in the liver producing two metabolites which are active. It might have been thought that hepatic impairment would affect the dosage but in chronic cirrhosis it has been found that although there are increased plasma levels of encainide there are correspondingly less active metabolites produced (Quart et al 1986, Bergstrand et al 1986).

Group 2. Beta-adrenergic blocking agents

Mackay et al (1985) have studied the effects of intrinsic sympathomimetic activity of cardioselective beta-adrenergic blocking agents. Atenolol, a selective beta-blocker without intrinsic sympathomimetic effects, was a potent hypotensive. It also reduced renal plasma flow and urinary sodium excretion. Epanolol, also a cardioselective beta-blocker but with intrinsic sympathomimetic activity, had no effect on renal plasma flow or urinary sodium excretion. Glomerular filtration was unchanged following either drug. It appears that intrinsic sympathomimetic activity is preferred in patients with impaired renal function.

Patakas et al (1983) found that propranolol produced bronchoconstriction on the large and small airways in asthmatics while pindolol only affected the small airways. However in a study of patients with chronic angina pectoris Northcote & Ballantyne (1986) showed there was a marked deterioration of respiratory function following the long term use of propranolol and this was significantly greater than that seen when pindolol was given. There was a significant fall in vital capacity (VC) and FEV_1 after a year of treatment.

Peri-operative administration. The peri-operative use of beta-adrenergic blocking drugs has been recommended prior to surgical procedures. In a study by Magnusson et al (1986) hypertensive patients undergoing cholecystectomy were pretreated with metoprolol for 2 weeks prior to surgery and then given 15 mg intravenously before induction of anaesthesia. Metoprolol significantly reduced the blood pressure during intubation, during the course of anaesthesia and during extubation. However the central venous pressure and the pulmonary arterial occlusion pressure increased markedly in response to surgical stimulation and the authors concluded this may have been due to inadequate anaesthesia. There was profound bradycardia following neostigmine.

Esmolol. An ultra-short-acting cardioselective beta-receptor blocking agent has been found to protect patients with coronary artery disease from fluctuations in blood pressure and heart rate during intubation (Reves & Flezzani 1985). The drug, esmolol is given in a loading dose of 500 μg/kg/min for 4 min followed by a maintenance dose of 300 μg/kg/min during induction and intubation and was found to attenuate tachycardia that results during laryngoscopy and intubation (Murphy et al 1986). The onset of action of esmolol is rapid and the duration short, with a half-life of 9 minutes, being rapidly destroyed by an esterase in the red cell. (Esmolol is available only in the USA from the American Hospital Supplies.)

Group 3. Amiodarone: bretylium

This group was discussed in detail in *Anaesthesia Review 4*. It should be noted that increased plasma levels of drugs such as warfarin may occur in patients being treated with amiodarone.

Group 4. Calcium antagonists

Calcium antagonist drugs interfere with the entry of calcium into cells and have little effect on the release of calcium from intracellular stores. Nifedipine reduces the contractility of smooth muscle especially blood vessels and is of value in the treatment of angina. Verapamil blocks calcium channels that are open or inactive and is effective at the SA and AV nodes. Verapamil is effective in supraventricular cardiac arrythmias whereas diltiazem is effective in both angina and cardiac arrhythmias (Snyder &

Reynolds 1985). Receptor interactions are also discussed in detail by Snyder & Reynolds (1985). Calcium-channel blocking agents are also effective in the treatment of hypertension, hypertrophic cardiomyopathy and pulmonary hypertension. Atrio-ventricular block and cardiac asystole have been reported in patients with pre-existing conduction defects and care must be taken with patients receiving beta-blocking agents. Other adverse effects include hyperglycaemia and hypokalaemia (Kenny 1985).

Gorven et al (1986) reported supraventricular tachycardia and hypotension during intubation in a patient receiving nifedipine and verapamil even though the drugs had been used to control the patient's blood pressure and heart rate prior to surgery. In another study Van Wezel et al (1986) compared nitroglycerine, verapamil and nifedipine in controlling hypertension following sternotomy in patients undergoing cardiac surgery. They concluded that nifedipine compared favourably with nitroglycerine for control of blood pressure but did not recommend the use of verapamil because of its negative inotropic effect and its depressant action on atrioventricular conduction. There are complex pharmacodynamic effects of verapamil especially in the elderly hypertensive. In the elderly there are decreases in heart rate whereas reflex tachycardia is common in the young. Prolongation of the PR interval is less in the elderly while as expected verapamil clearance is reduced (Abernethy et al 1986).

Calcium-channel inhibitors also increase the potency of anaesthetic drugs (Dolin & Little 1986).

A detailed account of the calcium messenger system is discussed in mechanism of disease by Rasmussen (1986a,b). A further account of the role of calcium and ischaemic injury is discussed by Cheung et al (1986). A complete supplement of the *British Journal of Clinical Pharmacology* is devoted to calcium antagonists and their future clinical potential (Reid et al 1986).

Pre-operative assessment

The assessment of cardiac risks and complications in patients requiring non-cardiac surgery was reviewed by Branthwaite (1985). In a further prospective study in geriatric patients undergoing non-cardiac surgery, Gerson et al (1985) found that the best predictor of peri-operative cardiac complications was an exercise test. The inability of the heart rate to rise above 90/min following 2 min of bicycle exercise was more reliable than the Goldman cardiac-risk index in this age group.

Antibiotics are often prescribed for patients who are susceptible to bacterial endocarditis especially for dental procedures but McShane & Hone (1986) have shown a 17% incidence of bacteraemia following nasal intubation and this rose to 21% if a cuffed endotracheal tube was used. The dental factors have been considered by Seldin (1985).

Cardiac surgery

Patients undergoing coronary artery bypass surgery had significantly more neurological changes compared with patients undergoing thoracic or major vascular surgery. This consists of nystagmus, failure of co-ordination, depressed reflexes or transient drowsiness. Psychological changes were present in both groups at 8 days and in a third of all patients this persisted for 8 weeks (Smith et al 1986). They were also concerned that deliberate peroperative hypotension may adversely affect postoperative cerebral blood flow.

In a follow-up study of patients who had developed early postoperative neurological disorders (61% of those having coronary artery bypass graft surgery) approximately 50% still had minor disability at 6 months (Shaw et al 1986). They concluded that long term prognosis following early neurological complications was favourable except for patients who had a major stroke.

Bleeding following cardiopulmonary bypass surgery may require re-exploration of the chest. The haemorrhagic tendency may be due to problems associated with clotting, such as a reduced platelet function or even the use of drugs such as heparin or protamine. Salzman et al (1986) introduced the use of desmopressin acetate (DDAVP), a synthetic analogue of vasopressin that has no vasoconstrictor activity, and found that it reduced the operative and early postoperative blood loss. They suggested this was due to the resulting increase in the plasma level of von Willebrand's factor following the administration of DDAVP.

During surgery for coronary artery bypass there are often episodes of hypertension possibly associated with a release of catecholamines or an increase in plasma renin activity (PRA). Intravenous nitroglycerine or isosorbide was successful in controlling the blood pressure in the pre-bypass phase and in the post-bypass phase while in the postoperative period, nitroglycerine was more effective. The effectiveness of isosorbide could be increased with a bolus dose prior to the infusion or by speeding up the rate of infusion (Thys et al 1986).

Pacemakers

Patients with pacemakers may have to be anaesthetised and it is important to recognise the type of pacemaker that has been inserted. The pacemaker is identified by a five letter code. See Bhatia & Goldschlager (1985), McConachie & Wilkinson (1986) and Shaw & Whistance (1986).

The first letter indicates the chamber that is being paced, e.g. V = Ventricle, A = atrium, D = dual.

The second letter indicates the chamber being sensed, e.g. V = ventricle, A = atrium, D = dual, O = no sensing.

The third letter indicates the mode of response, e.g. T = triggered, I = inhibited, D = dual, O = nil, R = reverse (pacemaker is activated at only fast rates).

The fourth letter indicates the programmable function, e.g. P = programmable for rate and/or output, M = multiprogrammable, C = communicating, O = none.

The fifth letter indicates the type of anti-arrhythmic function, e.g. B = bursts, N = normal rate competition, S = scanning, E = external.

During anaesthesia many authorities insist that diathermy should be limited to short periods only and that halothane and other similar agents should be avoided as they may affect pacemaker threshold. On demand pacemakers (VVI) may be converted to a fixed rate pacemaker by applying a powerful magnet over the pacemaker.

A pacemaker syndrome has been described when patients complain of dizzy spells, chest pain, fatigue, breathlessness, palpitations and postural hypotension. The syndrome occurs during ventricular pacing when there is atrial contraction during ventricular systole. Dual chamber pacing rarely results in the pacemaker syndrome (Ausubel & Furman 1985, Kenny & Sutton 1986).

Deep Venous Thrombosis (DVT)

The incidence of deep vein thrombosis diagnosed by fibrinogen uptake test was found to be 27% (Colditz et al 1986). The prophylactic use of heparin (2500 units before operation and 5000 units thereafter) twice daily for 5 days reduced the incidence to 9.6%. With the use of compression stockings deep vein thrombosis was reduced to 11% while the use of stockings and heparin further reduced the incidence to 6.3%. Low molecular weight heparin given postoperatively and continued for 14 days reduced the incidence of deep vein thrombosis in patients undergoing elective hip surgery without increasing the incidence of bleeding (Turpie et al 1986).

The pre-operative identification of patients liable to develop deep vein thrombosis following major abdominal surgery has been studied by Sue-Ling et al (1986). They produced a predictive index based on age and euglobulin lysis time (ELT) which was able to identify pre-operatively 93% of patients in whom DVT developed. The ELT is a measure of the fibrinolytic activity in the plasma. The use of a predictive index may be helpful in deciding which patients require the prophylactic administration of heparin or dextran which also increases the frequency of haemorrhagic complications.

There have been reports of reduced incidence of deep vein thrombosis following epidural or spinal anaesthesia for hip surgery. Bredbacka et al (1986) compared patients undergoing abdominal hysterectomy either under general anaesthesia or high epidural analgesia. In the patients having epidural analgesia the adrenocortical response was suppressed and the factor VIII complex showed less rise compared with patients having general anaesthesia.

The hypercoagulable state

Hypercoagulability may result from inherited abnormalities of coagulation, be secondary to acquired and be associated with other systemic disease. There are certain conditions where there is an increased incidence of thrombosis such as pregnancy, diabetes, postoperatively and following the use of oral contraceptives. The classification and paraphysiology of the hypercoagulable state have been reviewed by Schafer (1985). The primary coagulable states involve effects in the proteins or fibrinolytic systems. Congenital absence of antithrombin III is one of the most important of the congenital group and is characterised by recurrent attacks of deep vein thrombosis and pulmonary embolism.

Classification of hypercoagulable states

1. Primary
   Antithrombin III deficiency
   Protein C deficiency, protein S deficiency
   Disorders of the fibrinolytic system:
      Hyperplasminogenaemia
      Abnormal plasminogen
      Plasminogen activator deficiency
   Dysfibrinogenaemia
   Factor XII deficiency
   Lupus anticoagulant
2. Secondary
   Abnormalities of coagulation and fibrinolysis:
      Malignancy
      Pregnancy
      Use of oral contraceptives
      Infusion of prothrombin complex concentrates
      Nephrotic syndrome
   Abnormalities of platelets:
      Myeloproliferative disorders
      Paroxysmal nocturnal haemoglobinuria
      Hyperlipidaemia
      Diabetes mellitus
      Heparin-induced thrombocytopenia
   Abnormalities of blood vessels and rheology:
      Conditions promoting venous stasis (immobilisation, obesity, advanced age, postoperative state)

Artificial surfaces
Vasculitis and chronic occlusive arterial disease
Homocystinuria
Hyperviscosity (polycythaemia, leukaemia, sickle cell disease,
  leukoagglutination, increased serum viscosity)
Thrombotic thrombocytopenic purpura

The incidence of thrombosis in patients with malignancy varies between 5% and 50% and may be as high as 50% in prostatic carcinoma. There are increases in plasma levels of fibrinogen, factors VII, VIII, IX and XI, with decreased antithrombin III levels. There may be increased fibrinogen and an increase in fibrinolysis leading to disseminated intravascular coagulation. In the primary hypercoagulable state there is an increased resistance to antithrombotic therapy (Schafer 1985).

Kidney and diuretics

Studies continue to be undertaken on elucidating the mode of action of diuretics on renal function. The loop diuretics inhibit the means by which sodium, potassium and chloride cross cell membranes especially in the ascending loop of Henle. The diuretics inhibit Na-K-2Cl cotransport for which bumetanide has a greater affinity than frusemide. Bumetanide can be used in lower doses (40-fold lower on a mg basis), it has greater potential for improving tubular secretion in renal failure and is less likely to produce side effects such as hypokalaemia, hyperuricaemia, hyperglycaemia and ototoxicity (Feig 1986). Brater (1986) agreed with these findings. Bumetanide is absorbed more rapidly than frusemide and has a higher bioavailability. It has been suggested that bumetanide may reach the site of action via the bloodstream as opposed to the urine, which is of interest in renal failure.

The efficacy of response to frusemide was unaffected in chronic renal failure (Lau et al 1986). In fact those nephrons that are still active have an exaggerated effect to frusemide and there is no need to administer large doses (Brater et al 1986). Studies on the kinetics of bumetanide in patients with chronic renal failure reveal a low renal clearance with a high free fraction which correlated with a decrease in glomerular filtration. There was an increase in non-renal clearance probably by metabolism in the liver and an increase in biliary excretion with a prolonged elimination time ($t\frac{1}{2}$) as a result of increased volume of distribution. The renal failure probably decreased plasma protein binding of bumetanide (Pentikainen et al 1985).

In a review of haemodynamically mediated acute renal failure Myers & Moran (1986) referred to the protecting action of diuretics such as mannitol and frusemide which reduce the severity of renal failure if administered prior to the onset of ischaemic renal damage. Mannitol increased renal blood flow, increased glomerular infiltration rate and there was a high rate of tubular fluid flow. Frusemide lowered preglomerular vascular resistance and increased tubular fluid flow. Extensive hypoxic renal damage is reduced by frusemide (see Epstein 1985). The renal clearance of frusemide decreased in proportion to that of creatinine whereas non-renal clearance and volume of distribution were unchanged. However there was a reduction in the pharmacodynamic response with a reduction in urinary excretion of sodium which was much greater than the reduction in creatinine clearance (Villeneuve et al 1986).

Diuretics may be more effective during bed rest than normal daily activity. Ring-Larsen et al (1986) have shown that 1 mg of bumetanide given intravenously was more effective in supine patients than in those in the upright position. There was a greater sodium and potassium loss and the glomerular filtration rate was higher. The patients were suffering with cirrhosis and congestive cardiac failure and although the plasma concentrations of noradrenaline, renin and aldosterone were raised in the supine position a further significant rise occurred when the patients adopted the upright position.

Diuretics have been known to reduce blood pressure not only by their diuretic effect but also by direct vasodilator action. Not only are there differences of potency between frusemide and bumetanide there are vascular differences. Frusemide can cause significant reduction in forearm blood flow with increases in venous capacity and mean arterial blood pressure. Plasma renin activity increased after frusemide but was unaltered after bumetanide. Neither drug affected aldosterone concentrations (Johnston et al 1986).

There are many other factors controlling glomerular filtration rate, renal blood flow and electrolyte excretion including prostaglandin which is metabolised from arachidonic acid. There are also other products of lipoxygenase and cytochrome P-450 enzymatic activity (Morrison 1986). Drugs such as indomethacin affect the action of loop diuretics. Paracetamol decreased the diuretic effect of frusemide as well as the sodium loss (Abrams et al 1986).

The bioavailability and diuretic effect of frusemide is altered during long term treatment of chronic respiratory failure. The bioavailability was decreased due to enhanced glucuronidation and incomplete drug absorption, which may be associated with alterations in acid base status due to respiratory failure (Ogata et al 1985). Animal studies have shown that hypercarbia and respiratory acidosis together with hypoxaemia decrease the effectiveness of frusemide excretion of sodium and water (Babini & du Souich 1986).

Dopamine infusion in low doses causes an increase in renal blood flow and glomerular filtration rate with loss of sodium and water, the effect being due to stimulation of dopamine receptors in the kidney. Higher doses of dopamine cause an increase in heart rate and blood pressure and renal vasoconstriction affecting alpha and beta adrenoreceptors. Worth et al

(1985) have described a dopamine pro-drug, gamma-L-glutamyl-L-dopa, which is converted to dopamine in the kidney. Their observations also confirm previous studies that renin secretion in the kidney is inhibited by dopamine. Metoclopramide, a dopamine antagonist, in large doses (1–2.5 mg/kg) led to a decrease in renal plasma flow (Israel et al 1986). This finding may be of importance in patients receiving treatment with potentially nephrotoxic agents.

The dangers of diuretics have been repeatedly emphasised. Freis (1986) has suggested that the evidence for this is not supported by recent research studies although serum potassium is reduced by only small reductions in total body stores of potassium. In the absence of digoxin and obvious cardiac disease hypokalaemia does not lead to an increased incidence of ventricular arrhythmias and the prescribing of potassium replacement therapy is unnecessary. The fall in serum potassium may be due to an excess of catecholamines in the bloodstream seen after myocardial infarction. Another possible side effect of thiazide diuretics is a raised serum cholesterol but with long term treatment this reverts to normal. Maronde et al (1986) were concerned however with the low serum potassium following thiazide diuretics which often necessitated the need for supplements of 60–80 mg a day and furthered the use of potassium-sparing diuretics such as amiloride.

REFERENCES

See end of Chapter 2.

Medicine relevant to anaesthesia (2)

RESPIRATION

Assessment of pulmonary function

Pre-operative tests of lung function which would predict postoperative morbidity and mortality have been considered in detail by Gass & Olsen (1986). They confirmed that the incidence of pulmonary complications was greater in thoracic and upper abdominal surgery compared with those occurring after cardiac surgery. This may in part be due to the high degree of postoperative intensive care in most cardiac units. Postoperatively there are significant decreases in vital capacity (VC) even in fit patients but those with chronic obstructive pulmonary disease (COPD) are likely to develop postoperative complications. The maximal expiratory flow rate (MEFR) was considered to be the best spirometric test and levels below 200 l/min were considered to have a poor prognostic outlook. If the FEV_1:FVC was less than 65% and the FVC was less than 70% of the predicted value then the incidence of postoperative pulmonary complications was 100%. For thoracic surgery involving pneumonectomy, patients over 60 years of age with an FEV_1 of less than two litres and an FEV_1:FVC of less 50% also had a poor postoperative prognosis. Gass & Olsen (1986) referred to a study by Miller et al (1981) who were able to assess mortality rates from spirometric data for patients having operations ranging from limited resection of lung to total pneumonectomy. Lung scanning could predict postoperative pulmonary function and a FEV_1 of 0.8–1 litre was considered to be the lower limit of operability.

Breathing and sleep

Although oxygen saturation has been known to fall in patients with sleep apnoea syndrome, ventilation is reduced in a normal population during slow wave (SW) sleep and rapid eye movement (REM) sleep. During SW sleep there was less diaphragmatic contribution to ventilation but this returned to normal during REM sleep. The arterial oxygen saturation fell during both SW and REM sleep and was similar to that seen in patients with chronic airways obstruction (Stradling et al 1985).

Stradling & Phillipson (1986) have reviewed the effect of sleep on breathing in normal patients, in those with chronic obstructive airway disease and in patients with sleep apnoea syndrome. Flenley (1985) in a discussion paper confirmed that obstructive sleep apnoea syndrome can occur in patients with chronic bronchitis and emphysema while Fletcher & Brown (1985) showed that despite tracheostomy in these patients nocturnal oxygen desaturation could still occur. This may be due to long standing right heart strain and hypoxic vasoconstriction. Nasal breathing may be an important factor in maintaining the rhythmicity of ventilation as with increasing age there are more mouth breathers in men than women, and mouth breathing appears to be associated with apnoea during sleep (Gleeson et al 1986). There is a reduction in pharyngeal cross-section in those who snore and this is further reduced in those with sleep apnoea as lung volume falls (Bradley et al 1986).

Patients with idiopathic Parkinson's disease had reduced REM sleep, but hypoventilation did not occur (Apps et al 1985). In patients with Parkinson's disease with autonomic dysfunction, central and obstructive apnoea were frequently present.

Asthma

Asthmatic attacks may occur at night. Shapiro et al (1986) found that asthmatics on being awakened from REM sleep had reduced FEV_1 and reduced peak expiratory flow rates when compared with that when they had been awakened from non-REM sleep. They suggested that as muscle tone increases during rapid eye movement this might affect the tone of the bronchial muscles which is labile in the asthmatic. It is believed that leukotrienes C_4 and D_4 are released from mast cells causing bronchoconstriction and may be involved in the development of asthma (Adelroth et al 1986).

Bronchoconstriction is only one feature of asthma and there are other problems including oedema and inflammation of the bronchial walls, loss of elastic tissue, hypertrophy of the mucous glands, smooth muscle hypertrophy in the bronchi and loss of function of the cilia. Some of these features are associated with chronic airway obstruction (Reed 1986). Newhouse & Dolovich (1986) advocate the use of aerosols in the control of asthma. There are now more accurate aerosol generators producing particles of 1–5 μg provided the inspiratory flow rate is kept below 1 l/s. Prophylaxis with cromoglycate or even a sympathomimetic aerosol are satisfactory. The use of ipratropium, an anticholinergic, gives few side effects and may give greater response with an adrenoreceptor agonist than if the drugs are given separately. The use of steroids in aerosol form results in less adrenal suppression than when given orally and also avoids risk of osteoporosis, hyperglycaemia and fluid retention, features seen with prolonged oral steroid therapy. Easton et al (1986) when comparing the maximum dose of an anticholinergic such as ipratropium with a beta-2-adrenergic agonist (albuterol) found that there was no significant difference between the two in increasing airflow and reducing hyperinflation, and there was little advantage in using one after the other. However they did concede that there might be special circumstances where both agents could be used together.

Respiratory failure

Diaphragmatic function has been studied in patients who were being artificially ventilated for acute respiratory failure. The mean serum phosphorus level was 0.55 ± 18 mmol/l (normal 1.20 ± 0.10). The contractile properties of the diaphragm were reduced but following an infusion of 10 mmol of phosphorus (KH_2PO_4) the diaphragm regained its activity. Respiratory acidosis may have resulted in the low phosphate levels decreasing the activity of the diaphragm (Aubier et al 1985). It has been shown that chlorpromazine caused a marked and statistically significant reduction in breathlessness without affecting ventilation or causing sedation during a progressive exercise test. The use of chlorpromazine therefore offers a distinct advantage to patients dying from malignant disease with breathlessness (O'Neill et al 1985).

Respiratory paralysis following trauma

In patients who have respiratory paralysis following traumatic quadriplegia there is a reduced expiratory reserve volume. In an electromyographic study De Troyer et al (1986) were able to show that these patients accomplished this by maintaining the shoulders in abduction by the active use of the pectoral head of the pectoralis major muscle. They also suggested that by instructing patients to use muscles more efficiently there would be a reduced incidence of pulmonary complications as the effectiveness of coughing would be improved. Increased compliance of the abdominal wall is also a factor in limiting expansion of the lower rib cage (Goldman et al 1986).

Poliomyelitis

Muscle weakness may develop many years after recovery from acute paralytic poliomyelitis. Dalakas et al (1986) followed up 27 patients in whom new muscle weakness developed approximately 30 years after recovery from the initial paralysis. Detailed tests involving muscle biopsy, EMG, virology and immunology suggested that the 'post-polio syndrome' was not life threatening and was due to surviving motor neurones functioning less efficiently.

Pulmonary function and gastro-oesophageal reflux

Although reflux is not uncommon it is not appreciated that there are associated respiratory complications, both in adults and in children. In children apnoea, recurrent respiratory infections or asthma resistant to treatment may be the presenting features, whereas chronic bronchitis, recurrent pneumonia, pulmonary fibrosis and hoarseness can be seen in adults. There are two causes for the pulmonary complications, one being the aspiration of acid gastric contents and the other being reflex brochoconstriction due to irritation of the oesophageal mucosa. The paraphysiology, investigation and treatment are outlined by Barish et al (1985). The application of acid in the oesophagus on pulmonary function has been studied by Andersen et al (1986) who found that the application of 50 ml of 0.1 mol/l hydrochloric acid on the oesophagus resulted in a reduction in expiratory flow and an increase in airway resistance in patients with pre-existing oesophagitis and bronchial asthma. Pretreatment with atropine for 3 days (0.1 ml/kg b.d.) prevented these lung changes, indicating that the bronchoconstriction was mediated by the vagus.

Respiratory distress syndrome

Previous studies have suggested that activated neutrophils cause tissue injury in the lung possibly by producing oxygen metabolites. The neutrophils release lysozyme hydrogen peroxide, a volatile oxygen metabolite. This was measured in patients undergoing mechanical ventilation by Baldwin et al (1986) and found to be significantly raised as was the plasma lysozyme level. The measurement of breath condensate peroxide levels may be a useful test in confirming the diagnosis of adult respiratory distress syndrome (ARDS).

The ratio of oxygen availability to oxygen consumption has been compared in patients with pulmonary oedema from acute congestive heart failure or in those with adult respiratory distress syndrome. Despite the high ratio of oxygen availability to oxygen consumption, patients in the ARDS group died of multi-organ failure, especially renal failure, while those with congestive cardiac failure died of pump failure and low oxygen delivery. ARDS patients die of low oxygen extraction despite adequate cardiac function and availability of oxygen. In ARDS there is not only damage to the pulmonary capillaries but also metabolic problems possibly due to inhibition of enzyme release from the damaged tissues of the lung (Kariman & Burns 1985).

Propranolol

Intravenous propranolol (1–3 mg) led to an increase in arterial oxygen tension probably by decreasing venous admixture associated with a decrease in cardiac output. Propranolol significantly decreased pulmonary shunt in patients who were acutely hypoxic either with pulmonary oedema or atelectasis following surgery. However the depression of cardiac output following propranolol may depress the oxygen delivery to the tissues (Vincent et al 1985).

Peptic ulcer

Respiratory function has been studied in patients with peptic ulceration and it was found that the VC and FEV_1 were significantly reduced in patients with gastric ulcer whether they were smokers or not. Total lung capacity was lower only in smokers. Similar but less severe defects in respiratory function were present in patients with duodenal ulcer (Kellow et al 1986). The reductions in VC and FEV_1 would predispose patients to pulmonary complications following operation.

Crohn's disease

Patients with Crohn's disease may have reduced pulmonary function even though they are clinically free of symptoms. Bonniere et al (1986) found that a high proportion of patients had broncho-alveolar lavage lymphocytosis and had an increased physiological dead space in the upper part of the lung. They also showed that the alveolar macrophages caused an increased production of superoxide anion. Bonniere et al (1986) suggested that these may be the result of some immunological mechanism as lung abnormalities in Crohn's disease appear to be similar to those seen in sarcoid. There are differences as the serum angiotensin-converting enzyme is low in Crohn's disease.

Polycythaemia

The cause of polycythaemia is not often determined but intermittent hypoxic episodes may stimulate erythropoiesis. Five patients developed nocturnal hypoxaemia with the arterial oxygen saturation falling below 92%, the level at which hypoxia stimulates the production of red cells (Moore-Gillon et al 1986).

DIABETES

Diabetes is now considered to be an auto-immune disease and islet-cell antibody screening in combination with glucose tolerance tests is capable of identifying immunologically people with reduced beta cell function who presumably are liable to develop insulin-dependent diabetes (Srikanta et al 1985). In a more detailed review Eisenbarth (1986) suggested there were five stages in the auto-immune process. Stage 1 consisted of genetic susceptibility; stage 2 the triggering process involving either environmental factors or drugs; stage 3 active immunity; stage 4 progressive loss of glucose-stimulated insulin secretion; stage 5 overt diabetes.

There is a high mortality in diabetics following myocardial infarction and Clark et al (1985) have shown that this can be reduced by instituting a regime of continuous infusion of intravenous insulin following the infarction. The incidence of cardiac arrhythmias fell but the biggest improvement in morbidity and mortality was seen in those patients who had been previously on oral hypoglycaemic drugs.

There is impaired hyperaemic response to minor skin trauma in type I diabetes in that there was reduced skin blood flow following minor injury. In the initial stages of diabetes there is an increase in the microvascular perfusion but this later falls. There is capillary hypertension associated with changes in the vessel wall, loss of autoregulation and hyperglycaemia (Tooke 1986). The response was not influenced by diabetic control and may account for the high incidence of ulceration in diabetics following minor trauma (Rayman et al 1986).

During insulin-induced hypoglycaemia plasma volume decreased with an increased loss of intravascular albumin to the extravascular space. Skin temperature decreased significantly 2 hours after the onset of hypoglycaemia (Hilsted et al 1985). Insulin-induced hypoglycaemia also results in increased plasma levels of ACTH, beta-endorphin and cortisol but following cholinergic blockade with atropine (600 μg) the response of ACTH and beta-endorphin were enhanced but the cortisol level was unaffected (Evans et al 1986). The mechanism for the increase in ACTH was thought to be associated with catecholamine release but Cryer & Gerich (1986) questioned whether this is applicable in man.

Autonomic neuropathy

The incidence of diabetic autonomic neuropathy has been reported to be as high as 20–40% (Niakan et al 1986), but the condition may be improved by careful metabolic control and the use of continuous subcutaneous insulin infusion. After 10 days there was some improvement in parasympathetic activity as assessed by the Valsalva manoeuvre. After 4–8 months of treatment there was significant improvement in the response to Valsalva manoeuvre as well as in the response to sustained hand grip and amelioration of postural hypotension. After this time there was no further improvement (Fedele et al 1985).

Stress

Kemmer et al (1986) studied the effects of psychological stress in patients with type 1 diabetes. They found that although stress (such as public speaking or performing mental arithmetic) elevated the systolic and diastolic pressures, raised plasma adrenaline and noradrenaline and caused a rise in plasma cortisol, there were no changes in the circulating levels of glucose, ketones, free fatty acids, glucagon or growth hormone.

Surgery

Hjortrup et al (1985) assessed the influence of diabetes mellitus on operative risks in patients undergoing major vascular surgery, major abdominal surgery and surgery for fracture of the hip. Their findings did not endorse the belief that diabetes itself increases the risks of surgical procedures. Compared with a control group of patients there was no increased incidence of myocardial infarction, thrombosis or embolism, anastomotic leak or wound infection. In fact if anything the incidence was less in diabetic patients with a raised blood sugar compared to those with a blood sugar below 12 mmol/l. Minor surgery can be carried out safely in well controlled non-insulin-dependent diabetic patients without the use of insulin provided that intravenous glucose solutions are not administered during the course of operation (Thompson et al 1986).

Treatment

Mecklenburg et al (1985) assessed the value of insulin pumps over a long period by analysing the trends in glycosylated haemoglobin and concluded that metabolic control was satisfactory. However Knight et al (1985) reported diabetic keto-acidosis during treatment with continuous subcutaneous infusions of insulin, one case of cardiac arrest occurring from hyperkalaemia.

The problems of the 'brittle' diabetic and the management with insulin pumps were discussed in *Anaesthesia Review 4*. Tattersall (1985) has outlined many of the causes of instability of control and drawn attention to the possibility that patients may interfere with their treatment for emotional reasons and emphasised the need for psychiatric assistance. For a detailed study of the mechanisms of blood glucose control see Cryer & Gerich (1985).

Hypoglycaemia

Simonson et al (1985) found that during insulin pump treatment there was a reduced release of hormones that occurs in response to hypoglycaemia. When circulating glucose levels fall below 5–7 mmol/l there is an increased secretion of glucagon and adrenaline which restores glucose levels. The reduced response may be due to a lowering of the threshold at which hypoglycaemia occurs during insulin pump therapy and it may be difficult to detect asymptomatic hypoglycaemia. On the other hand nocturnal hypoglycaemia was noted by Pramming et al (1985) in patients receiving conventional treatment with insulin. Low glycosylated haemoglobin A_{1c} (HbA$_{1c}$) values were reduced and might be used as an indicator of possible hypoglycaemia.

Hypoglycaemia may occur in patients being treated with antimalarial drugs. Parenteral quinidine leads to the release of insulin which may cause hypoglycaemia especially in ill, fasting patients (Phillips et al 1986).

Hyperkalaemia

Hyperkalaemia occurs in untreated diabetic keto-acidosis and is thought to be a cause of death. Serum levels of greater than 6 mmol/l have been reported. The cause for the high serum potassium has usually been ascribed to the metabolic acidosis but it appears that the hyperglycaemia may cause a movement of potassium to the extracellular fluid following the increased cellular tonicity. It appears that the insulin deficiency is the main initiating factor in the hyperkalaemia (see Leading Article Lancet 1986c).

Insulin resistance

The management of the young diabetic on insulin may be beset by difficulties. Amiel et al (1986) found that insulin resistance occurred during puberty in both normal and diabetic children, the response to insulin being inversely related to the level of growth hormone. In addition at the various changes in the child's development the effect of insulin on glucose metabolism was always less in diabetic children. However in newly diagnosed type 1 diabetes in older patients there was often a partial recovery of endogenous insulin secretion leading to apparent clinical remission. Long term diabetic patients had varying degrees of insulin resistance (Yki-Jarvinen & Koivisto 1986). In patients with impaired liver function such as cirrhosis although fasting insulin secretion rates may be increased, the action of the hormone on peripheral tissue is impaired as well as its clearance by the liver (Taylor et al 1986).

Patients with non-insulin-dependent diabetes have been reported to develop resistance to endogenous insulin but a study by Firth et al (1986) concluded that treatment with sulphonylureas (tolazamide) or exogenous insulin showed an equal improvement in the action of insulin and the choice of either of these agents should therefore not be influenced by the possibility of insulin resistance.

Insulin-mediated glucose metabolism may be altered by hepatic microsomal enzymes. Phenobarbitone increased glucose metabolism by 30% while it decreased by almost 20% following cimetidine. These results may explain some of the instances of insulin resistance (Lahtela et al 1986).

Nephropathy

The renin-angiotensin system has been suggested as being involved in the production of diabetic nephropathy. Hommel et al (1986) found that angiotensin II did not influence glomerular filtration rate. In other studies Bjorck (1986) confirmed the value of the use of the angiotensin-converting enzyme inhibitor, captopril, in protecting the kidney from further renal damage. Nine days' treatment with captopril showed that the glomerular filtration was unchanged, whereas the renal plasma flow had increased. After 2 years' treatment the mean arterial blood pressure had fallen and the rate of deterioration of glomerular filtration rate had decreased. The use of drugs such as captopril offers a new line of treatment for diabetic patients on insulin with hypertension and renal damage.

Hypothermia

There is an increased risk of hypothermia developing in elderly patients with diabetes (Neil et al 1986). Although diabetic metabolic problems accounted for some of the episodes of hypothermia there were other causes such as cerebrovascular accident, respiratory tract infection, urinary tract infection and a fall. Other causes were concomitant hypothyroidism, Addison's disease, autonomic neuropathy, congestive cardiac failure and the use of benzodiazepines. The incidence of hypothermia excluding diabetic causes was higher than in the general population.

Diabetes and pregnancy

See Chapter 17.

CENTRAL NERVOUS SYSTEM

Epilepsy

Anticonvulsant therapy with phenytoin affected the half-life of cortisol in the plasma as anticonvulsant therapy resulted in microsomal enzyme induction (Evans et al 1985).

Carcinoid

Neurological complications

Neurological complications of carcinoid tumour occurred in 16% of patients in a series of 219 patients reported by Patchell & Posner (1986). Most of the complications were metastatic resulting in spinal cord compression. Other metastases were intracranial, affecting the meninges and peripheral nerves (the brachial plexus was involved by direct spread while the recurrent laryngeal nerve was affected by the secondaries in the lung). One patient was believed to have carcinoid myopathy. Some patients had encephalopathy associated with liver failure. It was also noted that the carcinoid syndrome was less common when there were metastases in the central nervous system but the secondaries usually responded favourably to radiotherapy.

Treatment

Many of the symptoms of carcinoid syndrome only arise when there are metastases in the liver which is unable to inactivate the excess of hormones released. Oates (1986) has summarised various attempts at treatment including the use of H_1 and H_2 histamine antagonists. Somatostatin is the growth-inhibiting hormone secreted by the pancreas. It is also secreted by the cells of the gastrointestinal tract and the pancreas inhibiting the secretion of insulin, glucagon and pancreatic peptides. Somatostatin was found to inhibit hypertension associated with stimulation of the carcinoid tumour as well as affecting diarrhoea, bronchoconstriction and flushing. Somatostatin had to be administered intravenously but a long acting analogue, SMS 201–995 (Sandoz), given subcutaneously, 150 μg three times a day relieved flushing and diarrhoea and decreased the urinary excretion of 5-hydroxyindoleacetic acid (5-HIAA). No serious side effects have been observed but the mode of action appears to be related to inhibition of serotonin release or synthesis and may possibly involve other amines (Kvols et al 1986). They also referred to the value of SMS 201–995 in preventing crisis during induction of anaesthesia and also the possibility that the drug may reduce the size of hepatic metastases.

Somatostatin analogue has also been used in postprandial hypotension and orthostatic hypotension associated with autonomic neuropathy (Hoeldtke et al 1986). It has also been advocated in the management of upper gastrointestinal haemorrhage, pancreatitis, short bowel syndrome, secretory diarrhoea and Zollinger-Ellison tumours (Mulvihill et al 1986).

Neuroleptic malignant syndrome

In a review of neuroleptic malignant syndrome (NMS) Guze & Baxter (1985) reported an incidence of 0.5–1% of all patients who are given neuroleptic drugs. The abrupt cessation of treatment with anti-Parkinsonian drugs or the use of those which deplete dopamine have been reported to produce NMS. It develops over a period of 24–72 hours and may last for 5 to 10 days even when the drug has been discontinued. The features include hyperthermia, hypertonicity of muscles, fluctuating level of consciousness and autonomic dysfunction. Increased muscle tone may produce rigidity even of the chest wall producing hypoventilation which may require respiratory assistance. The patients may be comatose or agitated. Rigidity is seen and occurs before the rise in temperature which may reach 41°C. Electrolyte levels may suggest dehydration. There is an increase in the white cell count as well as increased levels of transaminase, lactic dehydrogenase and alkaline phosphatase. The creatine kinase is elevated. Renal failure may develop from acute myoglobinuria. Mortality may range from 20% to 30% and is due to cardiovascular, respiratory or renal failure. The differential diagnosis includes heat stroke, catatonia, malignant hyperpyrexia, drug interactions with monoamine oxidase inhibitor or overdose of atropine. Treatment of NMS includes intravenous dantrolene (2–3 mg/kg/day) which may result in liver damage. Oher agents include bromocriptine, amantadine or L-dopa.

Blue et al (1986) described the successful treatment of NMS with sodium nitroprusside. They had a patient who developed NMS following fluphenazine or loxapine. She was treated with intravenous fluids and cooling measures to reduce the body temperature which had risen to 40.5°C. 150 mg of dantrolene were given intravenously every 6 hours with little effect on the patient's temperature. It was noted that the patient had marked peripheral vasoconstriction with a raised diastolic pressure. 3–4 μg/kg of sodium nitroprusside intravenously not only reduced the blood pressure but led to a fall in temperature and any attempt to decrease the amount of nitroprusside infused led to recurrence of the elevated temperature. The nitroprusside presumably reduced body temperature by increasing peripheral vasodilatation and heat loss.

Hyperventilation syndrome (HVS)

The neurological manifestations of the hyperventilation syndrome were reported by Perkin & Joseph (1986). The most frequent symptoms were giddiness, paraesthesia, loss of consciousness and visual disturbances (including blurring of vision, loss of vision, photophobia and flashing lights). Headache, ataxia, tremor and tinnitus were also noted. Dyspnoea and palpitations were frequent as was nausea. HVS may be mistaken for epilepsy but the loss of consciousness is of brief duration. The hypocapnia resulting from hyperventilation leads to cerebral vasoconstriction, alkalosis, a shift in the oxygen dissociation curve, and changes in calcium which lead to paraesthesia. Beta-blockers have been advocated in the treatment.

HISTAMINE (H$_2$) ANTAGONISTS

Ranitidine

Ranitidine is often used in the prophylaxis of stress ulceration. Quadriplegic patients appear to be resistant to the drug but there is no pharmacological reason for this. There is a possibility that injuries to the spinal cord may denervate the sympathetic nerve supply to the stomach allowing unopposed vagal action. The role of the sympathetic in inhibiting acid secretion is still unclear (More et al 1985).

In critically ill patients in intensive care units plasma clearance of ranitidine was reduced probably due to renal impairment. Despite this it was difficult in some patients to maintain the gastric pH above 4 and it may well be that some critically ill patients are resistant to treatment with ranitidine (Ilett et al 1986).

H_2 receptor antagonists are reputed to affect drugs with a high hepatic clearance. Robson et al (1985) have shown that ranitidine only causes a small reduction in splanchnic blood flow.

Cimetidine

Intravenous cimetidine (200 mg) results in a fall in blood pressure and this is due to a reduction in total peripheral resistance. The cause of the hypotension does not appear to be due to a histamine-receptor blocking effect but due to some possible vasodilator cholinergic receptor action in smooth muscle or blood vessels (Totterman et al 1985).

Cimetidine is known to interact with lignocaine and quinidine. The effect of pretreatment with cimetidine on drugs such as lignocaine which are rapidly cleared from the liver is not due to reduction in hepatic blood flow but to inhibition of lignocaine metabolism (Robson et al 1985). Mexiletine, a class I anti-arrhythmic similar to lignocaine given orally in the treatment of chronic ventricular arrhythmias has an incidence of side effects including nausea, vomiting, indigestion, hyperacidity. Oral cimetidine was found to reduce the gastric side effects of acidity without altering the plasma concentration or efficacy of mexiletine (Klein & Sami 1985).

Alcohol

Edwards (1985) has outlined in detail the problems associated with anaesthesia in alcoholics. There are problems associated with diminished adrenocortical response to stress, liver disease, cardiomyopathy and alcohol withdrawal syndrome. Cirrhosis may affect metabolism of drugs as well as affecting the prothrombin time. On the other hand alcoholics may be resistant especially to induction agents such as thiopentone. Close attention should be paid to electrolyte balance, the possibility of hyperkalaemia following suxamethonium and drugs used during the course of anaesthesia which depend on metabolism for their destruction. Postoperatively the alcohol withdrawal syndrome may require management with chlormethiazole or diazepam.

The alcohol withdrawal syndrome which is associated with seizures, hallucinations and delirium appears to have an autonomic component and may respond to beta-blockers such as atenolol (Kraus et al 1985).

REFERENCES

Abernethy D R, Schwartz J B, Todd E L, Luchi R, Snow E 1986 Verapamil
pharmacodynamics and disposition in young and elderly hypertensive patients. Annals of Internal Medicine 105: 329–336

Abrams S M L, Jackson S H D, Johnston A, Turner P 1986 Does paracetamol modify frusemide diuresis? British Journal of Pharmacology 89 (proceedings suppl): 718P

Adelroth E, Morris M M, Hargreave F E, O'Byrne P M 1986 Airway responsiveness to leukotrienes C_4 and D_4 and to methacholine in patients with asthma and normal controls. New England Journal of Medicine 315: 480–484

Ajayi A A, Campbell B C, Meredity P A, Kelman A W, Reid J L 1985; The effect of captopril on the reflex control heart rate: possible mechanisms. British Journal of Clinical Pharmacology 20: 17–25

Alabaster V A, Davey M J 1986 The alpha-1 adrenoceptor antagonist profile of doxazosin: preclinical pharmacology. British Journal of Clinical Pharmacology 21 (suppl 1): 9S–17S

Amiel S A, Sherwin R S, Simonson D C, Lauritano A A, Tamborlane W V 1986 Impaired insulin action in puberty: a contributing factor to poor glycemic control in adolescents with diabetes. New England Journal of Medicine 315: 215–219

Andersen L, Schmidt A, Bundgaard A 1986 Pulmonary function and acid application in the esophagus. Chest 90: 358–363

Apps M C P, Sheaff P C, Ingram D A, Kennard C, Empey D W 1985 Respiration and sleep in Parkinson's disease. Journal of Neurology, Neurosurgery and Psychiatry 48: 1240–1245

Aubier M, Murciano D, Lecocguic Y et al 1985 Effect of hypophosphatemia on diaphragmatic contractility in patients with acute respiratory failure. New England Journal of Medicine 313: 420–424

Ausubel K, Furman S 1985 The pacemaker syndrome. Annals of Internal Medicine 103: 420–429

Babini R, Du Souich P 1986 Furosemide pharmacodynamics: effect of respiratory and acid-base disturbances. Journal of Pharmacology and Experimental Therapeutics 237: 623–628

Baldwin S R, Grum C M, Boxer L A, Simon R H, Ketai L H, Devall L J 1986 Oxidant activity in expired breath of patients with adult respiratory distress syndrome. Lancet 1: 11–14

Barish C F, Wu W C, Castell D O 1985 Respiratory complications of gastroesophageal reflux. Archives of Internal Medicine 145: 1882–1888

Bergstrand R H, Wang T, Roden D M et al 1986 Ecainide disposition in patients with chronic cirrhosis. Clinical Pharmacology and Therapeutics 40: 148–154

Bhatia S, Goldschlager N 1985 Office evaluation of the pacemaker patient. Detection of normal and abnormal pacemaker function. Journal of the American Medical Association 254: 1346–1352

Bjorck S, Nyberg G, Mulec H, Granerus G, Herlitz H, Aurell M 1986 Beneficial effects of angiotensin converting enzyme inhibition on renal function in patients with diabetic nephropathy. British Medical Journal 293: 471–474

Blue M G, Schneider S M, Noro S, Fraley D S 1986 Successful treatment of neuroleptic malignant syndrome with sodium nitroprusside. Annals of Internal Medicine 104: 56–57

Bonniere P, Wallaert B, Cortot A et al 1986 Latent pulmonary involvement in Crohn's disease: biological, functional, bronchoalveolar lavage and scintigraphic studies. Gut 27: 919–925

Bradley T D, Brown I G, Grossman R F et al 1986 Pharyngeal size in snorers, nonsnorers, and patients with obstructive sleep apnea. New England Journal of Medicine 315: 1327–1331

Bradshaw M J, Edwards R T M 1986 Postural hypotension — pathophysiology and management. Quarterly Journal of Medicine 60: 643–657

Branthwaite M A 1985 Assessment of cardiac risks and complications for patients requiring non-cardiac surgery. In: Kaufman L (ed.) Anaesthesia review 3, Churchill Livingstone Edinburgh, 8–14

Brater D C 1986 Disposition and response to bumetanide and furosemide. American Journal of Cardiology 57: 20A–25A

Brater D C, Anderson S A, Brown-Cartwright D 1986 Response to furosemide in chronic renal insufficiency. Rationale for limited doses. Clinical Pharmacology and Therapeutics 40: 134–139

Bredbacka S, Blomback M, Hagnevik K, Irestedt L, Raabe N 1986 Per- and postoperative changes in coagulation and fibrinolytic variables during abdominal hysterectomy under epidural or general anaesthesia. Acta Anaesthesiological Scandinavica 30: 204–210

Cheung J Y, Bonventre J V, Malis C D, Leaf A 1986 Calcium and ischemic injury. New England Journal of Medicine 314: 1670–1676

Clark R S, English M, McNeill G P 1985 Effect of intravenous infusion of insulin in diabetics with acute myocardial infarction. British Medical Journal 291: 303–305

Cohn J N, Archibald D G, Ziesche S et al 1986 Effect of vasodilator therapy on mortality in chronic congestive heart failure. New England Journal of Medicine 314: 1547–1552

Colditz G, Tuden R, Ostler G 1986 Rates of venous thrombosis after general surgery: combined results of randomised clinical trials. Lancet 2: 143–146

Colucci, W S, Wright R F, Braunwald E 1986 New positive inotropic agents in the treatment of congestive heart failure. Mechanisms of action and recent clinical developments (first of two parts). New England Journal of Medicine 314: 290–299

Committee on safety of medicines — current problems 1986 Adverse reactions to enalapril. No 17

Cox D A, Leader J P, Milson J A, Singleton W 1986 The antihypertensive effects of doxazosin: a clinical overview. British Journal of Clinical Pharmacology 21 (suppl 1): 83S–90S

Cryer P E, Gerich J E 1985 Glucose counter regulation, hypoglycaemia, and intensive insulin therapy in diabetes mellitus. New England Journal of Medicine 313: 232–241

Cryer P E, Gerich J E 1986 The sympathochromaffin system and the pituitary-adrenocortical response to hypoglycemia. Science 231: 501

Dalakas M C, Elder G, Hallett M et al 1986 A long-term follow-up study of patients with post-poliomyelitis neuromuscular symptoms. New England Journal of Medicine 314: 959–963

De Troyer A, Estenne M, Hailporn A 1986 Mechanism of active expiration in tetraplegic subjects. New England Journal of Medicine 314: 740–744

Dolin S J, Little H J 1986 The effects of bay K 8644 on the general anaesthetic potencies of ethanol and argon. British Journal of Pharmacology 89 (proceedings suppl): 622P

Easton P A, Jadue C, Dhingra S, Anthonisen N R 1986 A comparison of the bronchodilating effects of a beta-2 adrenergic agent (albuterol) and an anticholinergic agent (ipratropium bromide), given by aerosol alone or in sequence. New England Journal of Medicine 315: 735–739

Edwards R 1985 Anaesthesia and alcohol. British Medical Journal 291: 423–424

Eisenbarth G S 1986 Type I diabetes mellitus. A chronic auto-immune disease. New England Journal of Medicine 314: 1360–1368

Epstein F H 1985 Hypoxia of the renal medulla. Quarterly Journal of Medicine 57: 807–810

Evans P J, Walker R F, Peters J R et al 1985 Anticonvulsant therapy and cortisol elimination. British Journal of Clinical Pharmacology 20: 129–132

Evans P J, Dieguez C, Rees L H, Hall R, Scanlon M F 1986 The effect of cholinergic blockade on the ACTH. B-Endorphin and cortisol responses to insulin-induced hypoglycemia. Clinical Endocrinology 24: 687–691

Fedele D, Bellavere F, Cardone C, Ferri M, Crepaldi G 1985 Improvement of cardiovascular autonomic reflexes after amelioration of metabolic control in insulin-dependent diabetic subjects with severe autonomic neuropathy. Hormone and Metabolic Research, 17: 410–413

Feig P U 1986 Cellular mechanism of action of loop diuretics: implications for drug effectiveness and adverse effects. American Journal of Cardiology 57: 14A–19A

Firth R G, Bell P M, Rizza R A 1986 Effects of tolazamide and exogenous insulin on insulin action in patients with non-insulin-dependent diabetes. New England Journal of Medicine 314: 1280–1286

Flenley D C 1985 Disordered breathing during sleep: discussion paper. Journal of the Royal Society of Medicine 78: 1031–1033

Fletcher E C, Brown D L 1985 Nocturnal oxyhemoglobin desaturation following tracheostomy for obstructive sleep apnea. American Journal of Medicine 79: 35–42

Freis E D 1986 The cardiovascular risks of thiazide diuretics. Clinical Pharmacology and Therapeutics 39: 239–244

Gass G D, Olsen G N 1986 Preoperative pulmonary function testing to predict postoperative morbidity and mortality. Chest 89: 127–135

Gerson M C, Hurst J M, Hertzberg V S et al 1985 Cardiac prognosis in noncardiac geriatric surgery. Annals of Internal Medicine 103: 832–837

Gleeson K, Zwillich C W, Braier K, White D P 1986 Breathing route during sleep. American Review of Respiratory Disease 134: 115–120

Goldman J M, Rose L S, Morgan M D L, Denison D M 1986 Measurement of abdominal wall compliance in normal subjects and tetraplegic patients. Thorax 41: 513–518

Gorven A M, Cooper G M, Prys-Roberts C 1986 Haemodynamic disturbances during anaesthesia in a patient receiving calcium channel blockers. British Journal of Anaesthesia 58: 357–360

Guazzi M D, Alimento M, Fiorentini C, Pepi M, Polese A 1986 Hypersensitivity of lung vessels to catecholamines in systemic hypertension. British Medical Journal 293: 291–294

Guze B H, Baxter L R 1985 Current concepts. Neuroleptic malignant syndrome. New England Journal of Medicine 313: 163–166

Hallstrom A P, Cobb L A, Ray R 1986 Smoking as a risk factor for recurrence of sudden cardiac arrest. New England Journal of Medicine 314: 271–275

Hilsted J, Bonde-Petersen F, Madsbad S et al 1985 Changes in plasma volume, in transcapillary escape rate of albumin and in subcutaneous blood flow during hypoglycaemia in man. Clinical Science 69: 273–277

Hjortrup A, Sorensen C, Dyremose E, Hjortso N C, Kehlet H 1985 Influence of diabetes mellitus on operative risk. British Journal of Surgery 72: 783–785

Hoeldtke R D, O'Dorisio T M, Boden G 1986 Treatment of autonomic neuropathy with a somatostatin analogue SMS-201–995. Lancet 2: 602–605

Hommell E, Parving H-H, Mathiesen E, Edsberg B, Nielsen M D, Giese J 1986 Effect of captopril on kidney function in insulin-dependent diabetic patients with nephropathy. British Medical Journal 293: 467–470

Ilett K F, Nation R L, Tjokrosetio R, Thompson W R, Oh T E, Cameron P D 1986 Pharmacokinetics of ranitidine in critically ill patients. British Journal of Clinical Pharmacology 21: 279–288

Israel R, O'Mara V, Austin B, Bellucci A, Meyer B R 1986 Metoclopramide decreases renal plasma flow. Clinical Pharmacology and Therapeutics 39: 261–264

Johnston G D, Nicholls D P, Kondowe, G B, Finch M B 1986 Comparison of the acute vascular effects of frusemide and bumetanide. British Journal of Clinical Pharmacology 21: 359–364

Kariman K, Burns S R 1985 Regulation of tissue oxygen extraction is disturbed in adult respiratory distress syndrome. American Review of Respiratory Disease 1132: 109–114

Kellow J E, Tao Z, Piper D W 1986 Ventilatory function in chronic peptic ulcer. Gastroenterology 91: 590–595

Kemmer F W, Bisping R, Steingruber H J et al 1986 Psychological stress and metabolic control in patients with type 1 diabetes mellitus. New England Journal of Medicine 314: 1078–1084

Kenny J 1985 Regular review: calcium channel blocking agents and the heart. British Medical Journal 291: 1150–1152

Kenny R A, Sutton R 1986 Pacemaker syndrome. British Medical Journal 293: 902–903

Klein A, Sami M H 1985 Usefulness and safety of cimetidine in patients receiving mexiletine for ventricular arrhythmia. American Heart Journal 109: 1281–1286

Knight G, Jennings A M, Boulton A J M, Tomlinson S, Ward J D 1985 Severe hyperkalaemia and ketoacidosis during routine treatment with an insulin pump. British Medical Journal 291: 371–372

Kraus M L, Gottlieb L D, Horwitz R I, Anscher M 1985 Randomized clinical trial of atenolol in patients with alcohol withdrawal. New England Journal of Medicine 313: 905–909

Kunis R, Greenberg H, Yeoh C B et al 1985 Coronary revascularization for recurrent pulmonary edema in elderly patients with ischemic heart disease and preserved ventricular function. New England Journal of Medicine 313: 1207–1210

Kvols L K, Moertel G, O'Connel M J, Schutt A J, Rubin J, Hahn R G 1986 Treatment of the malignant carcinoid syndrome. Evaluation of a long-acting somatostatin analogue. New England Journal of Medicine 315: 663–666

La Croix A Z, Mead L A, Liang K-Y, Bedell Thomas C, Pearson T A 1986 Coffee consumption and the incidence of coronary heart disease. New England Journal of Medicine 315: 977–982

Lahtela J T, Gachalyi B, Eksyma S, Hamalainen A, Sotaniemi E A 1986 The effect of liver microsomal enzyme inducing and inhibiting drugs on insulin mediated glucose metabolism in man. British Journal of Clinical Pharmacology 21: 19–26

Lau H S H, Hyneck M L, Berardi R R, Swartz R D, Smith D E 1986 Kinetics, dynamics and bioavailability of bumetanide in healthy subjects and patients with chronic renal failure. Clinical Pharmacology and Therapeutics 39: 635–645

Leading Article 1986a Intravenous beta-blockade during acute myocardial infarction. Lancet 2: 79–80

Leading Article 1986b A better outlook in primary pulmonary hypertension? Lancet 1: 1420–1421

Leading Article 1986c Hyperkalaemia in diabetic ketoacidosis. Lancet 2: 845–846

Mackay I G, Macnicol A M, Smith H J, Cumming A D, Watson M L 1985 Intrinsic sympathomimetic activity of cardioselective B-adrenoceptor blockers and effects on renal function. British Journal of Clinical Pharmacology 20: 197–203

McConachie I, Wilkinson K 1986 Pacemaker assessment for junior doctors. British Journal of Hospital Medicine 35: 197–199

McShane A J, Hone R 1986 Prevention of bacterial endocarditis: does nasal intubation warrant prophylaxis? British Medical Journal 292: 26–27

Magnusson J, Thulin T, Werner O, Jarhult J, Thomson D 1986 Haemodynamic effects of pretreatment with metoprolol in hypertensive patients undergoing surgery. British Journal of Anaesthesia 58: 251–160

Maronde R F, Chan L S, Vlachakis N 1986 Hypokalemia in thiazide-treated systemic hypertension. American Journal of Cardiology 58: 18A–21A

Mecklenburg R S, Benson E A, Benson J W et al 1985 Long-term metabolic control with insulin pump therapy: report of experience with 127 patients. New England Journal of Medicine 313: 465–468

Miller J I, Grossman G D, Hatcher C R 1981 Pulmonary function test criteria for operability and pulmonary resection. Surgery, Gynecology and Obstetrics 153: 893–895

Moore-Gillon J C, Treacher D F, Gaminara E J, Pearson T C, Cameron I R 1986 Intermittent hypoxia in patients with unexplained polycythaemia. British Medical Journal 293: 588–590

More D G, Watson C J, Boutagy J S, Shenfield G M 1985 Pharmacokinetics of raniditine in quadriplegics. British Journal of Clinical Pharmacology 20: 166–169

Morrison A R, 1986 Biochemistry and pharmacology of renal arachidonic acid metabolism. American Journal of Medicine 80 (suppl 1A): 3–11

Muller J E, Stone P H, Turi Z G et al 1985 Circadian variation in the frequency of onset of acute myocardial infarction. New England Journal of Medicine 313: 1315–1322

Mulvihill S, Pappas N, Passaro E, Debas H T 1986 The use of somatostatin and its analogs in the treatment of surgical disorders. Surgery 100: 467–473

Murthy M, Hwang T-F, Sandage B W, Laddu A R 1986 Esmolol and the adrenergic response to perioperative stimuli. Journal of Clinical Pharmacology 26 (suppl A): A27–A35

Myers B D, Moran S M 1986 Haemodynamically mediated acute renal failure. New England Journal of Medicine 314: 97–104

Neil H A W, Dawson J A, Baker J E 1986 Risk of hypothermia in elderly patients with diabetes. British Medical Journal 293: 416–418

Newhouse M T, M B Dolovich M B 1986 Current concepts: control of asthma by aerosols. New England Journal of Medicine 315: 870–874

Niakan E N, Harati Y, Comstock J P 1986 Diabetic autonomic neuropathy. Metabolism 35: 224–234

Northcote R J, Ballantyne D 1986 Influence of intrinsic sympathomimetic activity on respiratory function during chronic beta blockade: comparison of propranolol and pindolol. British Medical Journal 293: 97–99

Oates J A 1986 The carcinoid syndrome. New England Journal of Medicine 315: 702–704

Ogata H, Kawatsu Y, Maruyama Y, Machida K, Haga T 1985 Bioavailability and diuretic effect of furosemide during long-term treatment of chronic respiratory failure. European Journal of Clinical Pharmacology 28: 53–59

O'Neill P A, Morton P B, Stark R D 1985 Chlorpromazine — a specific effect on breathlessness? British Journal of Clinical Pharmacology 19: 793–797

Patakas D, Argiropoulou V, Louridas G, Tsara V 1983 Beta blockers in bronchial asthma: effect of propranolol and pindolol on large and small airways. Thorax 38: 108–112

Patchell R A, Posner J B 1986 Neurologic complications of carcinoid. Neurology 36: 745–749

Pentikainen P J, Pasternack A, Lampainen E, Neuvonen P J, Penttila A 1985 Bumetanide kinetics in renal failure. Clinical Pharmacology and Therapeutics 37: 582–588

Perkin G D, Joseph R 1986 Neurological manifestations of the hyperventilation syndrome. Journal of the Royal Society of Medicine 79: 448–450

Phillips R E, Looareesuwan S, White N J et al 1986 Hypoglycaemia and antimalarial drugs. Quinidine and release of insulin. British Medical Journal 292: 1319–1321

Quart B D, Gallo D G, Sami M H, Wood A J J 1986 Drug interaction studies and encainide use in renal and hepatic impairment. American Journal of Cardiology 58: 104C–113C

Pramming S, Thorsteinsson B, Bendtson I, Ronn B, Binder C 1985 Nocturnal hypoglycaemia in patients receiving conventional treatment with insulin. British Medical Journal 291: 376–379

Rasmussen H 1986a The calcium messenger(a). New England Journal of Medicine 314: 1094–1101

Rasmussen H 1986b The calcium messenger(b). New England Journal of Medicine 314: 1164–1170

Rayman G, Williams S A, Spencer P D, Smaje L H, Wise P H, Tooke J E 1986 Impaired microvascular hyperaemic response to minor skin trauma in type I diabetes. British Medical Journal 292: 1295–1298

Reed C E 1986 Aerosols in chronic airway obstruction. New England Journal of Medicine 315: 888–889

Reid J L, Prichard B N C, Bridgman K M (ed.) 1986 Calcium antagonists and their future clinical potential. British Journal of Clinical Pharmacology 21 (suppl 2): 93S–204S

Reves J G Flezzani P 1985 Perioperative use of esmolol. American Journal of Cardiology 56: 57F–62F

Ring-Larsen H, Henriksen J H, Wilken C, Clausen J, Pals H, Christensen N J 1986 Diuretic treatment in decompensated cirrhosis and congestive heart failure: effect of posture. British Medical Journal 292: 1351–1353

Robson R A, Wing L M H, Miners J O, Lillywhite K J, Birkett D J 1985 The effect of ranitidine on the disposition of lignocaine. British Journal of Clinical Pharmacology 20: 170–173

Roden D M, Woosley R L. 1986a Drug therapy: tocainide. New England Journal of Medicine 315: 41–45

Roden D M, Woosley R L 1986b Drug therapy: flecainide. New England Journal of Medicine 315: 36–41

Salzman E W, Weinstein M J, Weintraub R M et al 1986 Treatment with desmopressin acetate to reduce blood loss after cardiac surgery. A double-blind randomized trial. New England Journal of Medicine 314: 1402–1406

Schafer A I 1985 The hypercoagulable states. Annals of Internal Medicine 102: 814–828

Seldin E B 1985 Dental factors in infective endocarditis. Circulation 71: 1093–1094

Semenkovich C F, Jaffe A S 1985 Adverse effects due to morphine sulfate. Challenge to previous clinical doctrine. American Journal of Medicine 79: 325–330

Shapiro C M, Catterall J R, Montgomery I, Raab G M, Douglas N J 1986 Do asthmatics suffer bronchoconstriction during rapid eye movement sleep? British Medical Journal 292: 1161–1164

Shaw D, Whistance T 1986 Clever pacemakers. Hospital Update 12: 843–852

Shaw P J, Bates D, Cartlidge N E F et al 1986 Neurological complications of coronary artery bypass graft surgery: six month follow-up study. British Medical Journal 293: 165–167

Simonson D C, Tamborlane W V, Defronzo R A, Sherwin R S 1985 Intensive insulin therapy reduces counter regulatory hormone responses to hypoglycemia in patients with type 1 diabetes. Annals of Internal Medicine 103: 184–190

Smith P L C, Treasure T, Newman S P et al 1986 Cerebral consequences of cardiopulmonary bypass. Lancet 1: 823–825

Smits P, Thien T, Laar A Van't 1985 The cardiovascular effects of regular and decaffeinated coffee. British Journal of Clinical Pharmacology 19: 852–854

Synder S H, Reynolds I J 1985 Calcium-antagonist drugs: receptor interactions that clarify therapeutic effects. New England Journal of Medicine 313: 995–1002

Srikanta S, Ganda O P, Rabizadeh A, Soeldner J S, Eisenbarth G S 1985 First-degree relatives of patients with type I diabetes mellitus: islet-cell antibodies and abnormal insulin secretion. New England Journal of Medicine 313: 416–464

Stradling J R, Chadwik G A, Frew A J 1985 Changes in ventilation and its components in normal subjects during sleep. Thorax 40: 364–370

Stradling J R, Phillipson E A 1986 Breathing disorders during sleep. Quarterly Journal of Medicine 58: 3–18

Sue-Ling H M, Johnston D, McMahone M J, Philips P R, Davies J A 1986 Pre-operative identification of patients at high risk of deep venous thrombosis after elective major abdominal surgery. Lancet 1: 1173–1178

Tattersall R 1985 Brittle diabetes. British Medical Journal 291: 555–556

Taylor R, Johnston D G, Alberti G M M 1986 Glucose homoeostasis in chronic liver disease. Clinical Science 70: 317–320

Thompson J, Husband D J, Thai A C, Alberti K G M M 1986 Metabolic changes in the non-insulin-dependent diabetic undergoing minor surgery: effect of glucose-insulin-potassium infusion. British Journal of Surgery 73: 301–304

Thys D M, Sivak G, Kaplan J A 1986 The role of isosorbide dinitrate in the treatment of perioperative hypertension. American Heart Journal 110: 273–276

Tooke J E 1986 Microvascular haemodynamics in diabetes mellitus. Clinical Science 70: 119–125

Totterman K, Kupari M, Paakkari I, Nieminen M S 1985 Acute cardiovascular effects of intravenous cimetidine. Acta Medica Scandinavica 217: 277–280

Turpie A G G, Levine M N, Hirsh J et al 1986 A randomized controlled trial of a low-molecular-weight heparin (enoxaparin) to prevent deep vein thrombosis in patients undergoing elective hip surgery. New England Journal of Medicine 315: 925–929

Van Wezel H B, Bovill J G, Schuller J, Gielen J, Hoeneveld M H 1986 Comparison of nitroglycerine, verapamil and nifedipine in the management of arterial pressure during coronary artery surgery. British Journal of Anaesthesia 58: 267–273

Villeneuve J-P, Verbeeck R K, Wilkinson G R, Branch R A 1986 Furosemide kinetics and dynamics in patients with cirrhosis. Clinical Pharmacology and Therapeutics 40: 14–20

Vincent J-L, Lignian H, Gillet J-B, Berre J, Contu E 1985 Increase in PaO_2 following intravenous administration of propranolol in acutely hypoxemic patients. Chest 88: 558–562

Worth D P, Harvey J N, Brown J, Lee M R 1985 Gamma-L-glutamyl-L-dopa is a dopamine pro-drug, relatively specific for the kidney in normal subjects. Clinical Science 69: 207–214

Yki-Jarvinen H, Koivisto V A 1986 Natural course of insulin resistance in type 1 diabetes. New England Journal of Medicine 315: 224–230

3

Psychiatric aspects of surgical operations

A surgical operation is clearly a major event in the life of most people. It has complex emotional connotations. There is the diagnostic build-up, often with procedures which are still ill-understood by the patient, and the involvement in the mysterious environment of the hospital. It involves sudden, new systems of relationships and adjustments to existing ones within the family. It involves the awareness of the threat to life of the disease as well as the disquiet of trusting one's life to the anaesthetist and surgeon. It involves the concern and fantasies about loss, death, mutilation and pain. There is concern about the length of suffering, the prognosis and the ability to cope with the resumption of daily life. Pertinently it involves trust in institutions as well as members of the caring professions, which is all too easy to destroy and difficult to reconstitute. Perhaps it is therefore surprising and encouraging that so many people undergo surgery with so few seemingly severe psychiatric difficulties. According to Knox (1961) one in 1500 surgical procedures are followed by a severe psychiatric reaction, suggesting that if anything surgery acts as a precipitant and not the cause of a disturbance. Nevertheless when psychiatric disturbance does occur pre- or postoperatively staff find themselves taken by surprise and bewildered as to the best treatment. Equally it may be that some patients' problems might have been anticipated and treated more effectively, thereby reducing the burden on the patient and his family.

It is no surprise that major life events can precipitate psychiatric illness. A little reflection however will indicate how difficult this is to prove, for the life event, and this may apply to surgery in particular, may be part of the total crisis through which the patient is going. A few examples may illustrate this. People involved in road traffic accidents have an increased likelihood of having a high blood alcohol and also have an excess of hostility as far as can be measured. Thus the road traffic accident with its trauma and surgery, in itself a major life event, may be compounded with the life difficulties which led to alcohol consumption and increased anger. This, in turn, may be traced back to, say, an unhappy marital situation, and in turn could be related to the onset of a psychiatric change in the patient. The unravelling of these problems is difficult and time consuming. Equally, at crisis points in a patient's life there is a greater incidence of disease, several of which will include those requiring surgery. Certain surgical procedures may indeed be sought at times of emotional disturbance, for example plastic operations on the face or breasts. It has been suggested too, that even operations for varicosities are performed at times of marital stress rather than at times of worsening of the varicose veins. It should be stressed that whatever the medical 'reality' about the severity of the operation, it is probably the patient's concept of the operation that is most often pertinent. What may be a minor, 'routine' procedure to the nursing or medical profession can be endowed with terror for the patient.

Therefore, although there must be little doubt that the surgical intervention produces its own physiological and psychological disturbance, it may be part of a more general psychiatric problem which may, unfortunately, only become overt postoperatively. It follows that it is important to look not only at the 'effect of the operation' on the patient as though this was a random and independent outside stimulus, but also to examine some of the psychiatric illnesses and personality traits which may contribute not only to the production of the abnormality requiring surgery, but also shape the patient's response to it. This last will be the major concern of this review.

SURGERY AS A STRESSFUL LIFE EVENT

There has been an increasing awareness that significant life events such as marriage, a new job, having a child and bereavement precede the onset of illness. Early work revealed this association for psychosomatic illness (Paykel 1974) and subarachnoid haemorrhage (Penrose 1972). This is not the place to review the psychological mechanisms behind this, but to draw attention to the possibility that surgery may act in a similarly stressful way to precede the onset of other illness such as depression, schizophrenia and psychosomatic disorders. Predictably therefore the reduction, however minimal, of the physical and emotional aspects of operations will reduce postoperative morbidity, and would decrease the disease effect of the operation for several months. 'No one can practice medicine without being almost appalled at the number of times thinking back on an organic physical illness, how often some emotional or mental upset has occurred which has seemed to trigger off this illness' (Anderson 1977). It is vital therefore that the emotional and mental upset of surgical treatment is minimised, not only to reduce physical disease in the months following operation, but also psychiatric disorders. For the majority of people the onset of an abnormal bodily sensation, a symptom to be complained about, has two aspects. First the degree of unpleasantness in the symptom, i.e. the severity of the pain or vertigo or haemorrhage, and second the fear engendered by the imaginative leap into self diagnosis. Often these are inversely related — the more severe the pain the more it 'concentrates the mind' leaving little room for fear, only a longing for relief. The pain that occasionally nags may leave more time for cancerophobic speculation. Anxious feelings are therefore an integral part of illness for most people. This will of course be related to the fantasies about the disease. The late Clark-Kennedy always asked the outpatient what he himself thought was wrong, and in this way began to tap the patient's worries and concerns. These will increase with the time taken for investigation to be performed and processed, and in response to doubts expressed overtly or covertly by the doctors and nurses, especially if the patient detects a real or apparent divergence of opinion. All these factors clearly must influence the extent and duration of the stressful experience. It is in this context that the efficiency of the hospital service becomes of paramount importance, the speed at which information about investigations is made available to the medical team and the facility with which communication occurs between members of that team. These are very much related to the general ward atmosphere and Ley (1977), in a discussion about patient's compliance with drug therapy in particular, pointed out that the anxieties, expectations and diagnosis should all be discussed in a friendly and discursive way. From an analogous situation in psychiatry it seems best to try and incorporate the patient in the team grappling with the problems that beset him. There is little doubt, however, that patients are often relieved at being able to put all their anxious doubts onto the doctor, adopting the role of helplessness in the face of the all powerful, all knowing medical profession. Although this may produce an immediate lessening of the anxious feelings, it may then result in angry resentment later that no consultation occurred and that the hospital 'did not tell me anything'. It may progress further so that the patient becomes quite regressed in behaviour, in this way engendering another fear, that of the loss of control over his own emotional state. All these aspects in behaviour, which can be observed in response to illness, can be exacerbated by the prospect of surgery. The fear of loss of control is a particularly worrying aspect of anaesthesia to many patients. It can, however, be quite reassuring to see that none of these events occurs in others of the ward group, and once again this is where the milieu within the ward becomes of paramount importance. Given, therefore, a supportive communicating ward group the Nightingale Ward can be an advantage over the isolated cubicle. The converse however can equally be true, and it is uncertain how many 'disturbing patients' in a ward group can be assimilated without a lowering of morale. The morale of the ward depends greatly on the nursing staff and the support given by the medical staff. The ward will often throw up a leader from the patients, someone perhaps who has been around longest, and through him the folklore of the ward will be distributed, very like the group leader in group psychotherapy. He will give first opinions as to the nature of the diseases, the effect of investigations, and perhaps more pertinently, what to say to staff in order to get privileges or more analgesics or sedatives. At the other extreme it is often the very isolated patient who may be the source of most considerable concern to the staff, particularly because of the absence of visitors and the absence of outside support. The reaction of a patient's family to surgery, and the interaction between the patient and the family may be very pertinent to his recovery. The anxious feelings in the family may manifest themselves in an equivalent variety of forms, ranging from over-solicitous visiting to a joking denial. In addition other factors come to play an important part. The relatives often feel guilt — did they in some mysterious way contribute to the illness, did the wife run up too many debts or press her husband too hard? The illness may exacerbate marital discord but it is more likely, at least temporarily, to increase the harmony. The illness, in itself, may alter the balance of dominance and submissiveness in the marriage and also produce resentment at the intrusiveness of the illness in the previous life style. This in turn will produce guilty feelings. The patient too will have been alienated from the family, particularly if the illness is prolonged. His world now centres around the hospital and the operation, and the ward and the patients, rather than his family with whom it is less easy to communicate. The relatives often feel even more remote from decisions concerning treatment and the risks involved, and they often consider they have less opportunity to discuss problems with the staff. They may even be protected from doing so by the patient who fears they may either irritate the staff, therefore putting him at a disadvantage, or find out something that he would rather not be aware of.

Most of these general factors are observed universally among patients. There are special problems related to the age of the patients. The elderly patient, perhaps a survivor from an age when surgical intervention was more hazardous, may have an over-pessimistic view of the risks of anaesthesia and operation. They may have lived long enough to have accumulated stories of unfortunate results of surgical intervention. The young child may, in addition, have other misapprehensions and fears which may require special skills in anaesthetic counselling (for a review see Pinkerton 1981).

EXAGGERATED REACTIONS TO ANAESTHESIA AND SURGERY

a) Anxiety

It is impossible to determine the degree to which anxious feelings are acceptable, or tolerated pre-operatively. Early work by Janis (1959) suggested that 'extreme anxiety' or absence of normal fear, presumably by a mechanism of denial, led to difficulties postoperatively when compared to a normal level of anxiety. Clearly excessive levels of catecholamines as a result of anxiety will increase, amongst other things, the risk of dysrhythmias. The history of the patient's personality and reaction to illness will reveal the patients who are particularly anxious pre-operatively, and it may be because of some particular apprehension concerning the operation which will respond to explanation and reassurance, or it may determine that the patient is an anxious personality responding almost to any stress with extreme anxiety, and hence probably in need of some heavy pre-operative sedation — for example with lorazepam 2.5 mg t.d.s. or diazepam 5–10 mg t.d.s. A few questions will often determine the patient's responses to earlier stressful life events and help in the diagnosis. Several studies have related the pre-operative emotional state to the postoperative need for analgesia, and there are many suggestions in the literature that pre-operative explanation and discussion, by lessening anxious feelings, reduce the postoperative demand for analgesia (Egbert et al 1964, Johnson et al 1970, Leigh et al 1977). The pre-operative anxiety proceeding an acute emergency will obviously require tranquillisation in addition to the use of analgesia. For elective surgery, however, and with childhood problems, relaxation exercises, meditation or even acupuncture may be a useful pre-operative adjunct, and sometimes much more acceptable to the patient. It is a characteristic of some patients that they deal with extreme anxiety by a process of denial. A patient does not appear to care at all about the illness or its severity; the prospect of anaesthesia or surgery does not appear to worry him at all. This denial indeed may have prevented him seeking help early (Aitken-Swan & Paterson 1955). It may be causative in a refusal to accept advice and treatment, leading sometimes to difficulties between the patient and the medical staff. The patient often becomes quite a leader in the ward in terms of his flippant and jovial attitude towards even the most distressing of investigations or surgical procedures. It is clear, however, that this denial is very frequently a fragile defence, and if punctured suddenly may lead to quite a disastrous psychological reaction, mainly of a depressive sort. On the other hand some authors have maintained that a degree of denial, particularly as a defence against the disasters of some situations in which the patient finds himself, is an advantage (Hackett & Cassem 1974).

b) Obssessional personalities

The neat, tidy, rigid, meticulous and methodical type of personality responds badly to any interruption to their usual life style. They take poorly to any change in the environment, be it a holiday or a surgical operation. They need precise answers to questions, and will be irritated if these are not forthcoming. They are used to checking repeatedly their own actions, and will wish to do that to those of the medical team. Discrepant shades of medical opinion will be queried exhaustively. It is my experience that this group of patients dislikes the effect of cerebral depressant drugs: they need constantly to be in control of their thinking and behaviour. They fear the loss of control induced by anaesthesia. These patients will be particularly perturbed by any personal uncleanliness consequent upon faecal or urinary incontinence. Underlying many obsessional personalities is the need to control feelings of anger and resentment, and these feelings can be

exacerbated by the 'disruption' or inconvenience of the illness and operation. These feelings are communicated to the medical team, and often
produce an angry irritation on the part of doctors and nurses. Pre-operative
detailed explanations often prevent postoperative anger and disappointment
and recrimination by the patient. Closely allied to this group are the
patients who have always prided themselves on their physical fitness; that
they should require surgery is an affront to their personal pride and it is
not tolerated well. These problems often result in anger directed towards
the medical team or inwards in terms of depression postoperatively. There
seems to be, in practice, a group of obsessional patients who take unkindly
to any form of medical or surgical intervention. In addition to the obsessional traits they have a deep distrust of medical activity and will quote
untoward actions to most attempts at treatment. They seem to be persistent
'negative placebo' reactors, and indeed do seem to suffer the unfortunate
side effects or toxic effects of most medical preparations. They often seem
to manage better if encouraged to suggest their own analgesia or premedication 'from bitter experience'. At least, including them in the decision
making process with regard to analgesia, sedatives and tranquillisers is
paramount.

c) Hysterical personality and conversion symptoms

It is useful in clinical practice to consider these complex and confusing
problems under two conceptual headings. The hysterical personality with
its well recognised description of lifelong histrionics, egocentricity, role
playing, hypochondriacal and attention-seeking traits; and the hysterical
conversion symptoms with fits, or faints, or paralysis or somatic pain. It
is generally accepted that these two problems are related in so far as the
hysterical personality has a greater propensity towards conversion symptoms. Anaesthesia and surgery therefore have an increased risk of producing
conversion symptoms in the hysterical personality, although not exclusively
so.

It is not uncommon for the hysterical personality to greet the prospect
of surgical intervention with what amounts to almost joy. At last the long
saga of problems is to be resolved and there will be visible proof of disease.
The drama of the surgical theatre needs no additional histrionics and the
patient is truly the centre of attention. Hopefully, however, the surgery is
fully indicated, and not performed as an ultimate attempt to help the
unfortunate patient, for if it is so it may subsequently act as a focus for all
the patient's concern — 'everything was all right until I had that operation'
— and another sheaf of notes becomes incorporated in the fat folder that
is carried around by the patient.

In a proportion of the hysterical personalities an operation may precipitate conversion symptoms such as paralysis, fits, chronic pain, abnormal
movements, vomiting and sensory symptoms. In general the more sophis-

ticated the patient, the more difficult and subtle becomes the diagnosis. It is evident too, that although a 'pre-operative' hysterical personality is quite likely to produce a conversion symptom, many patients have conversion symptoms without necessarily much evidence of a pre-existing personality problem.

The prognosis too is related to this. A sudden monosymptomatic conversion symptom with well recognised precipitant and understandable aetiology, in motivational terms, will quickly resolve given the satisfactory or partial resolution of the aetiological problem; usually a resolution of a conflict. If, however, the conversion symptom is one episode in a lifelong style of response then the prognosis is poor.

It is not uncommon for a patient with a defined psychiatric illness to need surgery and often a good deal of anxiety is engendered among the medical and nursing staff of the surgical ward with regard to the management of the patients. In general, however, these patients are often easier to manage successfully than the grossly disturbed personality disorder. It is useful to review the clinical pictures of manic depressive illness and schizophrenia briefly, emphasising those somatic manifestations and complaints that may often complicate the surgical picture.

The depressed patient often has a gradual onset to the depression or occasionally it may come quite suddenly. The patient will describe it as though it were a cloud descending on him. There is a lack of feeling, a lack of interest, an apathy, an inertia, a tiredness, a weariness for life, the gloomy outlook and in particular despair about the future. This may progress to a lack of feeling about things which may be even more distressing than the sadness with which the illness starts. Sleep is impaired and often is the first sign of a depressive illness. Characteristically the depressed patient has little difficulty in getting off to sleep, but wakes in the early hours of the morning when everybody else is asleep and there is little else to do but to ruminate depressively about life and the future. In severe depression food may sometimes comfort but not often and most patients lose their appetite and with it a considerable amount of weight. The patient will begin to look quite emaciated and with lack of food intake, there is often a complaint of severe constipation or even a delusional idea that the bowels are 'stopped up'.

Often in the elderly, depressive illness is characterised by extreme restlessness, an agitated depression. The patient will constantly pace up and down the ward whilst wringing his hands and often moaning repetitively about his condition. Weight clearly will be increasingly lost in this state. Hypochondria is of course a frequent symptom in the depressed patient and sometimes it may become delusional. Sometimes the patient will complain that his bowels are 'stopped up', that he is afraid to eat or swallow as a consequence. They may be convinced that they have an incurable disease and that no surgery or any other treatment will help. They may be certain that they will die under the anaesthetic and expect to because they have been so wicked. Interestingly enough this does not seem to affect the prognosis following surgery in quite a number of patients.

Sometimes the depressed patient has a constant nagging pain as a symptom of the depressive illness. Sometimes this is abdominal or thoracic but often facial. Not only will this make surgical diagnosis difficult on occasions, but the patient may be so importunate that operative treatment may be undertaken when perhaps conservative management might be more indicated.

Depression is not taken into account often enough in the management of medical and surgical cases, even though its treatment is certainly effective and would appreciably improve the 'quality of life' following an operation. For example Maguire et al (1985) performed a controlled trial of psychiatric versus non-intervention following mastectomy, and found significantly less depression in the treated group.

In depression concomitant with cancer chemotherapy or advanced malignant disease, an antidepressant drug was effective (Costa et al 1985).

Drugs used in the treatment of depression may present problems for the anaesthetist but they are beyond the scope of this review. In general, however, antidepressant drugs, it must be remembered, have a relatively slow onset of antidepressant action. It is most unlikely for improvement to take place in less than a week or so. The 'physiological' response, however, is more rapid in onset. The anticholinergic and cardiovascular effects therefore are seen quite quickly. When stopping medication for whatever reason, the reduction of dosage should be slow, if possible over a week or so. In emergency situations it is my experience that a short cessation of medication does not produce an immediate relapse. On occasions, however postoperatively, the antidepressant is not re-introduced and the patient gradually declines into despair. Tricyclic antidepressants which are effective in treating depression may complicate surgical procedures by precipitating glaucoma and diminish motility of the bowel adding to the risk of ileus (Clarke 1971). Some degree of urinary retention may also be induced, particularly in patients with large prostates.

The relationship between physical disease and self-destructive episodes is complex in depressive illnesses. Physical illness undoubtedly contributes to the act of suicide and attempted suicide (Dropat et al 1968).

Very often the 'successful' suicide is the isolated middle-aged man with a chronic painful physical disability. If in addition to this the patient has the characteristic features of anxious agitation and more complaints with less tolerance of pain, then he is more likely to attempt suicide (Farberow et al 1966).

Mania is totally disruptive to the patient and the surgical ward alike. The patient is often garrulous, demanding, restless, grandiose and paranoid if restrained. He will be intolerant of the restrictions of both his illness and the ward routine. Postoperatively phenothiazines are useful often in large dosage, eg. 100–200 mg t.d.s. of chlorpromazine or 5–10 mg t.d.s. of haloperidol. These doses may even need to be increased. If the patient was receiving lithium treatment before operation care must be taken to ensure adequate urinary output and an absence of dehydration, otherwise lithium toxicity is easily induced with a serum level of 1.5 mmol/l or above. Symptoms of marked tremor, ataxia, and dysarthria may progress towards coma in lithium toxicity.

The schizophrenic patient is often no problem at all to the surgical ward, often taking the surgery seemingly in his stride with an incongruous lack of concern. Medication can usually be continued and apart from occasional bizarre or asocial activities cause little concern in the short term.

Surgical diagnosis may be hampered by lack of co-operation or fleeting delusional ideas concerning bodily functions. Equally the surgical team has to be prepared for impulsive decisions for or against particular procedures. Persistence and patience, however, usually result in an acceptance. It is worth remembering that the psychotropic drugs used may very rarely cause a malignant neuroleptic reaction with high fever and stupor, which may be difficult to diagnose postoperatively.

Patients dependent on alcohol may pose a considerable problem: preoperatively as the alcohol is withdrawn, during operation because of the anaesthetic difficulties and in particularly postoperatively as the withdrawal for the first time becomes apparent. The extent of alcohol consumption is often denied and the initial tremulousness which may start as soon as 6 hours after cessation of alcohol intake, may be attributed to anxiety. The nausea, vomiting, weakness, tachycardia and sweating may confuse the diagnostic picture. In many cases atypical responses may occur with mild organic mental impairment or marked irritability as the main feature. It is often at this stage that pre-operative sedation is given, and this added to the sedation obtained during anaesthesia or postoperatively may interrupt the development of a full blown alcohol withdrawal syndrome. Up to 4–5 days postoperatively, therefore, may pass before delirium ensues. Consciousness is clouded, perception abnormal and the patient is confused and incoherent.

PSYCHIATRIC PROBLEMS ASSOCIATED WITH PARTICULAR SURGICAL PROCEDURES

So far the effect of the particular personality type on the outcome of the surgery has been explored and the particular problems associated with specific psychiatric disease. The influence of different surgical procedures and the psychiatric state of the patient is clearly a matter of considerable concern.

Open heart surgery

Early observations suggested a high incidence of postoperative psychiatric problems following open heart surgery. Abram (1971) for example, pointed out that one in 1500 general surgical postoperative convalescents was impaired by a psychotic illness, but 15% of closed heart operations and as high as 57% of open heart operations had this complication.

Others confirm this picture (Silverstein & Krieger 1960, Heller et al 1970, Tufo et al 1970). The symptoms occurred against a background of neurological damage which even recent studies suggest may be as high as 30% (Brever et al 1981), or even in some series 61% (Shaw 1986). Naturally the more sensitive the test of dysfunction the higher the incidence of abnormality recorded. Savageau et al (1982) subjected patients pre-operatively and again postoperatively on two occasions to a battery of tests. They found deterioration in three of the four battery tests involved and went a considerable way towards defining the situations pre-operatively and during operation that might be correlated with diminished psychometric performance. The predisposing features proposed were advanced age and pre-operative presence of neurological or cerebrovascular disease. During operation they noted the adverse effects of hypothermia, biochemical changes, extended duration of extracorporeal circulation and possible inadequate cerebral perfusion. They also noted the adverse effect of beta blockers and benzodiazepines. There was a clear relationship between poor performance postoperatively on psychometric tests and postoperative psychiatric disturbance. More recently it has been postulated that multiple small infarcts may be causative and induced by heparin (Mikhailidis et al 1986). The evidence indicates that the psychometric tests returned to normal in the great majority after about 6 months. Nevertheless it is within this time that psychiatric symptoms may arise. It is of interest that there was considerable enthusiasm early on for the results of coronary artery surgery. For example, Jenkins et al (1983) found that the physical and psychological and social, as well as sexual functioning, all improved following coronary artery bypass graft operation. These results were later tempered by the realisation that many patients failed to return to work after the operation.

Hoffmeister et al (1986) found a decrease in the numbers returning to work after the operation of between 21% and 81% and only 51% returned to a presurgery level of household activity. Hoffmeister et al in their discussions point out that 'the symptomatic and functional improvement after coronary bypass surgery correlates poorly with improvement in psychosocial status, with return to work and with the general resumption of pre-illness life style'. It may be, therefore, that the psychiatric morbidity is related to the subtle disturbance in cerebral function, which may recover after 6 months but which nevertheless leaves the patient lacking in self confidence and motivation.

Investigating this further Bass (1984) studied the psychosocial outcome in 36 patients receiving bypass surgery. He found that the operation did not increase the likelihood of unemployed patients resuming work and about a quarter of those employed pre-operatively, failed to return to work.

Impotence was reported in five of the 34 patients, but the majority of patients had pre-existing sexual difficulties. Pre-operative neurotic traits were associated with adverse psychiatric outcome.

It would seem, therefore, as though the open cardiac surgery for coronary artery disease can produce postoperative psychiatric disturbance in a significant proportion of patients. This may be related to the transient disturbance of brain function following the operation. Present research does not suggest that pre-operative psychiatric assessment is an accurate enough prediction to detect any but the most personality disturbed patients. Nevertheless a return to pre-operative work pattern may be encouraged by counselling as well as physical rehabilitation. These findings, of course, must be measured against the as yet mainly unresolved debate concerning the psychological characteristics of coronary patients in general. A recent paper (Tennant & Langeluddecke 1985) reviewed the conflicting literature regarding personality types, particularly type A with its aggressiveness, its hostility, a sense of urgency and a competitive striving for achievement. The majority of workers suggesting that type A personalities are more prone to coronary artery disease, but it does not seem to be correlated with coronary angiographic changes. Certainly hostility and depression would be likely consequences of the limitations produced by cardiac disease, rather than the cause of it. Once again, therefore, the effect of surgery alone is difficult to assess in patients with pre-existing personality problems that may be correlated with the disease and who also show a reaction shaped more by the illness, than by the surgery.

Cardiac transplantation has been studied in depth from the psychiatric point of view. The not infrequent use of psychological denial, as discussed above, which is apparent in many patients with cardiac disease, is very prominent in patients receiving transplants. Dimsdale & Hackett (1982) in their study in men with heart disease, found that denial was useful in some patients promoting quick recovery and rehabilitation, whereas in others it seemed to prevent adequate care and co-operation with medical advice. Mai et al (1986) studied transplant patients and understandably found a high level of pre-operative anxiety and depression. They did not find that this appreciably altered the decisions to proceed to surgery. Brief counselling and the occasional use of mild sedation were required. Six of the 33 patients who received grafts had delirious episodes, which was lower than in some earlier reports of postoperative delirium in open heart surgery (Kornveld et al 1965). The authors suggested support, encouragement and 'destimulation' as immediate measures in combating the acute organic mental syndrome, and only resorted to psychotropic drugs if restlessness, agitation and psychotic phenomena were severe. Three patients remained extremely anxious postoperatively and responded to supportive psychotherapy and benzodiazepines. Once again, however, it was the patients with pre-existing behavioural and psychosocial problems of extreme degree, who were the most difficult to help postoperatively.

Open heart surgery would still seem, therefore, to have an increased risk of postoperative psychiatric illness. Most work shows that this is a transient phenomenon related to acute or organic mental syndromes, but sometimes precipitating a psychiatric illness. Abram (1971) wrote 'If one considers postoperatively, a frightened individual having experienced a procedure which symbolically and realistically threatens his very existence, a clouded sensorium, being in physiological imbalance and in a vivid science fiction like environment, a break with reality does not seem too untenable'. This still seems very pertinent in most of the more recent literature and care to avoid, so far as possible, both the physical and psychological precipitants of cerebral dysfunction will improve the postoperative return to full activity.

The patient recovering from open heart surgery will be nursed in an intensive care unit and the psychological distress brought about by the unfamiliar, highly technical environment, has been repeatedly studied (Lazarus & Hagens 1968). Conflicting needs have to be resolved. Patients and staff alike are reassured by the intensive nursing and medical coverage in an intensive care unit (Cay et al 1970). On the other hand, this represents for others a continuing anxiety about their clinical condition and for patients to witness suffering or death of others, will lead to a suggestion that single rooms are best. This will also however lead to sensory isolation and difficulties for nursing observation. In the end the stress for the patient is more likely to reflect staffing anxieties and failure of communication, rather than the mechanics which should be kept as unobtrusive as possible.

Kidney transplants

The number of patients having postoperative psychiatric problems was high in a survey done by Penn et al (1971). Pre-operatively 17% were considered to have psychiatric problems and postoperatively this figure had risen to 32%. At first sight this appears an alarming increase, but the postoperative course during which psychiatric disturbance might manifest itself was up to 8 years in this study. Penn et al attempted to avoid sensory deprivation and isolation, by returning the patient to the familiar surroundings of his own hospital room and there was no restriction on visiting. The patients were kept well informed of their progress and supportive psychotherapy in a group was undertaken. The authors suggested that the psychiatric morbidity was less with transplant patients than with dialysis. In dialysed patients the authors underline the stressful boredom of repetitious visits to hospital and the reminder each time of the tenuous hold that they have on life. Similarly the family are constantly reminded of the seriousness of the patient's plight. Schreiber & Huber 1985, pointed out that dialysis had a far less distressing effect when performed at home than in the hospital. Work on the neuropsychiatric sequelae of dialysis must take into account not only the emotional responses but also the profound psychiatric change following the disequilibrium syndrome due possibly to cerebral oedema which is reversible. In addition the chronic encephalopathy which may be due to aluminium intoxication has to borne in mind (Kogeorgos 1983). Once again the most difficult postoperative behavioural problems are found in those patients with severe personality disorders.

Surgery for carcinoma of the breast

Major changes have taken place over the past two decades in the surgical treatment of the carcinoma of the breast. Originally a radical mastectomy was performed with considerable physical limitation, as well as severe disfigurement. Recently far less radical procedures have been developed, often with chemotherapy and radiation in addition. That psychiatric morbidity is high is not surprising, but it is important to determine if the psychological distress is due to the knowledge that a cancer is present, to the disfigurement of surgery or to the confidence which more extensive surgery may produce, as well as the effect of chemotherapy and radiation.

Early workers for example (Renneker & Cutler 1952) tended to describe postmastectomy patients in terms of persistent depression, increased anxiety, worthless feelings, shame and suicidal ideas. Interpretations were generally made about the effect of the operation on femininity as a major contributory factor to the syndrome. To test this hypothesis Worden & Weisman (1977) compared 40 women postmastectomy with a group with operations for other types of cancer. They reported an 18% to 20% incidence of depression, low of self-esteem and loss of energy, in both groups, suggesting that the concern was with the carcinoma rather than with the mastectomy itself. They found that marital problems, lack of support, previous psychiatric symptoms, pessimism, and pre-existing feelings of worthlessness were important in predicting the outcome. Interestingly enough a similar proportion of about 20% to 50% of patients were found by Morris et al (1977) to have a more persistent depression postmastectomy. Once again the patients most judged to be at risk were those with pre-operative depression and sexual difficulties, and were ascertained to be more emotionally labile pre-operatively. Maguire et al (1978), again found that approximately 25% of the mastectomy patients had significant anxiety or depression or both. This was in comparison with only 10% of the control group with benign breast disease. An equivalent increase and the incidence of sexual problems were also noted. Hughes (1982) examined 44 patients before mastectomy and on three occasions following it. She found that 35 expressed emotional distress and eight developed symptoms of depressive illness proper. Five of the severely depressed patients clearly felt themselves to be severely mutilated by the operation. Of interest, however, is the fact that the patients in the group who received chemotherapy thought it was 'as bad or worse than the mastectomy itself'. Sanger & Reznikoff (1981) tried to compare the psychiatric morbidity following breast saving procedures with modified radical mastectomy treatment. They interestingly found no difference between the two groups in psychological adjustment, but the radical group had no awareness of alternative treatment pre-operatively, and some of the more distressed patients were not included in the analysis. Steinberg et al (1985) compared 46 patients who underwent mastectomy compared with 21 patients who underwent lumpectomy and radiation. After over a year the mastectomy patients felt less attractive and feminine. They perceived their husbands' sexual interest as having declined and they were less socially at ease. On the other hand there was no evidence of any marked difference in anxiety or severe depression between the groups. The difficulties of many studies were discussed, as many may be to a certain extent self-selecting for a particular type of surgery and of course as a consequence not randomly allocated nor strictly comparable.

The paper by Alagaratnam & Kung (1986) from Hong Kong, compared 23 mastectomy survivors with 34 survivors of surgery for other malignancies. The patients all had a high incidence of depression (47%) which persisted for several years, but they found no greater incidence than in those suffering other forms of malignancies.

It would, therefore, seem that the incidence of postoperative depression is high following operation of carcinoma of the breast. Most surveys, however, suggest the major contributory factor to the depressive reaction is the awareness of the existence of cancer rather than the type of operation performed. There are indications, however, that lumpectomy and radiation, particularly in those self-selected women produced far less postoperative emotional distress, but no real difference in the incidence of defined depressive disease.

Some women however become quite distressed at having to make a decision themselves about which form of surgery to undergo, they 'fear that they may be compromising survival for appearance or vanity' (Holland & Jacobs 1986). Certainly it would seem important to include a counselling service as part of any oncology practice either to substitute for or encourage the continuation of good interpersonal relationships as this is one well documented finding which is correlated with longer survival (Weisman & Worden 1975). With counselling there is also much less likelihood of being grossly crippled by the disease psychologically or socially (Mages et al 1981).

Hysterectomy

The likelihood of having a hysterectomy seems to depend more on the country of residence than on the disease present. In the USA and Australia nearly every second woman will have her uterus removed by the age of 65 (Roeske 1979). Clearly therefore the indications are not absolute and depend to an extent on the availability of medical resources. Hysterectomy is often requested to reduce perceived heavy menstrual loss. Ryan &

Dennerstein (1986) suggested it may be due to an intolerance of methods other than the contraceptive pill and when this is considered inadvisable hysterectomy may be requested. The psychological problems of patients are certainly often present before hysterectomy and may be as high as 55–57% (Martin et al 1977). This however, does not seem to be particularly specific for those patients requiring hysterectomy for Byrne (1984) found that 46% of a group of women attending the general gynaecology clinic had psychiatric problems. Both these results are significantly different from the incidence of psychiatric morbidity in women. It is against this background that the possibility of psychiatric disorder induced by the hysterectomy must be assessed and as many of the early studies were retrospective, no comparison could be made of the post- and prehysterectomy psychiatric status. In these early reports the general conclusions seemed to be that the incidence of psychiatric complaints after hysterectomy was perhaps a major complication. In contrast however, Gath et al (1982) in a careful study of patients undergoing hysterectomy for menorrhagia of benign origin found a significant improvement in psychiatric morbidity within the first 6 months and the improvement was found to be maintained at 18 months. Psychosexual functioning improved as well. They also found that hysterectomy seldom if ever led to psychiatric disorder and that the clearest indicator of posthysterectomy psychiatric illness was the presence of psychological problems before operation. Roeske in 1979 gave a remarkable list of pre-operative psychosocial problems which indicated a poor prognosis postoperatively. They included poor gender identity, adverse reactions to stress particularly depressive episodes, previous depressive or mental illness incidence in the family, multiple physical complaints especially chronic low back pain, numerous hospital admissions, age of less than 35, a wish for pregnancy and children and anticipation that surgery will produce a loss of sexual interest and satisfaction. They also included a negative attitude on the behalf of the spouse, marital dissatisfaction and instability, a lack of vocational involvement and a disapproval either based upon cultural or religious attitudes. They pointed out that the patients seemed to be vulnerable between 3 months and 3 years postoperatively. Nowhere would it seem more important therefore that the pre-operative psychiatric status of women considered for hysterectomy should be reviewed and as much help given before operation as possible. It may be that in this way the number requiring operation may be reduced particularly in those societies with a high rate of hysterectomy, and in addition the postoperative psychiatric morbidity might be lessened.

Colostomy

Once again earlier reports seemed to indicate a high psychiatric morbidity following colostomy operations (Sutherland et al 1952, Druss et al 1968). In 1971 Devlin et al found that 23% were severely psychiatrically disturbed and a further 59% mildly disturbed after colostomy and these figures seemed to compare most unfavourably with only 2% severe and 30% mildly disturbed after restorative surgery. Once again many of the studies were rectrospective but Thomas et al (1984) point out that it is difficult to study patients with colostomy prospectively because quite a number of patients arrive as emergencies. They however performed a psychosocial assessment shortly after admission and again after 3 months. They found evidence for definite psychiatric morbidity following stoma surgery amounting to more than 50% of the subjects. Many of the disturbances were mild and although patients operated upon for carcinoma had a greater psychological distress, this was not significantly more than the others. Survey of the results however, indicates that the same overall psychiatric morbidity seemed to occur before the operation as postoperatively, so the effects of stoma surgery are still somewhat in doubt. Sexual disturbance was early noted to be common and Foster et al (1985) reviewed by questionnaire a large number of patients with stomal operations; 1 year after operation 69% of the patients with colostomies and 83% of the patients with ileostomies were 'fully integrated in their professions, and acceptance by family and friends was good, but sexual problems were prominent — 33% of the male and 13% of the female patients reported major problems in this area'.

Aesthetic surgery

Nowhere is the co-operation between psychiatrist and surgeon more important than in plastic surgical attempts to alter the appearance of patients. There is no doubt that many patients undergoing rhinoplasties, mammaplasties and face-lifts survive well without postoperative psychiatric illness. Nevertheless the number with severe postoperative psychiatric disorders is high. Gipson & Connolly (1975) studied 194 patients 10 years after rhinoplasty: they pointed out that only 8% of the patients who came to surgery following disease or trauma of the nose had severe psychiatric disturbance whereas many as 38% of those who had 'purely aesthetic deformities' had postoperative disturbance. It probably follows that the more severe bodily deformities which are readily appreciated by the family, friends and professional advisers have a much greater likelihood of successful outcome than those patients in whom the abnormality 'is in a sense often in the eye of the beheld rather than in the eye of the beholder' (Goin & Goin 1986). Nevertheless it is those patients who consider themselves to be unattractive who most persistently demand surgery. Indeed it is often this group who attribute all and every difficulty in their lives to the supposed abnormality. It is unrealistic of a patient to expect that every aspect of their life will be benefited by a slight rearrangement of their physical appearance.

It is evident however, that the problem is not simple. It is the aesthetic judgement of the patient compared with that of the rest and it is not surprising that many patients complain bitterly that it is *their* disfigurement, *they* are aware of it and that nobody else can appreciate how *they* feel about it. If there is an obvious discrepancy between the patient's judgement of the defect and those who behold it then the term dysmorphophobia can be applied. This symptom often indicates the beginning of a schizophrenic syndrome or other severe psychiatric disturbance. Using the figures tabulated by Thomas et al (1984) it is apparent that in various studies, between 50% and 100% of the dysmorphophobic patients suffered from or developed severe psychiatric syndromes. As a rule of thumb therefore a patient too importunate about the surgical correction of a minimal abnormality should be referred for psychiatric assessment as should those who fantasise that all their problems may be resolved by surgery and hence are never satisfied with the result and often resort to litigation.

CONCLUSION

This review has concentrated on three major aspects of the interface between surgery and psychiatry — the problems facing patients undergoing surgery, their expectations and anxieties and ways of attempting to reduce these. In addition an account has been given of the commonly encountered eccentricities of personality which colour the response to operation. Finally, it necessarily briefly surveyed some operations of special concern psychiatrically. It is clear that adequate information, discussion and communication before surgery not only makes the trauma less in a psychiatric sense, but also speeds satisfactory convalescence. Like childbirth, marriage, divorce or bereavement a surgical operation is undoubtedly a major life event; the former life events often receive adequate psychiatric input while surgical operations rarely seem to command this. Liaison work with surgical teams, group work and perhaps individual treatment before and after surgery may influence the prognosis considerably. With an elective operation it should be possible to establish such help for the patient. Knowledge by interview and even questionnaire of the personality of the patient will enable some predictions however imprecise to be made concerning the emotional reaction to the operation, but this needs close collaboration between surgeon and psychiatrist. In discussing various surgical procedures a pattern seems to emerge of initial concern at the number of postoperative psychiatric problems encountered, followed by a more careful reappraisal which often indicates clearly that postoperative disturbance is more correlated with premorbid psychiatric abnormality than the nature or extent of the operative interference. It therefore seems pertinent to involve psychiatric colleagues in assessments of the risks of surgery when at all possible.

> 'Success is influenced far more by the state of the patient's constitution than by the severity of an operation or by the mechanical dexterity with which the surgeon performs it, though individuals with different antecedents be placed under exactly the same hygienic circumstances after the performance of an operation yet the results will probably be very dissimilar influenced as they must be by their past rather than by their present condition' (Erichsen 1872).

REFERENCES

Abram H S 1971 Psychotic reactions after cardiac surgery: a critical review. In: Castelnuovo-Tedesco P (ed.) Psychiatric aspects of organ transplantation. Grune Stratton, London pp 70–78

Aitken-Swan J, Paterson R 1955 The cancer patient: delay in seeking advice. British Medical Journal 1: 623

Alagaratnam T T, Kung N Y T 1986 Psychosocial effects of mastectomy: is it due to mastectomy or to the diagnosis of malignancy. British Journal of Psychiatry 149: 296–299

Anderson F 1977 Brain failure in old age. Age and Ageing (suppl. 6): 1–3

Bass C 1984 Psychosocial outcome after coronary artery bypass surgery. British Journal of Psychiatry 145: 526–532

Brever A C, Furlan A J, Hanson A R et al 1981 Neurologic complications of open heart surgery: computer assisted analysis of 531 patients. Cleveland Clinic Quarterly 48: 205–206

Byrne P 1984 Psychiatric morbidity in a gynaecology clinic: an epidemiological survey. British Journal of Psychiatry 144: 28–34

Cay E L, Velter N J, Phillip A E, Dugard P 1970 Psychological reactions to a coronary care unit. Scandinavian Journal of Rehabilitative Medicine 28: 78–84

Clarke I N C 1971 Adynamic ileus and amitriptyline. British Medical Journal 2: 531

Costa D, Mogos I, Toma T 1985 Efficacy and safety of mianserin in the treatment of depression of women with cancer. Acta Psychiatrica Scandinavica 72 (Suppl. 320): 85–92

Devlin B H, Plant J A, Griffin M 1971 Aftermath of surgery for ano-rectal cancer. British Medical Journal 3: 413–418

Dimsdale J E, Hackett T P 1982 The effect of denial on cardiac health and psychological assessment. American Journal of Psychiatry 139: 1477–1480

Dropat T L, Anderson W F, Ridley H S 1968 In: Resnick H L P (ed.) Suicidal behaviour, Little & Brown, Boston

Druss R S, O'Connor J F, Prudden J F, Stern I O 1968 Psychologic response to colectomy. Archives General Psychiatry 18: 53–59

Egbert L D, Battit G E, Welch C E, Bartlett N K 1964 Reduction of post-operative pain by encouragement and instruction of patients. New England Journal of Medicine 270: 825–827

Erichsen J E 1872 The science and art of surgery. Longman Green & Co, London, p 3

Farberow N L, McKelligott J W, Cohen S, Darbonne A 1966 Suicide among patients with cardiorespiratory disease. Journal of American Medical Association 195: 422–428

Foster C, Refenacht R, Varga L, Halten F 1985 Psychosoziale adaptation bei kundstecker darmausgang. Schweize Medizine Wochenschrift 115: 987–993

Gath D, Cooper P, Day A 1982 Hysterectomy and psychiatric disorder. I. Levels of psychiatric morbidity before and after hysterectomy. British Journal of Psychiatry 140: 335–350

Gipson N, Connolly F H 1975 The incidence of schizophrenia in severe psychological disorders in patients 10 years after cosmetic rhinoplasty. British Journal of Plastic Surgery 28: 155

Goin M K, Goin J M 1986 Psychological effects of aesthetic facial surgery. Advances in Psychosomatic Medicine 15: 84–108

Hackett T P, Cassem N H 1974 Development of a qualitative rating scale to assess denial. Journal of Psychosomatic Research 18: 93–100

Heller S S, Frank K A, Malm J R et al 1970 Psychiatric complication of open heart surgery, a reexamination. New England Journal of Medicine 283: 1015–1020

Hoffmeister J M, Grüntzig A R, Wenger N K et al 1986 Long term management of patients following successful percutaneous transluminal coronary angioplasty and coronary artery bypass grafting. Cardiology 73: 323–332

Holland J C, Jacobs E 1986 Psychiatric sequelae following surgical treatment of breast cancer. Advances in Psychosomatic Medicine 15: 109–123

Hughes J 1982 Emotional reaction to the diagnosis and treatment of early breast cancer. Journal of Psychosomatic Research 26: 277–283

Janis I L 1959 Psychological stress. John Wiley, Chichester

Jenkins C D, Stanton B-A, Savageau J A et al 1983 Coronary artery bypass surgery: economical, ethical and social issues. Journal of American Medical Association 250: 782–788

Johnson J E, Dabbs J M, Leventhal H 1970 Psychosocial factors in the welfare of surgical patients. Nursing Research 19: 18–28

Knox S J 1961 Severe psychiatric disturbance in the postoperative period. Journal of Mental Sciences 107: 1078

Kogeorgos J 1983 Psychiatry and the artificial kidney. British Journal of Psychiatry 143: 87–88

Kornveld D S, Zimberg S, Malm J R 1965 Psychiatric complications of open heart surgery. New England Journal of Medicine 273: 287–292

Lazarus H R, Hagens S H 1968 Prevention of psychosis following open heart surgery. American Journal of Psychiatry 124: 1190–1195

Leigh J M, Walker J, Janaganathan P 1977 Effect of preoperative anaesthetic visit on anxiety. British Medical Journal 2: 987–989

Ley P 1977 Patient's compliance: a psychologist's viewpoint. Prescribers Journal 17: 1

Mages N L, Castro J R, Fobair P et al 1981 Patterns of psychosocial response to cancer: can effective adaptation be predicted? International Journal of Radiation Oncology, Biology, Physics 7: 385–392

Maguire G P, Lere E S, Bevington D J et al 1978 Psychiatric problem in the first year after mastectomy: a two year follow up study. British Medical Journal 1: 163–165

Maguire P, Hopwood P, Tarrier N, Howell T 1985 Treatment of depression in cancer patients. Acta Psychiatrica Scandinavica 72 (suppl. 320): 81–84

Mai F M, McKenzie F N, Kostuk W J et al 1986 Psychiatric aspects of heart transplantation: preoperative evaluation and post-operative sequelae. British Medical Journal 1: 311–313

Martin R L, Roberts W V, Clayton P J, Wetzel R 1977 Psychiatric illness and non-cancer hysterectomy. Diseases of the Nervous System 38: 974–980

Mikhailidis D P, Greenbaum R, Barradas M A, Evans T R, Dandona P 1986 Neurological dysfunction following coronary artery bypass graft surgery. Journal of Royal Society of Medicine 79: 496

Morris T, Greer H J, White P 1977 Psychological and social adjustment to mastectomy. Cancer 40: 2381–2387

Paykel E S 1974 Recent life events and clinical depression. In: Gunderson E K, Rake R H (eds) Life stress in psychiatric illness. Charles C Thomas, Springfield, Illinois, pp 134–163

Penn I, Bunch D, Olenik D, Abovna G 1971. In: Castelnuovo-Tedesco P (ed.) Psychiatric aspects of organ transplantation. Grune Stratton, New York pp 133–144

Penrose R J J 1972 Life events before a subarachnoid haemorrhage. Journal of Psychosomatic Research 16: 329–333

Pinkerton P 1981 Preventing psychotrauma in childhood anaesthesia. In: Jackson Rees G, Cecil Gray T (eds) Paediatric anaesthesia. Butterworths, London pp 1–18

Renneker R, Cutler M 1952 Psychological problems of adjustment to cancer of the breast. Journal of the American Medical Association 148: 833–839

Roeske N C 1979 Hysterectomy and the quality of a woman's life. Archives of Internal Medicine 139: 146–147

Ryan M, Dennerstein L 1986 Hysterectomy and tubal ligation. Advances in Psychosomatic Medicine 15: 186–198

Sanger C K, Reznikoff M 1981 A comparison of the psychological effects of breast saving procedures with the modified radical mastectomy. Cancer 48: 2341–2346

Savageau J A, Stanton B A, Jenkins C D et al 1982 Neuropsychological dysfunction following elective cardiac operation. Journal of Thoracic & Cardiovascular Surgery 84: 585

Schreiber W K, Huber W 1985 Psychological situation of dialysis patients and their families. Dialysis — Transplantation 14: 696–698

Shaw P J 1986 Neurological morbidity following coronary artery bypass graft surgery. Journal of The Royal Society Medicine 79: 130–131

Silverstein A, Krieger H P 1960 Neurologic complications of cardiac surgery. Archives of Neurology 3: 601–605

Steinberg M D, Juliano M A, Wise L 1985 Psychological outcome of lumpectomy versus mastectomy in the treatment of breast cancer. American Journal of Psychiatry 142: 34–39

Sutherland A M, Orbach C E, Dyk R S, Bard M 1952 The psychological impact of cancer and cancer surgery. Cancer 5: 857–872

Tennant C G, Langeluddecke P M 1985 Psychological correlates of coronary heart disease. Psychological Medicine 15: 581–588

Thomas C, Madden F, Jehu D 1984 Psychosocial morbidity in the first three months following stoma surgery. Journal of Psychosomatic Research 28: 251–257

Tufo H M, Ostfeed A M, Sjele E R 1970 Central nervous system dysfunction following open heart surgery. Journal of the American Medical Association 212: 1333–1340

Weisman A D, Worden J W 1975 Psychosocial analysis of cancer deaths. Omega 6: 61–75

Worden J W, Weisman A D 1977 The fallacy in postmastectomy depression. American Journal of Medical Science 273: 168–175

The autonomic nervous system

INTRODUCTION

Familiarity with the autonomic nervous system is important to the anaesthetist:

(1) in understanding the physiology of the cardiovascular system
(2) for skilful use of agonist and antagonist drugs acting on the sympathetic and parasympathetic systems
(3) in management of patients with impaired autonomic function
(4) in assessing anaesthetic depth
(5) in performing diagnostic and therapeutic nerve blocks

The autonomic system was first described by Langley in 1921, as an efferent system of nerves controlling the body's internal environment. Thirty years ago von Euler (1956) showed noradrenaline to be the substance released from postganglionic sympathetic nerves. Adrenergic receptors were subsequently subdivided by physiological responses to various agonist and antagonist drugs, and another group of receptors responding to dopamine were discovered, while, at the same time, investigators probed the intracellular 'second messenger' responses to receptor activation. In the last 10 years, radioligand-binding techniques, using radioactively labelled hormone and drug derivatives, have helped characterise and quantify adrenergic and dopaminergic receptors, and considerable information has come to light about prejunctional receptor modulation. This review attempts to pull together some current concepts of adrenergic and dopaminergic receptors, and to discuss their relevance, along with that of the autonomic system in general, to the anaesthetist.

SOMATIC AND AUTONOMIC REFLEXES

A three-neuron *somatic* spinal reflex has an afferent neuron with its cell body in the dorsal root ganglion, a connector neuron terminating in the ventral horn and a ventral horn effector cell which transmits the efferent impulse to the skeletal muscle. A comparable *visceral* reflex starts with an afferent from an internal organ. This synapses with the connector cell. As the autonomic effector cell has migrated out of the central nervous system to an autonomic ganglion, the connector axon leaves the CNS in a white ramus (medullated B fibres) to reach it. The effector cell then transmits its impulse to the target organ through a grey ramus (non-medullated C fibres). In the autonomic system, connector cells are not uniformly distributed throughout all segments of the nervous system. They occur in:

(1) the brain, in connection with the nuclei of cranial nerves III, VII, IX, X,
(2) the whole of the thoracic region and first two lumbar segments of the spinal cord, and
(3) the second, third and fourth sacral segments of the spinal cord.

SYMPATHETIC vs PARASYMPATHETIC SYSTEMS

Anatomy

The sympathetic system has connector cell bodies in the thoracolumbar region. Their axons travel to the sympathetic trunk where they may synapse with their effector cells. Alternatively, they may pass directly through to synapse at a more distant ganglion. The sympathetic trunk is a ganglionated nerve chain which extends from the base of the skull to the coccyx, lying about one inch from the midline of the vertebral column throughout its length. As a result of fusion, there are approximately three cervical, eleven thoracic, two to four lumbar and four sacral ganglia. The higher and lower ganglia, not receiving white rami directly, receive their preganglionic supply from medullated fibres which pass through their corresponding ganglion without synapse.

In the parasympathetic system, of cranio-sacral origin, the ganglia are distant from the CNS and, in contrast to the sympathetic chain, there is no interconnecting system. Consequently, the medullated preganglionic fibres synapse with the effector neurons close to, or actually in the wall of, the viscera supplied.

Function

The sympathetic system is concerned with an often widespread 'fight or flight' response to stress, while the parasympathetic deals with the more discrete adjustments of relaxed homeostasis. Some organs are stimulated by one division only (e.g. uterus, adrenal medulla and most arterioles from the sympathetic only; glands of the stomach and pancreas from the parasympathetic only). Others have dual innervation, which produces antagonistic effects in the target organs.

Pharmacology

Acetylcholine is the ganglionic neurotransmitter for all autonomic nerves. At the target organ, noradrenaline is the neurotransmitter of the sympathetic system and acetylcholine of the parasympathetic. Sweat glands are exceptional, being anatomically sympathetic but having acetylcholine as the postganglionic neurotransmitter. The adrenal medulla is essentially a sympathetic ganglion in which the postganglionic cells have lost their axons and secrete directly into the bloodstream.

CENTRAL AUTONOMIC CONTROL

The autonomic ganglia are relay stations without independent activity, central control coming from the medulla, pons, hypothalamus and limbic system. Even after the cord is severed from the brain, however, the connector cells continue to show tonic activity (Keele et al 1982). Thus, for example, some degree of vasoconstriction is maintained in tetraplegia, keeping the blood pressure at a somewhat stable, if low, level.

SYMPATHETIC RECEPTORS

Peripherally, most sympathetic postganglionic fibres release noradrenaline and are called 'adrenergic', while, centrally, dopamine and adrenaline also act as neurotransmitters. Each nerve terminal is extensively branched, a single postganglionic sympathetic nerve innervating as many as 25 000 receptors. This is consistent with the diffuse response to sympathetic stimulation. Noradrenaline is synthesised in the nerve terminal from the amino acid tyrosine in a series of enzyme-controlled steps. It is inactivated primarily by re-uptake into the sympathetic nerve ending, where a small amount is de-aminated in the cytoplasm by monoamine oxidase, while most of it is taken up in storage granules. A small amount of noradrenaline escapes re-uptake and enters the circulation. This is metabolised by monoamine oxidase and catechol-O-methyltransferase, mostly in the liver and kidneys. Adrenaline, released by the adrenal medulla, is inactivated in the same way.

The detailed physiology of the sympathetic nerve ending has been comprehensively reviewed by Langer and Hicks (1984).

Relationship of receptors to effector systems

Catecholamines, key regulators of many physiological processes, initiate target cell responses by binding to specific receptor sites. At present, it appears likely that there are two α-adrenergic, two β-adrenergic and two dopaminergic subtypes (Molinoff 1984, Stoof & Kebabian 1984). These conclusions are based on differing responses to various sympathomimetic drugs, and on differing intracellular biochemical changes leading to the cellular physiological response to sympathetic stimulation. Although the biochemistry associated with receptor activation is not yet fully understood, specific receptor subgroup stimulation may have the consequences outlined below.

Calcium has been suggested as a second messenger for stimulation of α_1-receptors although earlier events are probably responsible for transmission of receptor-mediated information across the cell membrane. Breakdown of phosphoinositide, a relatively minor membrane constituent, seems to be associated with increased release of cytosolic Ca^{2+} from internal stores. This increased intracellular Ca^{2+} binds with calmodulin and the resulting complex appears to generate the appropriate physiological response through activation of a protein kinase. Alternatively, a second breakdown product of phosphoinositide and increased intracellular Ca^{2+} results in phosphorylation of a Ca^{2+} phospholipid-dependent protein kinase, followed by the cellular response. In contrast, stimulation of α_2-adrenergic receptors results in decreased cyclic-AMP activity and inhibition of noradrenaline release. The mechanisms involved in α-adrenergic phenomena have been comprehensively reviewed by Exton (1985).

As originally suggested by Sutherland et al (1965) most, but not all, of the effects of catecholamines at β receptors are mediated through activation of adenyl cyclase and increases in cyclic-AMP accumulation.

Dopamine is a catecholamine which appears to have more importance as a transmitter in the central than the peripheral nervous system. As yet there is no definite proof, in man, that dopamine, a precursor of noradrenaline, acts as a peripheral neurotransmitter, although, in the dog, stimulation of sympathetic fibres accompanying the renal artery is followed by the release of large amounts of dopamine (Lee 1982). Dopaminergic receptors appear to be the least well understood of all the sympathetic system receptors. Most studies point to the existence of two subtypes, each of which may exist in two affinity states (Stoof & Kebabian 1984), but this concept is not accepted by all investigators (Seeman 1981, Martres et al 1984), and it remains to be resolved whether central and peripheral subtypes are the same. Stimulation of the peripheral DA-1 dopamine receptor results in activation of adenyl cyclase and increased cyclic-AMP, while activation of the DA-2 dopamine receptor leads to a reduction in the release of the transmitter noradrenaline (Cavero et al 1982a).

Function

The tissue locations and responses of the various receptors are outlined in Table 4.1. It was initially thought that α_1- and α_2-receptors could be distinguished by location; α_1 being postjunctional, and α_2 prejunctional, inhibiting the release of noradrenaline. This concept now appears too simplistic as α_2-receptors also occur postjunctionally in smooth muscle,

Table 4.1 Locations and responses of sympathetic receptors

Receptor	Location	Response
α_1-Adrenergic	Smooth muscle (vascular, iris, ureter, uterus, gastrointestinal and bladder sphincters)	Contraction
	Smooth muscle (gastrointestinal)	Relaxation
	Liver	Glycogenolysis
	Heart	Inotropism
	Salivary gland	Secretion (K^+, H_2O)
	Kidney (proximal tubule)	Gluconeogenesis, Na^+ reabsorption
α_2-Adrenergic	Peripheral adrenergic nerve endings (prejunctional)	Inhibition of noradrenaline release
	Sympathetic ganglia	Hyperpolarisation
	Platelets	Aggregation
	Adipose tissue	Inhibition lipolysis
	Endocrine pancreas	Inhibition insulin release
	Vascular smooth muscle	Contraction
	Kidney	Inhibition renin release
β_1-Adrenergic	Heart	Increased rate, contractility, conduction velocity
	Adipose tissue	Lipolysis
β_2-Adrenergic	Liver	Glycogenolysis, gluconeogenesis
	Skeletal muscle	Glycogenolysis, lactate release
	Smooth muscle (bronchi, uterus, vascular, detrusor, gastrointestinal)	Relaxation
	Endocrine pancreas	Insulin secretion
	Salivary glands	Amylase secretion
DA-1 dopaminergic	Vascular smooth muscle (renal, mesenteric)	Relaxation
	Kidney	Natriuresis
DA-2 dopaminergic	Peripheral adrenergic nerve endings (prejunctional)	Inhibition of noradrenaline release

mediating contraction. On the basis of differing dose-response alterations with specific agonist and antagonist drugs, Davey (1986) has theorised that α_1-adrenoceptors provide the background level of sympathetic tone, based both on the local release of noradrenaline and on circulating catecholamines, while postjunctional α_2-adrenoceptors are most sensitive to circulating catecholamines and amplify cardiovascular responses during stress or disease states. The concept that α_1-receptors are intrajunctional whereas α_2 vascular receptors are extrajunctional and not involved in the mediation of responses to sympathetic nerve stimulation (Langer et al 1980), while appealing, is probably an oversimplification (Gardiner & Peters 1982, Kou et al 1984). The possibility that α_2-receptor mechanisms might be altered in hypertension has been examined in detail by Lokhandwala & Eikenburg (1983).

The role of prejunctional α_2-adrenoceptors in the regulation of the release of the transmitter noradrenaline through a negative feedback mechanism is well established, and it has been proposed that prejunctional β-adrenoceptors may exist, the stimulation of which facilitates the release of noradrenaline (Langer 1980, Majewski et al 1982). The finding that adrenaline may preferentially activate these prejunctional β-receptors might be of relevance in the pathogenesis of some forms of hypertension, and suggests a mechanism for the clinical efficacy of β-adrenergic blocking drugs in their treatment (Majewski & Rand 1981, Misu & Kubo 1983).

At present, understanding of dopaminergic receptor function has been limited by a lack of highly specific agonists and antagonists. Theoretically at least, pure dopaminergic agonists, free of other adrenergic effects, could be useful antihypertensive agents, either through direct smooth muscle relaxation via postjunctional DA-1 receptors or through the reduction of the neuronal release of noradrenaline resulting from activation of DA-2 receptors on ganglionic bodies or sympathetic nerve terminals (Cavero et al 1982b). Clinically, dopamine also produces a natriuresis by an effect on tubular transport mechanisms. Whether dopamine is normally formed in the kidney from circulating L-dopa or released from dopaminergic nerves, or both, is not yet clear (Lee 1982).

Regulation of the sensitivity of catecholamine receptor systems

The altered response to catecholamines under various circumstances — with age, disease or during drug administration, for example — has prompted an assessment of adrenergic receptors in these situations. Although adrenergic receptors are widely distributed throughout the body, most studies have been performed using platelets and lymphocytes, for the ready accessibility of α- and β-receptors, respectively. As the receptors on blood cells are exposed only to circulating catecholamines, they do not necessarily react in the same way as receptors exposed to neuronally derived catecholamines. Nevertheless, the results of quantitative studies using human lymphocytes suggest that receptor density is affected by prolonged exposure to agonist and antagonist drugs.

Administration of a β-receptor antagonist, such as propranolol, leads to an increase in receptor density (Aarons et al 1980). This may account for the observed hypersensitivity to catecholamines which follows abrupt discontinuation of therapy (propranolol withdrawal syndrome), since it takes several days for the receptor density to return to normal. A similar increase in β-adrenergic receptor density follows autonomic denervation (Davies 1983). In contrast, prolonged stimulation with the β-agonist terbutaline has led to decreased receptor density (Aarons et al 1983), which may account for loss of efficacy of this and other sympathomimetics with long term therapy.

Evidence for α-receptor alteration in response to pharmacological manoeuvres (Molinoff 1984) is less clear than that relating to β-receptors.

However, in autonomic failure, increased numbers of platelet α-adrenoceptors are found. In this situation, there are often low plasma levels of noradrenaline and this supports the theory that adrenergic receptor number may be regulated in part by the amount of agonist to which the tissue receptor population is exposed. Additionally, in the presence of a phaeochromocytoma and the resulting high levels of circulating noradrenaline, platelet α-receptors are markedly decreased (Davies 1983).

Lee et al (1978) have described increased numbers of postsynaptic dopamine receptors in the corpora striata of post-mortem brains from Parkinsonian patients, suggesting that the same regulatory mechanism may apply to dopamine receptors.

Cholinergic receptors

Acetylcholine (ACh) is the transmitter substance of cholinergic nerves. It is synthesised in the cytoplasm of the cholinergic nerve terminals and stored in synaptic vesicles. As a result of constant passage of nerve impulses at low frequency (tonic activity), ACh is released continuously at cholinergic nerve terminals. Cholinergic receptors have been subdivided into two types: muscarinic, at postganglionic parasympathetic terminals, and nicotinic, at autonomic ganglia and skeletal muscle, each subtype being activated by a different region of the ACh molecule. Most cholinergic receptors in the central nervous system are muscarinic. The excitatory effects of ACh on postsynaptic membranes are due to increases in permeability to Na^+ and Ca^{2+}. After denervation, nicotinic cholinergic receptors, normally confined to the motor end-plate, spread to other parts of the muscle membrane, resulting in denervation hypersensitivity. It is not certain if this occurs with muscarinic receptors.

ANAESTHESIA AND THE AUTONOMIC SYSTEM

Pharmacological alteration

Drugs may alter autonomic transmission and thus interfere with the maintenance of blood pressure and cardiac output under anaesthesia. These may form part of a regular therapeutic regimen or might be administered by the anaesthetist. Modes of action include:

(1) Ganglionic blockade, e.g. trimetaphan
(2) Interference with noradrenaline synthesis
    a. inhibition of rate-limiting enzyme
    b. synthesis of false transmitter e.g. α-methyldopa
    c. inhibition of dopa decarboxylase e.g. carbidopa
(3) Prevention of noradrenaline release e.g. guanethidine
(4) Interference with noradrenaline re-uptake e.g. cocaine

Table 4.2   Examples of agonists and antagonists of autonomic nervous system receptors

Receptor	Agonist	Antagonist
α_1-Adrenergic	Methoxamine	Prazosin
α_2-Adrenergic	Clonidine	Yohimbine
β_1-Adrenergic	Adrenaline★	Metoprolol
β_2-Adrenergic	Salbutamol	Butoxamine
DA-1 dopaminergic	Dopamine★	Metoclopramide★
DA-2 dopaminergic	Bromocriptine	Haloperidol
Muscarinic	Acetylcholine★	Atropine
Nicotinic	Nicotine	Hexamethonium (autonomic ganglia)
		Curare (motor end-plates)

★ = non-specific

(5) Interference with noradrenaline breakdown e.g. monoamine oxidase inhibitors
(6) Stimulation or blockade of receptors (see Table 4.2)

Decreased autonomic function

Dysautonomia may be primary, idiopathic or due to systemic disease such as diabetes, amyloidosis, rheumatoid arthritis, carcinomatosis or Chagas' disease. Diabetes is the most common cause of autonomic neuropathy (Watkins & Edmonds 1983) with 20% of randomly selected diabetics showing cardiovascular reflex abnormalities (Ewing 1983). Tests of autonomic function may remain normal for years or decline unpredictably and irreversibly. The development of symptoms such as postural hypotension or gastroparesis is associated with a 50% 3-year mortality. Parasympathetic denervation of the heart is usually the earliest sign of dysautonomia, with sympathetic denervation occurring at a later stage. Abnormalities of respiratory control have been associated with diabetic autonomic dysfunction (Page & Watkins 1978, Rees et al 1981). These authors concluded that this group of patients may be at increased risk of sudden death during sleep, following anaesthesia, or in association with severe respiratory infections.

Familial dysautonomia (Riley-Day syndrome) occurs most commonly in children. In adults, progressive autonomic failure is usually insidious in onset with postural hypotension (a fall of more than 20 mmHg systolic pressure on standing) as the cardinal feature, although in some cases bladder symptoms or apparent Parkinsonism appear first. Case reports concerning the anaesthetic management of patients with autonomic impairment have stressed the difficulties involved in maintaining a stable blood pressure and have noted a hypersensitivity to sympathomimetic agents (Bartels & Mazzia 1970, Meridy & Creighton 1971). It is now understood that in dysautonomias associated with degeneration of the peripheral autonomic nervous system, circulating levels of noradrenaline are low and α-receptors are present in increased numbers. A different situation is encountered in the tetraplegic with decentralisation of autonomic function, although supersensitivity to catecholamines is demonstrable (see below). Patients presenting with autonomic failure are not a homogeneous group and may have limited or widespread disease with a spectrum of central and peripheral involvement. Case reports have suggested that fentanyl used in high (Beilin et al 1985) or low (Stirt et al 1982) doses conveys cardiovascular stability in these patients. A pre-operative trial of α-agonist to determine individual sensitivity, has been advised by Beilin et al (1985). Abnormal respiratory control has been noted in primary autonomic failure, both awake (Eisele et al 1971) and in association with general anaesthesia (Sweeney et al 1985). In this non-homogeneous group of patients it is difficult to anticipate individual cardiovascular and respiratory responsiveness without specific testing.

In tetraplegia the autonomic impairment is different from that in primary autonomic failure because, although the spinal cord is isolated from the cerebral sympathetic centres, sympathetic reflexes at the spinal level persist. At rest there is little sympathetic activity, with low plasma noradrenaline concentrations, but stimulation of sympathetic activity (i.e. from bladder distension) leads to outpouring of noradrenaline from peripheral nerves and a marked increase in plasma noradrenaline. It is felt that this periodic exposure to large amounts of catecholamines accounts for the normal numbers of α-receptors observed in chronic tetraplegics (Bannister et al 1981). Chronic tetraplegics are, nevertheless, very sensitive to intravenous noradrenaline. This is probably due to a defective baroreflex, in which the only compensatory mechanism left, a vagally mediated bradycardia, is unable to restore the blood pressure towards normal (Davies 1983). This autonomic hyper-reflexia may be detrimental, both because of the very severe hypertension that can occur and the bradyarrythmias which may ensue. Several investigators (Alderson 1983, Barker et al 1985) have successfully abolished the hyper-reflexic response to bladder distension while maintaining a stable, if somewhat lower, blood pressure, with low dose spinal anaesthesia, although not all reports are enthusiastic (Fraser & Edmonds-Seal 1982).

As reviewed by Motulsky & Insel (1982), adrenergic responses are altered in a variety of clinical disorders. Ageing is associated with a decrease in baroreflex sensitivity, but adrenergic receptor numbers are probably unchanged. Patients with cystic fibrosis have abnormal autonomic regulation being more sensitive to α stimulation and less sensitive to β stimulation than normal.

Diagnosis of autonomic dysfunction can often be accomplished with simple bedside tests as summarized by Ewing (1983). These either assess primarily the parasympathetic system, by noting heart rate responses to the Valsalva manoeuvre, to standing, and ordinary beat to beat variability, or the sympathetic system, by observing blood pressure changes that occur on standing or during sustained handgrip.

Increased autonomic function

Phaeochromocytoma, the classic example of autonomic hyperactivity, has been well reviewed by Kaufman (1982) and Desmonts & Marty (1984). Sympatho-adrenal hyperactivity is a feature of tetanus as well, and the chief cause of death in this condition (Kerr et al 1968). A direct effect of tetanic toxins on the sympathetic nervous system is likely, with neurogenic releasing mechanisms causing the high plasma catecholamine levels of predominantly noradrenaline (Keilty et al 1968). Infusions of intravenous labetalol (Domenighetti et al 1984) or epidural local anaesthetics (Lindahl et al 1985) have both proved effective in the management of severe cases. Hyperthyroidism resembles a hyperadrenergic state but plasma levels of catecholamines are not increased. Motulsky & Insel (1982) suggest that thyroid hormone may regulate adrenergic receptors as increased numbers of β-adrenergic receptors are found in hyperthyroidism. Similarly, hypertension might appear to be due to sympathetic overactivity, yet it is associated with only slight increases in the concentration of catecholamines. Changes in adrenergic receptors have been sought here too, as discussed earlier.

Anaesthetic-induced impairment

General anaesthesia can depress the peripheral sympathetic nervous system at several sites along its pathway and, to some extent, the signs of autonomic activity can be used to gauge the depth of anaesthesia. Halothane, for example, decreases preganglionic release of acetylcholine as well as postganglionic release of noradrenaline. It also depresses the baroreceptor reflex (Duke et al 1977), although there appears to be a rapid return to normal during anaesthetic recovery (Carter et al 1986). However, even the large doses of analgesics required to abolish the stress response to conventional surgery are not enough to eliminate the endocrine changes of maximally stressful conditions, such as cardiopulmonary bypass.

Spinal and epidural anaesthesia interrupt the sympathetic nervous system in proportion to the height of the sensory block. Previously, the zone of differential sensory/autonomic blockade was believed to be about two segments (Green 1958). Recent work by Chamberlain & Chamberlain (1986) using thermographic imagery suggests that the zone of differential blockade is probably six segments or more, and that blockade of cardiac sympathetic fibres during spinal anaesthesia is much more common than previously thought.

The effects of isolated high level sympathectomy, accomplished by cervico-thoracic epidural block, have been examined by Takeshima & Dohi (1985) and Dohi et al (1986). They found no alteration in ventilation, either resting or in response to CO_2, compared to control. Also, apart from slight suppression of the cardio-accelerator response, acute sympathetic denervation of the central organs did not appear to interfere with reflex circulatory responses to the Valsalva manoeuvre or to moderate blood pressure changes. They speculate that sympathetic control of heart rate functions as an inhibitor of the vagus, rather than an active cardiac accelerator.

SUMMARY

Understanding of the autonomic nervous system has improved a great deal, recently, as adrenergic receptors and their modifying influences have come under scrutiny. The definition of the properties, distribution and regulation of the adrenergic and dopaminergic receptors has been aided by the development of the radioligand-binding technique and the creation of new, more specific agonist and antagonist drugs. At present, it seems likely that a cause for hypertension may be found in disordered adrenergic receptor function, and that receptor abnormalities may eventually prove to be associated with other diseases, hyperthyroidism for instance. Certainly, adrenergic and dopaminergic receptors form a fluid population, capable of changing in number in various circumstances.

Recent case reports remind us that patients with dysautonomia are a diverse group who can exhibit severe cardio-respiratory instability under anaesthesia. The report of a six-segment sensory/sympathetic differential during intrathecal blockade will prompt reassessment of previous studies which assumed that a sensory level below T6 spares the cardiac sympathetic fibres. As Green (1981) has pointed out, spinal anaesthesia is unique in producing pure sympathetic denervation with minimal interference from circulating local anaesthetic agent, and, as such, this technique should continue to provide valuable information in clinical studies.

REFERENCES

Aarons R D, Nies A S, Gal J, Hegstrand L R, Molinoff P B 1980 Elevation of β-adrenergic receptor density in human lymphocytes after propranolol administration. Journal of Clinical Investigation 65: 949–957
Aarons R D, Nies A S, Gerber J G, Molinoff P B 1983 Decreased beta adrenergic receptor density on human lymphocytes after chronic treatment with agonists. Journal of Pharmacology and Experimental Therapeutics 224: 1–6
Alderson J D 1983 Spinal cord injuries. Anaesthesia 38: 605
Bannister R, Davies I B, Frankel H L et al 1981 Platelet alpha-receptor properties and pressor responses to noradrenaline in tetraplegia compared with multiple system atrophy. Journal of Physiology, 312: 25P–26P
Barker I, Alderson J, Lydon M, Franks C I 1985 Cardiovascular effects of spinal subarachnoid anaesthesia. Anaesthesia 40: 533–536
Bartels J, Mazzia V D B 1970 Familial dysautonomia. Journal of the American Medical Association 221: 318–319
Beilin B, Maayan Ch, Vatashsky E, Shulman D, Vinograd I, Aronson H B 1985 Fentanyl anesthesia in familial dysautonomia. Anesthesia and Analgesia 64: 72–76
Carter J A, Clarke T N S, Prys-Roberts C, Spelina K R 1986 Restoration of baroreflex control of heart rate during recovery from anaesthesia. British Journal of Anaesthesia 58: 415–421
Cavero I, Massingham R, Lefevre-Borg F 1982a Peripheral dopamine receptors, potential

targets for a new class of antihypertensive agents. Part I: Subclassification and functional description. Life Sciences 31: 939–948

Cavero I, Massingham R, Lefevre-Borg F 1982b Peripheral dopamine receptors, potential targets for a new class of antihypertensive agents. Part II: Sites and mechanisms of action of dopamine receptor agonists. Life Sciences 31: 1059–1069

Chamberlain D P, Chamberlain B D L 1986 Changes in the skin temperature of the trunk and their relationship to sympathetic blockade during spinal anaesthesia. Anesthesiology 65: 139–143

Davey M J 1986 Overview of α-receptors. Clinical Science 70 (suppl 14): 33S–39S

Davies B 1983 Adrenergic receptors in autonomic failure. In: Bannister R (ed) Autonomic failure. Oxford University Press, Oxford, p 174

Desmonts J M, Marty J 1984 Anaesthetic management of patients with phaeochromocytoma. British Journal of Anaesthesia 56: 781–789

Dohi S, Takeshima R, Naito H 1986 Ventilatory and circulatory responses to carbon dioxide and high level sympathectomy induced by epidural blockade in awake humans. Anesthesia and Analgesia 65:9–14

Domenighetti G M, Savary G, Stricker H 1984 Hyperadrenergic syndrome in severe tetanus: extreme rise in catecholamines responsive to labetalol. British Medical Journal 288: 1483–1485

Duke P C, Fownes D, Wade J G 1977 Halothane depresses baroreflex control of heart rate in man. Anesthesiology 46: 184–187

Eisele J H, Cross C E, Rausch D C, Kurpershoek C J, Zelis R F 1971 Abnormal respiratory control in acquired dysautonomia. New England Journal of Medicine 285: 366–368

von Euler U S 1956 Noradrenaline: chemistry, physiology, pharmacology and clinical aspects. Charles C Thomas, Springfield

Ewing D J 1983 Practical bedside investigation of diabetic autonomic failure. In: Bannister R (ed) Autonomic failure. Oxford University Press, Oxford, p 371

Exton J H 1985 Mechanisms involved in α-adrenergic phenomena. American Journal of Physiology 248 (Endocrinology Metabolism 11): E633–E647

Fraser A, Edmonds-Seal J 1982 Spinal cord injuries. Anaesthesia 37: 1084–1098

Gardiner J C, Peters C J 1982 Postsynaptic alpha$_1$- and alpha$_2$-adrenoceptor involvement in the vascular responses to neuronally released and exogenous noradrenaline in the hind limb of the dog and cat. European Journal of Pharmacology 84: 189–198

Greene N M 1958 The area of differential block during spinal anesthesia with hyperbaric tetracaine. Anesthesiology 19: 45–50

Greene N M 1981 Preganglionic sympathetic blockade in man: a study of spinal anaesthesia. Acta Anaesthesiologica Scandinavica 25: 463–469

Kaufman L 1982 Phaeochromocytoma. In: Kaufman L (ed) Anaesthesia review 1. Churchill Livingstone, Edinburgh, p 21

Keele C A, Neil E, Joels N 1982 The autonomic nervous system. In: Samson Wright's applied physiology. Oxford University Press, Oxford, p 405

Keilty S R, Gray R C, Dundee J W, McCullough H 1968 Catecholamine levels in severe tetanus. Lancet ii: 195–198

Kerr J H, Corbett J L, Prys-Roberts C, Crampton-Smith A, Spalding J M K 1968 Involvement of the sympathetic nervous system in tetanus. Studies on 82 cases. Lancet ii: 236–241

Kou K, Ibengwe J, Suzuki H 1984 Effects of alpha adrenoceptor antagonists on electrical and mechanical responses of the isolated dog mesenteric vein to perivascular nerve stimulation and exogenous noradrenaline. Naunyn-Schmiedeberg's Archives of Pharmacology 326: 7–13

Langer S Z 1980 Presynaptic regulation of the release of catecholamines. Pharmacological Reviews 32: 337–362

Langer S Z, Hicks P E 1984 Physiology of the sympathetic nerve ending. British Journal of Anaesthesia 56: 689–700

Langer S Z, Massingham R, Shepperson N B 1980 Presence of postsynaptic α$_2$-adrenoceptors of predominantly extrasynaptic location in the vascular smooth muscle of the dog hind limb. Clinical Science 59 (suppl 6): 225S–228S

Langley J N 1921 The autonomic nervous system. Heffer Cambridge

Lee M R 1982 Dopamine and the kidney. Clinical Science 62: 439–448

Lee T, Seeman P, Rajput A, Farley I, Hornykiewicz O 1978 Receptor basis for dopaminergic supersensitivity in Parkinson's disease. Nature, London 273: 59–61

Lindahl S G E, Dahlgren N, Lundberg D, Norden N 1985 Adrenergic hyperactivity and epidural block in severe tetanus. Acta Anaesthesiologica Scandinavica 29: 87–89

Lokhandwala M F, Eikenburg D C 1983 Presynaptic receptors and alterations in norepinephrine release in spontaneously hypertensive rats. Life Sciences 33: 1527–1542

Majewski H, Rand M J 1981 Adrenaline mediated hypertension: a clue to the antihypertensive effect of β-adrenoceptor blocking drugs. Trends in Pharmacological Sciences 2: 24–26

Majewski H, Tung L H, Rand M J 1982 Adrenaline activation of prejunctional beta-adrenoceptors and hypertension. Journal of Cardiovascular Pharmacology 4: 99–106

Martres M P, Sokoloff P, Schwartz J C 1984 Dopaminergic binding sites in rat striatal slices and the action of guanyl nucleotides. Naunyn-Schmiedeberg's Archives of Pharmacology 325: 116–123

Meridy H W, Creighton R E 1971 General anaesthesia in eight patients with familial dysautonomia. Canadian Anaesthetists' Society Journal 18: 563–570

Misu Y, Kubo T 1983 Presynaptic β-adrenoceptors. Trends in Pharmacological Sciences 4: 506–508

Molinoff P B 1984 α- and β-adrenergic receptor subtypes. Properties, distribution and regulation. Drugs 28 (suppl 2): 1–15

Motulsky H J, Insel P A 1982 Adrenergic receptors in man. New England Journal of Medicine 307: 18–29

Page M M, Watkins P J 1978 Cardiorespiratory arrest and diabetic autonomic neuropathy. Lancet 1: 14–16

Rees P J, Prior J G, Cochrane G M, Clark T J H 1981 Sleep apnoea in diabetic patients with autonomic neuropathy. Journal of the Royal Society of Medicine 74: 192–195

Seeman P 1981 Brain dopamine receptors. Pharmacological Reviews 32: 229–313

Stirt J A, Frantz R A, Gunz E F, Conolly M E 1982 Anesthesia, catecholamines, and hemodynamics in autonomic dysfunction. Anesthesia and Analgesia 61: 701–704

Stoof J C, Kebabian J W 1984 Two dopamine receptors: biochemistry, physiology and pharmacology. Life Sciences 35: 2281–2296

Sutherland E W, Oye I, Butcher R W 1965 The action of epinephrine and the role of the adenyl cyclase system in hormone action. Recent Progress in Hormone Research 21: 623–646

Sweeney B P, Jones S, Langford R M 1985 Anaesthesia in dysautonomia: further complications. Anaesthesia 40: 783–786

Takeshima R, Dohi S 1985 Circulatory responses to baroreflexes, Valsalva maneuver, coughing, swallowing, and nasal stimulation during acute cardiac sympathectomy by epidural blockade in awake humans. Anesthesiology 63: 500–508

Watkins P J, Edmonds M E 1983 Clinical presentation of diabetic autonomic failure. In: Bannister R (ed) Autonomic failure. Oxford University Press, Oxford, p 337

P. J. Simpson

Immunology and anaesthesia

INTRODUCTION

During the past decade, the inter-relationships between the immune system and anaesthesia have become increasingly apparent. The influence of anaesthesia upon the immune system and conversely the involvement of the immune system in adverse reactions to anaesthetic agents have become increasingly recognised. Anaesthetic agents may affect the production of a normal immune response during and after surgery in specific and non-specific ways. Various agents, both volatile and intravenous, have been shown to affect lymphocyte function, related particularly to the production of specific antibody. The non-specific influence of anaesthesia and surgical stress has also been studied extensively both in terms of cell distribution and numbers and in its effect on the complement system and the acute phase inflammatory response.

The main area in which the immune system affects anaesthesia is in the increasingly frequent occurrence of adverse responses to anaesthetic agents, largely confined to drugs administered intravenously. The importance of such reactions lies chiefly in their relative unpredictability together with the increasing severity seen on repeat exposure. While many agents will produce moderate histamine release with localised, usually cutaneous, manifestations on first exposure, the severe reactions seen on second or subsequent exposure to the drug, usually antibody-mediated, are associated with bronchospasm, cardiovascular collapse and even death.

Although some overlap exists in these two main areas of interaction between anaesthesia and the immune system, it is more logical to consider them totally separately.

THE EFFECTS OF ANAESTHESIA UPON THE IMMUNE SYSTEM

The integrity of the immune system is essential to the production and maintenance of resistance to foreign substances and invading organisms. This involves both specific and non-specific mechanisms. Specific immunity is concerned with the production of either sensitised lymphocytes (cell-mediated) or freely circulating antibodies (humoral), while non-specific mechanisms include the involvement of the acute phase proteins and the complement cascade in the inflammatory response, together with the non-specific production and migratory activity of macrophages.

Specific immunity

Antibody production follows two separate pathways depending upon the immune system involved. The bone marrow stem cells mature into lymphocytes which are 'processed' either by the thymus gland (T lymphocytes) or by the mammalian equivalent of the avian 'bursa of Fabricius' (B lymphocytes). Antigenic exposure then stimulates T lymphocytes to mature into lymphoblasts producing antibody-coated cells responsible for cell mediated immunity, and lymphocytes to become plasma cells, producing humoral antibody which freely circulates in plasma.

The effects of anaesthesia upon the development and efficacy of specific cell-mediated immunity have largely been investigated using tests of lymphocyte function. These are broadly divided into three main areas concerned with the effects of anaesthetic agents on:

1. The response of lymphocytes to specific antigen (mitogen) stimulation.
2. The migratory activity of sensitised lymphocytes.
3. The relative distribution of T and B lymphocyte populations, in relation to the efficiency of cell-mediated or humoral immunity.

1. Mitogen stimulation of peripheral lymphocytes (lymphocyte transformation tests)

These involve the activation of specific lymphocytes by antigenic exposure, thereby testing functional immune competence. The antigens used are usually plant mitogens, commonly either phytohaemagglutinin (PHA), concanavalin-A (Con-A) or pokeweed (PWM). All react non-specifically with the lymphocyte cell surface inducing the same cellular events as does an antigen, but, unlike specific antigens, which only affect certain lymphocyte subgroups, all cells are sensitive. PHA and Con-A are predominantly T lymphocyte specific mitogens, while PWM stimulates both T and B lymphocytes. Serial tests, therefore, using several different mitogens distinguish between the effects of anaesthesia upon cell-mediated and humoral immunity.

Although such investigations would appear to provide a repeatable method of distinguishing between the effects of anaesthesia on various different lymphocyte subgroups and, indeed, animal studies have shown some anaesthetic depression of mitogen stimulation, especially related to halothane (Salo 1978a), thiopentone and pentobarbitone (Formeister et al 1980), human studies show a wide variation between individual patients and also between in vitro and in vivo results (Doenicke et al 1981, Salo 1978b). While halothane has been shown to have a depressant effect upon both T and B lymphocyte stimulation, other agents and techniques, including opioid/relaxant and lumbar epidural, induced no change (Edwards et al 1984). The T cell population tends to be reduced during and after anaesthesia and surgery in a non-specific way, the depression appearing to be more closely related to the degree of surgical stress than to the anaesthetic employed. The cause for this is uncertain, although Walton (1979) has suggested that the high levels of circulating corticosteroids involved in the hormonal and metabolic response to stress, depress T cell reactivity in a non-specific way.

A further test which looks non-specifically at the relative proportion of T and B lymphocytes and the effect of anaesthesia upon this is the sheep red blood cell rosette formation test. This relies upon a non-immune, non-specific property of human T lymphocytes to produce spontaneous rosettes on exposure to sheep red blood cells. It therefore provides an indication of the proportion of T lymphocytes able to form rosettes expressed as a percentage of the total lymphocyte population, indicating the relative proportions of T and B lymphocytes. In addition, sheep red blood cells can be coated with particular substances such as IgG, or the C3 complement component to form specific rosettes predominantly in this case with B rather than T lymphocytes.

Using this test, it is difficult to demonstrate specific anaesthetic-related alterations in the T and B lymphocyte pool in man. Major surgery is associated with a leucopenia and a relative reduction in T cells (Salo 1978a) but these reductions appear to be related more to the degree of operative stress than to the anaesthetic technique involved. Edwards et al (1984) found no statistical difference in non-specific rosette production between halothane, opioid/relaxant or regional anaesthesia. In this study, however, lack of alteration in the total lymphocyte pool was thought to be due to the low degree of operative trauma involved during inguinal herniorrhaphy.

The importance of lymphocyte transformation test in the investigation of allergy to various anaesthetic agents, as opposed to their general depressant effect during surgery, is included in a recent review (Assem 1984) concerned with methods of detection of such responses during anaesthesia.

2. Cellular migration

Anaesthesia in general and certain agents in particular, may affect the migration of leucocytes rather than their ability to synthesise antibody in response to antigenic stimulation. Inadequate migration of leucocytes may lead to impaired resistance to infection due to an inability to engulf foreign material and to release vasoactive substances. These tests are unstimulated and simply measure the random migration of leucocytes. General anaesthesia with either halothane or morphine/relaxant appears to diminish this response together with the more specific chemotactic response, to a greater extent than lumbar epidural anaesthesia (Stanley et al 1976, Edwards et al 1984).

Migration inhibition factor is produced in response to antigenic stimulation by cells of peritoneal exudate from sensitised guinea pigs. If specific antigen is present in sufficient quantity, migration inhibition factor, a lymphokine, is produced, localising the fan-shaped spread of macrophages from the open end of a capillary tube. The degree of inhibition is assessed from the area of the macrophage fan obtained in the presence of antigen expressed as a percentage of that in a control. This correlates with the intensity of the delayed (cell-mediated) hypersensitivity state. Since a small lymphocyte population obtained from peritoneal exudate in this way is able to induce migration inhibition when considerably diluted by macrophages, the latter are acting as non-specific indicators of the reaction between antigen and specifically sensitised lymphocytes and, therefore, measure the reactivity of the T cell (cell-mediated) immunity.

The production of migration inhibition factor is depressed by volatile agents, resulting in reduced phagocytosis and increased lymphocyte movement (Walton 1979). The effect of these changes is difficult to quantify but it seems likely that they increase susceptibility to infection due to inadequate phagocytosis particularly in the postoperative period. It is questionable whether the anaesthetic-induced depression of phagocyte activity in vivo is significant, particularly by comparison with the far greater changes induced by surgical stress (Cullen & van Belle 1975).

3. Effect of anaesthesia on cell numbers and cell division

For several years halothane has been known to inhibit division of hamster fibroblasts (Sturrock & Nunn 1975) and halothane (Nunn et al 1971), nitrous oxide (Kieler 1951) and trichloroethylene and chloroform (Ostergren 1944) have been shown to arrest mitosis at the metaphase stage. The clinical significance of these results has yet to be fully demonstrated. As a result of the initial anxiety over the possible carcinogenicity of isoflurane, Baden et al (1977) studying the mutagenic effects of the commonly used volatile agents found that none of those tested induced mutation in salmonella microsomes.

In terms of cell numbers, minor surgery with little stress, for example inguinal herniorrhaphy produces a neutrophil leucocytosis irrespective of anaesthetic technique either general or regional (Edwards et al 1984). More major surgery, however, is associated with a leucopenia, probably due more to surgical stress than to prolonged anaesthesia. Halothane and nitrous oxide have both been shown to depress or even arrest development of bone marrow stem cells (Bruce et al 1972). Overall numbers and activity of T lymphocytes are depressed by anaesthesia and surgery (Slade et al 1975), greater reductions being associated with more severe surgical stress. In general, T lymphocyte function appears to be affected to a greater extent by these non-specific mechanisms than does humoral (B cell) immunity.

Specific humoral immunity

Freely circulating humoral antibodies are produced by antigenic stimulation of B lymphocytes to become plasma cells, producing five main classes of antibody (Tables 5.1, 5.2). There is considerable variation between the immunoglobulins, both in terms of molecular size, plasma concentration and complement-binding activity. Those of greatest importance in the production of normal immune response in the peri-operative period are IgA, IgG and IgM. Although halothane and nitrous oxide both decrease the numbers of humoral-antibody producing cells within the spleen, there is little evidence that immunoglobulin concentrations change in peripheral blood. This is mainly due to the long half-life of the immunoglobulins concerned, 2.5 days for IgE, and 21 days for IgG. In vitro depression of IgG, IgM and IgA synthesis lasts for 6 to 7 days after cardiopulmonary

Table 5.1 Classification of antibodies

Immunoglobulin	IgG	IgA	IgM	IgD	IgE
Molecular weight ($\times 10^3$)	150	160	900	185	200
Heavy chains	Gamma	Alpha	Mu	Delta	Epsilon
Light chains	Kappa Lambda	Kappa Lambda	Kappa Lambda	Kappa Lambda	Kappa Lambda
Serum concentration (mg.ml^{-1})	8–16	1.4–4	0.5–2	0–0.4	17–450 (ng.ml^{-1})
Complement fixation	+	–	+++	?	–
Mast cell and basophil fixation	–	–	–	–	++

Table 5.2 Main antibody actions

IgG	Most abundant antibody in body fluids Particularly extravascular Anti-microorganisms and toxins
IgA	Sero-mucous secretions Protects external body surfaces
IgM	Agglutinating antibody Produced early in immune response Anti-A, anti-B
IgD	Lymphocyte surface antibody in newborn
IgE	Reaginic antibody Atopy, allergy

bypass (Salo et al 1981), but this has not been demonstrated after general surgery and anaesthesia.

Non-specific immunity

Activation of non-specific immune mechanisms by antigen-antibody reactions is an integral part of the inflammatory response and involves increased production and activity of the acute-phase proteins and complement. Acute inflammation associated with infection induces an acute-phase response, the proteins and vasoactive substances released being involved in increased vascular permeability, cell lysis and phagocytosis. Peak concentrations of the different acute-phase proteins occur at varying intervals after surgery (Crockson et al 1966, Aronsen et al 1972, Colley et al 1983). Maximum concentrations of C-reactive protein and alpha-1 antitrypsin tend to occur within 48 hours, while orosomucoid and fibrinogen levels do not peak until 3 to 4 days postoperatively (Crockson et al 1966).

Although C-reactive protein responds in most types of inflammatory response (Fischer et al 1976), changes in the concentrations of certain other proteins have been particularly associated with distinct conditions. C3 complement activation for example is seen in gram-negative septicaemia (Whaley et al 1979), fibrinogen and fibronectin concentrations are changed in disorders of coagulation and fibrinolysis (Mosher & Williams 1978), alpha-1 antitrypsin levels are markedly increased in active hepatitis and cirrhosis (Milford-Ward 1978) and orosomucoid is raised dramatically in pancreatitis, peritonitis and gastrointestinal infections (Whicher et al 1981). By contrast, the initiation of the acute-phase response following elective cholecystectomy under general anaesthesia does not appear to be significantly influenced by the anaesthetic agent used, although only fentanyl and halothane were included in this study (Simpson et al 1987). Increased capillary permeability and migration of macrophages, however, do appear to be altered by both halothane and opioid/relaxant anaesthesia (Edwards et al 1984).

Postoperative infection is due to numerous causes, the generalised immunosuppression caused by volatile agents being an important factor. Halothane has also been shown to increase morbidity and mortality in mice caused by experimentally induced bacterial and viral infections (Bruce 1967). Non-specific phagocytosis is depressed both by surgical and non-surgical factors, appearing to be primarily related to the severity of the stress (Walton 1979).

THE INVOLVEMENT OF THE IMMUNE SYSTEM IN ANAESTHESIA

This is almost entirely concerned with adverse responses to intravenous anaesthetic agents and is of particular importance because of the apparent unpredictability of such reactions. Although only a small proportion of the overall number of adverse reactions to intravenous anaesthetics are due to hypersensitivity, the incidence is increasing. This is largely due to the general increase in both the number and magnitude of surgical operations in recent years, which has inevitably resulted in a considerable increase both in the number of anaesthetics administered and more important, the frequency of repeat anaesthesia. In one study of 5500 routine anaesthetics (Clarke et al 1978) the most important factor in the development of an anaphylactoid response was the prior administration of the same anaesthetic.

Immunological mechanisms of hypersensitivity

Under normal conditions, exposure to an antigen produces a primary response, usually undetectable, leading to the production of specific antibody. Subsequent exposure to the same agent usually only produces a localised secondary response, which is limited by the antibody present and which also stimulates further antibody production. Hypersensitivity reactions, resulting from an abnormal secondary response can arise in a number of ways which may or may not be associated with complement activation (Gell et al 1975).

Type I. Immediate hypersensitivity

Antigens react with specific reaginic antibody, usually IgE bound to the surface of mast cells causing degranulation and the release of histamine and other vasoactive amines (e.g. slow reacting substance of anaphylaxis (SRSA), bradykinin, serotonin, prostaglandins).

Type II. Cytotoxic-type hypersensitivity

Antibodies bind to an antigen on the cell surface, producing phagocytosis, which may be enhanced by opsonic or immune adherence, or by K-cell-mediated, non-phagocytic extracellular cytotoxicity. Activation of the classical complement pathway then produces cell lysis.

Type III. Immune-complex-mediated hypersensitivity

Formation of immune complexes between antigen and humoral antibody, leading to classic complement pathway activation. This may produce a diffuse response (serum sickness) if there is an antigen excess or a localised response (Arthus) if there is antibody excess.

Type IV. Cell-mediated (delayed) hypersensitivity

T lymphocytes, with specific surface receptors are stimulated by antigen contact to release factors (lymphokines) which mediate delayed hypersensitivity.

Complement

Activation of the classical pathway is mediated through complement components C1, C4 and C2. The resulting activation of C3 then triggers the remaining components of the pathway, C5–9, resulting in cell lysis. Complement also has the important functions of immune adherence, agglutination and is one of the acute-phase proteins involved in acute inflammation. Classical pathway activation is triggered by antigen-antibody combination producing antigen destruction by cell lysis or phagocytosis.

Hypersensitivity reactions involving complement are either type II (cell surface antigens) or type III (immune complex formation). The antibodies involved are either IgM or IgG, both of which bind complement (Tables 5.1, 5.2). IgE on the other hand, is not a complement-binding antibody. Reactions involving IgM tend to be severe, involving agglutination, loin pain, haemoglobinuria, renal failure and even death. Since such reactions are very rarely seen in reactions to intravenous anaesthetics, it is likely that antibodies to such drugs, which precipitate complement activation are of the IgG group.

Activation of both the classical and alternate complement pathways also results in the formation of C3a and C5a, both anaphylatoxins involved in histamine release from mast cells. These produce increased vascular permeability allowing phagocytes to pass extravascularly and reach the foreign antigens.

Direct activation of the alternative complement pathway may occur in response to endotoxin, aggregated IgA and some drugs, e.g. intravenous anaesthetic agents such as Althesin. This may result in a hypersensitivity response in certain conditions with C3a and C5a leading to histamine release, bronchospasm, vasodilatation, hypotension and tachycardia. It has been suggested that direct C3 activation is more likely in conditions associated with complement abnormalities, e.g. pregnancy and disseminated carcinoma, when the normal inhibitors of cyclical C3 activation are reduced or absent.

Unlike the classical pathway, pre-formed antibodies to the antigen are not necessary for activation and so prior exposure to the drug or endotoxin is unnecessary. Unless the trigger responsible is in high titre or persistent, the majority of hypersensitivity reactions mediated through direct C3 activation are of a milder nature than those occurring as a result of classical pathway activation (Radford et al 1982).

MECHANISMS OF ANAPHYLACTOID REACTIONS TO INTRAVENOUS ANAESTHETIC AGENTS

In the case of intravenous anaesthetic agents the earlier classification of hypersensitivity needs to be modified because many of the normal protective mechanisms e.g. skin, gastrointestinal mucosa and alveolar-capillary membrane are inevitably bypassed by direct intravenous injection. Anaphylactoid reactions resulting from the direct, rapid intravenous administration of large doses of anaesthetic agents are probably better classified as below.

1. Direct pharmacological effect

A non-specific effect of many intravenous anaesthetic agents and neuromuscular blocking drugs, producing immediate release of vasoactive amines, probably histamine.

2. Classical complement pathway activation

Hypersensitivity following intravenous injection of an agent which has previously been administered uneventfully, usually within the past few weeks. Although specific antibodies may not have been demonstrated, such a reaction implies that this has occurred and therefore that this is either a type II or III reaction. Cross-sensitisation between drugs containing a common constituent e.g. cremophor EL may produce this type of reaction (Dye & Watkins 1980).

3. Alternative complement pathway activation

Hypersensitivity occurring on first exposure to the agent, but which involves direct activation of C3, histamine release and symptoms of anaphylaxis.

4. Type I. Immediate hypersensitivity

This is reaginic antibody-mediated immediate hypersensitivity, involving IgE-coated mast cell degranulation, histamine release and anaphylaxis.

Histamine release is associated with adverse reactions to almost all intravenous anaesthetic agents in man (Lorenz 1975), with the exception of etomidate (Doenicke et al 1973), and may be the result of any of these four mechanisms. Antibody formation, necessitating prior exposure to the agent, is essential in 2 and 4, but in the other two, hypersensitivity can occur on first exposure to the drug. The term anaphylactoid is conventionally applied to cases of hypersensitivity suggestive of anaphylaxis, but in which no antibody has been isolated.

Although these four mechanisms encompass the vast majority of adverse reactions to intravenous anaesthetic agents, several more have been suggested (Watkins 1979). The two main reasons for this are probably the use of intravenous administration, mentioned earlier and also the possibility of mixed reactions or cross-sensitisation (e.g. Althesin, propanidid).

Many drugs (e.g thiopentone, d-tubocurarine, suxamethonium, alcuronium) frequently produce either local or generalised histaminoid reactions. Most tend to be mild and unassociated with the more severe symptoms of tachycardia, hypotension and bronchospasm. The association of both thiopentone anaphylaxis and d-tubocurarine-induced hypotension with histamine release would appear to confirm this. IgE mediated immediate hypersensitivity does not conventionally bind complement, these reactions being the direct result of antigen combination with reaginic antibody coating mast cells. The resulting degranulation leads to the release of histamine and other vasoactive amines and the production of bronchospasm, vasodilatation and hypotension.

Like classical pathway activation, antibody production is specific, depending upon prior, uneventful exposure to the antigen. Certain individuals (atopic) have higher than normal levels of circulating IgE, produced in response to certain common antigens, e.g. house dust, pollens, etc. Measurements of total IgE are therefore not specifically related to the antigen thought to have precipitated the hypersensitivity reaction, but are simply indicative of a 'highly tuned' situation, e.g. atopy.

Possible mechanism of adverse reactions

Thiopentone

Although hypersensitivity reactions to barbiturates and in particular thiopentone are comparatively rare, they are often severe. Their incidence is significantly reduced by the avoidance of the drug in atopic patients with chronically elevated levels of IgE. Most available reports (Fox et al 1971, Etter et al 1980, Lilly & Hoy 1980) suggest involvement of IgE in thiopentone anaphylaxis, in the absence of complement pathway activation, at least in a primary capacity. It is thought that the rare cases in which IgE and complement are both involved, probably occur due to secondary activation of complement as a result of hypotension leading to metabolic derangement.

Reactions to thiopentone at the site of injection have already been discussed and are seldom severe unless the drug is inadvertently injected into an artery. Pain on injection is a variable feature, but tends to occur in the nervous vasoconstricted patient and seldom results in prolonged venous sequelae. Since large numbers of patients are uneventfully exposed to repeated doses of thiopentone, the incidence of antibody production must be remarkably low and is presumably related to the relative lack of antigenicity of the barbiturate molecule.

Althesin

In contrast to thiopentone, repeated exposure to Althesin frequently resulted in antibody production leading to hypersensitivity reactions. These fell into two discrete groups, those occurring on first and those following repeat exposure to the drug (Radford et al 1982).

Those occurring on first exposure tended to be relatively mild and were mediated in one of two ways.

a. Direct activation of the alternative complement pathway via C3, resulting in the release of anaphylatoxin C3a. Such reactions appeared to be more common in patients with pre-existing, transient complement abnormalities such as pregnancy and were possibly related to the absence of inhibitor enzymes.

b. *A direct pharmacological effect of the drug*, presumably on mast cells, resulting in histamine release. These reactions were impossible to predict and were unassociated with pre-existing disease.

Uneventful first exposure to Althesin appeared to sensitise a significant number of patients to the drug, leading in some cases to a hypersensitivity reaction on second or subsequent exposure. These reactions invariably involved classical complement pathway activation and were frequently severe, particularly if the interval between exposures was short, i.e. less than 2 months (Radford et al 1982). Although histamine is involved as a mediator of the anaphylactoid response, IgE involvement was not demonstrated.

Cremophor EL

Cremophor was included as a solubilising agent in both Althesin, propanidid and in the original preparation of propofol (ICI 35868). Reports indicated that a degree of cross-sensitivity might occur in patients repeatedly exposed to one or more of these agents (Dye & Watkins 1980, Briggs et al 1982). Since the common factor was the solubilising agent cremophor EL, this alone was investigated in the minipig animal model (Glen et al 1979). Although repeat exposure to cremophor did induce hypersensitivity and histamine release, implying antibody formation, similar experiments using alphaxolone or the complete Althesin preparation produced similar results, implying perhaps an additive effect of the individual constituents of the preparation. Certainly it would appear that any drug solubilised in cremophor is likely to possess antigenic potential.

Etomidate, propofol

To date, no reports of hypersensitivity reactions directly related to either of these two drugs have appeared. This is perhaps a little surprising since both are insoluble in water. Etomidate is dissolved in propylene glycol and propofol in soya-bean oil and purified egg phosphatide. Localised pain on injection is the only minor adverse effect to be reported.

Incidence of adverse reactions

Although the reported incidence of severe or even fatal hypersensitivity reactions to intravenous anaesthetic agents is extremely small by comparison to the number of anaesthetics administered annually, their apparent unpredictability and occurrence in previously healthy patients makes even these small numbers important. Considerable variations occur between comparative studies of the frequency of hypersensitivity reactions to intravenous

Table 5.3 Comparative incidence of adverse reactions to intravenous anaesthetics

Intravenous anaesthetic	Incidence of reaction
Thiopentone	1:14 000–1:20 000
Althesin	1:400–1:2000
Methohexitone	1:7000
Propanidid	1:500–1:1700
Etomidate	—
Propofol	—

anaesthetic agents. This is probably largely due both to differences in reporting and to the significance attached to clinical observations recorded. Table 5.3 has been constructed from data from various sources (Evans & Keogh 1977, Clarke et al 1978, Beamish 1979, Fisher & More 1981, Radford et al 1982).

Although the incidence of reactions to Althesin was undoubtedly high, a large number of these were mild. Severe reactions, particularly on first exposure, were rare (Radford et al 1982) and only two possible fatalities were reported (Avery & Evans 1973, Vanezis 1979).

The incidence of reactions to propanidid was remarkably similar to those following Althesin supporting the theory that cremophor EL, common to both preparations, was responsible. Similarly, when ICI 35868 was dissolved in cremophor, a single report (Briggs et al 1982) suggested the possibility of cross-sensitivity between this drug and propanidid in a patient who had been previously exposed uneventfully to the latter. At first sight, drugs which are insoluble in water, necessitating formulation with solubilising agents such as cremophor, would seem most likely to cause hypersensitivity. While this may be a significant factor when considering complement-mediated anaphylaxis, other drugs which are water-soluble, e.g. thiopentone, may also produce histamine release, albeit by a different mechanism. Moreover, neither etomidate nor propofol appears to induce hypersensitivity at least as far as early reports indicate.

Although hypersensitivity reactions to thiopentone occur less frequently than those due to either Althesin or propanidid, they tend to be more severe, the proportion of fatalities being significantly greater than with other agents.

Reactions to methohexitone are apparently rare, only one report having been published (Driggs & O'Day 1972). Perhaps this is a drug which should be re-examined more closely, particularly for use in patients who have previously been exposed to other agents.

PREDISPOSING FACTORS TO THE DEVELOPMENT OF ADVERSE REACTIONS

Many clinicians believe that certain predisposing factors are important in the development of adverse, and particularly hypersensitivity reactions to intravenous anaesthetic agents. These can be broadly divided into patient-dependent and pharmacological factors.

Patient factors

Age

Although adverse reactions are comparatively rare in children, there is a steady increase in reports of hypersensitivity occurring in the young, particularly related to the use of Althesin (Radford et al 1982). When one considers that repeated exposure to any agent is probably the most important factor in the development of hypersensitivity, it is perhaps not surprising that reactions tend to occur when the drug is used on a subsequent occasion in the older child. The widespread use of phenothiazine premedication in children, with its associated antihistaminic properties, may well contribute significantly to the prevention of reactions in this age group.

Sex

Although hypersensitivity reactions appear to be more common in young females, this is probably related to the far greater number of short general anaesthetics administered to this age group for minor gynaecological surgery and to the large number who are coincidentally pregnant (vide infra). Significant numbers of reactions have been reported in males undergoing repeated anaesthesia, usually for orthopaedic procedures following trauma.

Atopy

As Clarke et al (1978) have shown, the incidence of hypersensitivity reactions is higher in atopic individuals than in the normal population. This increase, however, is small in comparison to that occurring on repeat exposure to the same anaesthetic agent. Two important clinical conclusions can be drawn.

1. Any atopic patient is more likely than an unaffected individual to suffer a hypersensitivity reaction to any intravenous anaesthetic agent.
2. Those agents thought to produce IgE-mediated hypersensitivity i.e. thiopentone, d-tubocurarine and alcuronium are contra-indicated in atopic individuals. Agents producing complement-mediated reactions, which therefore do not involve IgE, should not precipitate hypersensitivity in these patients with anything more than the generally increased incidence associated with atopy.

Pre-existing complement abnormalities

The absence of certain inhibitory proteins within the complement pathway, e.g. Cl esterase inhibitor in hereditary angioneurotic oedema (HANE), may itself produce signs of hypersensitivity, particularly oedema and broncho-spasm. Whether this and other similar conditions are likely to be precipitated by intravenous anaesthetics is not yet well understood. Anaesthesia in this situation is probably best achieved with an inhalational technique, preceded by antihistamine premedication and possibly the use of disodium chromoglycate (Intal) to stabilise mast cells and prevent histamine release.

Pregnancy

Pregnancy appears to be associated with an unusually high incidence of adverse reactions on first or subsequent exposure to intravenous agents. The widespread use of Althesin for vaginal termination of pregnancy and evacuation of retained products (ERPC) resulted in many unpredictable reactions. Comparison with other agents is difficult since no other single drug has been used so frequently, but a comparative study between pregnant and non-pregnant patients, exposed to Althesin for the first time, confirmed an increased incidence of adverse reactions in the pregnant group (Simpson et al 1982).

Previous exposure

Previous exposure to any intravenous anaesthetic agent is likely to predispose to the development of hypersensitivity on subsequent administration of either the same drug or to another with similar constituents (Dye & Watkins 1980). In the case of Althesin, Radford et al (1982) demonstrated a high incidence of reactions on second or subsequent exposure, all of which when investigated, indicated antigen-antibody combination initiating classic complement pathway activation. Of far greater clinical importance, however, was the high incidence of severe reactions (systolic blood pressure less than 60 mmHg) in this group, particularly when the interval between exposures was short.

Stress

Many clinical anaesthetists feel that 'reactions' are far more likely to occur in the highly stressed, nervous and often unpremedicated patient, and recommend the use of pre-operative anxiolytic drugs together with heavy premedication in susceptible patients. Adrenaline is certainly able to induce complement activation which may explain one way in which such reactions are mediated.

Pharmacological effects

These are largely unpredictable, although some patients will volunteer that they 'react' to many drugs either by the development of mild skin rashes or simply by 'feeling funny'. While such symptoms cannot specifically contra-indicate any particular intravenous anaesthetic agent, the use of antihistamine premedication and the avoidance of pre-operative stress already mentioned, may be of considerable importance.

Total dose and dose rate of administration

Although these have often been considered as factors likely to predispose particularly to a 'pharmacological' reaction, there is little evidence to support this. Methods of administration vary from rapid bolus injection of drugs to intravenous infusion, and reactions have occurred in all groups. Simpson et al (1982) were unable to demonstrate any difference in the incidence of reactions in two groups of patients, both pregnant and non-pregnant, given different doses and dose rates of Althesin.

The incidence of reactions to Althesin following intravenous infusion either for anaesthesia or continuous sedation was remarkably low and it is possible that a very slow infusion rate may have minimised pharmacological reactions.

Preservatives and solubilising agents

The inclusion of these agents in numerous intravenous anaesthetics and other drugs makes the incidence of inadvertent repeat exposure to them more likely. Cremophor-related cross-sensitivity has been documented (Dye & Watkins 1980) and other reports may follow if the use of these additives continues. It is important to remember that cremophor is still included in several non-anaesthetic intravenous preparations, for example vitamin K1 (Konakion), miconazole (Daktarin) and cyclosporin (Sandimmun).

PREVENTION OF ADVERSE REACTIONS TO INTRAVENOUS ANAESTHETIC AGENTS

Although many of the reactions, particularly those occurring on first exposure to the drug are apparently unpredictable, a number of possible predisposing factors do exist which may allow preventative measures to be employed. These may include:

1. The use of *local* rather than general anaesthesia, although the agents used should be of the amide rather than the ester type, since hypersensitivity to the latter is not uncommon.
2. If *general* anaesthesia is to be used, the use of adequate pre-operative anxiolysis and premedication to minimise stress.

3. Pre-operative prophylaxis.
   a. Sodium chromoglycate to stabilise mast cells and prevent histamine release.
   b. Salbutamol to prevent bronchospasm.
   c. Hydrocortisone.
   d. Antihistamine premedication, e.g. promethazine which can be incorporated into the normal pre-operative preparation and which is prob ably the most useful and important of these four suggested alternatives.
4. The avoidance of drugs to which the patient has been previously exposed, particularly within recent weeks or months. If no anaesthetic records are available, it should be assumed, if appropriate, that the patient has been given one of the more 'reactogenic' drugs.
5. If possible use an inhalational induction to avoid the use of intravenous induction agents.
6. Avoid the use of plasma expanders such as dextran and haemaccel, both of which are associated with hypersensitivity reactions.

TREATMENT OF ADVERSE REACTIONS

Many of the mild adverse reactions require no treatment other than, if the drug is still being administered, discontinuation of the infusion. If the patient is awake and either cutaneous symptoms of flushing or pruritis are troublesome, intravenous chlorpheniramine (Piriton) should be all that is necessary.

The most important aspects of treatment relate to the more severe reactions involving bronchospasm and hypotension. The cardiovascular symptoms are almost invariably related to relative hypovolaemia secondary to profound vasodilatation. Initial treatment should include the administration of oxygen, with or without endotracheal intubation according to the severity of the collapse, intravenous fluid therapy and posturing the patient in the head-down position.

In the early stages, restoration of intravascular volume is essential and crystalloid fluid replacement (Hartmann's solution or physiological saline) is sufficient. In cases requiring prolonged resuscitation, plasma expanders will be required to maintain intravascular volume. In this case plasma protein fraction (HPPF) is probably the best solution since many of the others are liable to produce hypersensitivity in their own right.

Drug therapy will also vary according to the severity of the reaction so that in the case of cardiac arrest, symptomatic treatment dependent upon cardiac rhythm will be necessary. Specific therapy in the initial stages of treatment should include intravenous chlorpheniramine (Piriton) and possibly hydrocortisone. The use of subcutaneous or intravenous adrenaline may also be necessary in severe cases. The need for other drugs will depend upon clinical symptoms, for example:

1. Aminophylline, isoprenaline or salbutamol for bronchospasm.
2. Isoprenaline, adrenaline or atropine for bradycardia.
3. Dopamine, ephedrine or adrenaline for persistant peripheral vasodilatation.

It is also important not to forget to take blood samples as soon as is reasonably practicable for subsequent laboratory investigation. Subsequent counselling should include an interview with the patient to explain the sensitivity, to reassure them that they can still receive anaesthesia provided the particular agent is avoided and to introduce them to MedicAlert or another similar organisation maintaining a central register of susceptible patients. A clear summary of the patient's reaction and the results of subsequent laboratory tests should appear in the case notes and be sent to the patient's general practitioner.

REFERENCES

Aronsen K–F, Ekelund G, Kindmark C–O, Laurell C B 1972 Sequential changes of plasma proteins after surgical trauma. Scandinavian Journal of Clinical Laboratory Investigation 29 (suppl 124): 127–136
Assem E S K 1984 Allergic responses during anaesthesia: methods of detection. In: Kaufman L (ed) Anaesthesia review 2. Churchill Livingstone, Edinburgh, p 49
Avery A F, Evans A 1973 Reactions to Althesin. British Journal of Anaesthesia 45: 301–302
Baden J M, Kelley M, Wharton R S et al 1977 Mutagenicity of halogenated ether anaesthetics. Anesthesiology 46: 346–350
Beamish D 1979 Adverse response to Althesin. Anaesthesia 34: 683
Briggs L P, Clarke R S J, Watkins J 1982 An adverse reaction to the administration of disoprofol (Diprivan). Anaesthesia 37: 1099–1101
Bruce D L 1967 Effect of halothane anaesthesia on experimental salmonella peritonitis in mice. Journal of Surgical Research 7: 180
Bruce D L, Lin H S, Bruce W R 1972 In: Fink R (ed) Cellular biology and toxicity of anesthetics. Williams and Wilkins, Baltimore, p 251
Clarke R S J, Fee J H, Dundee J W 1978 Hypersensitivity reactions to intravenous anaesthetics. In: Watkins J, Ward A M (eds) Adverse response to intravenous drugs. Academic Press, London, p 41
Colley C M, Fleck A, Goode A W, Muller B R, Myers M A 1983 Early time course of the acute phase protein response in man. Journal of Clinical Pathology 36: 203–207
Crockson R A, Payne C J, Ratcliff A P, Soothill J F 1966 Time sequence of acute phase reactive proteins following surgical trauma. Clinica Chimica Acta 14: 425–441
Cullen B F, van Belle G 1975 Lymphocyte transformation and changes in leukocyte count: Effects of anesthesia and operation. Anesthesiology 43: 563
Doenicke A, Lorenz W, Beigl R et al 1973 Histamine release after intravenous application of short-acting hypnotics. British Journal of Anaesthesia 45: 1097–1104
Doenicke A, Grote B, Suttmann H et al 1981 Effects of halothane on the immunological system in healthy volunteers. Clinical Research Reviews 1: 23
Driggs R L, O'Day R A 1972 Acute allergic reaction associated with methohexital anaesthesia: report of six cases. Journal of Oral Surgery 30: 906–909
Dye D, Watkins J 1980 Suspected anaphylactic reaction to cremophor EL. British Medical Journal 280: 1353
Edwards A E, Gemmell L W, Mankin P P, Smith C J, Allen J C, Hunter A 1984 The effects of three differing anaesthetics on the immune response. Anaesthesia 39: 1071
Etter M S, Helrich M, Mackenzie C F 1980 Immunoglobulin E fluctuation in thiopental anaphylaxis. Anesthesiology 52: 181–183

Evans J M, Keogh J A M 1977 Adverse reactions to intravenous anaesthetic induction agents. British Medical Journal 275: 735–736

Fischer C L, Gill C, Forrester M G, Nakamura R 1976 Quantitation of 'acute-phase proteins' postoperatively. American Journal of Clinical Pathology 66: 840–846

Fisher M McD, More D G 1981 The epidemiology and clinical features of anaphylactic reactions in anaesthesia. Anaesthesia and Intensive Care 9: 226–234

Formeister J F, MacDermott R P, Wickline D et al 1980 Alteration of lymphocyte function due to anaesthesia: in vivo and in vitro suppression of mitogen-induced blastogenesis by sodium pentobarbital. Surgery 87: 573

Fox G S, Wilkinson R D, Rabow R I 1971 Thiopental anaphylaxis: a case and method for diagnosis. Anesthesiology 35: 655–657

Gell P G H, Coombs R R A, Lachmann P 1975 Clinical aspects of immunology. 3rd edn. Blackwell Scientific, Oxford

Glen J B, Davies G E, Thomson D S, Scarth S C, Thompson A V 1979 An animal model for the investigation of adverse responses to intravenous anaesthetic agents and their solvents. British Journal of Anaesthesia 51: 819–829

Kieler J 1951 The cytotoxic effect of nitrous oxide at different oxygen tensions. Acta Pharmacologica Toxicologica 13: 301

Lilly J K, Hoy R H 1980 Thiopental anaphylaxis and reagin involvement. Anesthesiology 53: 335–337

Lorenz W 1975 Histamine release in man. Agents Actions 5: 402–416

Milford-Ward A 1978 Alpha-1-antitrypsin. In: Immunochemistry in clinical laboratory medicine (Proceedings of a symposium held at Lancaster University). MTP, Lancaster, p 183

Mosher D F, Williams E M 1978 Fibronectin concentration is decreased in plasma of severely ill patients with disseminated intravascular coagulation. Journal of Laboratory and Clinical Medicine 91: 729–735

Nunn J F, Lovis J D, Kimball K L 1971 Arrest of mitosis by halothane. British Journal of Anaesthesia 43: 524

Ostergren G 1944 Colchicine mitosis, chromosome contractions, narcosis and protein chain folding. Hereditas 30: 429

Radford S G, Lockyer J A, Simpson P J 1982 Immunological aspects of adverse reactions to Althesin. British Journal of Anaesthesia 54: 859–863

Salo M 1978a Effect of anaesthesia and surgery on the number of and mitogen-induced transformation of T- and B-lymphocytes. Annals of Clinical Research 10: 1

Salo M 1978b Effect of anaesthesia and open-heart surgery on lymphocyte responses to phytohaemagglutinin and concanavalin A. Acta Anaesthesiologica Scandinavica 22: 471

Salo M, Eskola J, Viljanen M K, Ruuskanen O (1981) B-Lymphocyte activation during anaesthesia and open-heart surgery. Abstract Acta Anaesthesiologica Scandinavica 25 (suppl 72): 67

Simpson P J, Radford S G, Lockyer J A, Sear J W 1982 Some factors predisposing to Althesin hypersensitivity. British Journal of Anaesthesia 54: 1131

Simpson P J, Radford S G, Lockyer J A 1987 The influence of anaesthesia on the acute phase protein response to surgery. Anaesthesia 42: 690–696

Slade M S, Simmons R L, Yunis E, Greenberg L J 1975 Immunodepression after major surgery in normal patients. Surgery 78: 363

Stanley T H, Hill G E, Portas M R, Hogan N A, Hill H R 1976 Neutrophil chemotaxis during and after general anaesthesia and operation. Anesthesia and Analgesia 55: 668–673

Sturrock J E, Nunn J F 1975 Mitosis in mammalian cells during exposure to anaesthetics. Anesthesiology 43: 21

Vanezis P 1979 Death after Althesin. The Practitioner 222: 249–251

Walton B 1979 Effects of anaesthesia and surgery on immune status. British Journal of Anaesthesia 51: 37

Watkins J 1979 Anaphylactoid reactions to intravenous substances. British Journal of Anaesthesia 51: 51–61

Whaley K, Yee Khong T, McCartney A C, Ledingham I McA 1979 Complement activation and its control in gram-negative endotoxic shock. Journal of Clinical and Laboratory Immunology 2: 117–124

Whicher J T, Bell A M, Southall P J 1981 Measurements in clinical management. Diagnostic Medicine July/August: 62–80

The endocrine system

This chapter only considers certain aspects of the endocrine system and this includes the endocrine response to surgery, the atrial natriuretic peptide and hyponatraemia. The rest of the chapter is concerned with advances on the mode of action of arginine vasopressin (AVP).

ENDOCRINE RESPONSE TO SURGERY

Peripheral surgery

There are still many studies being undertaken on the endocrine response to surgery. Seitz et al (1986) compared halothane, nitrous oxide, oxygen anaesthesia with epidural analgesia (without hypotension) produced by 0.5% bupivacaine for operations on the knee joint. There were significant rises in ACTH, beta-lipotropin, cortisol and dehydroepiandrosterone (DHA) during general anaesthesia but these were absent following epidural analgesia. The increased renin and ACTH levels which occurred appeared to be responsible for the increase in aldosterone.

Abdominal surgery

In another study patients undergoing elective cholecystectomy under general anaesthesia were compared with patients having in addition, extradural bupivacaine 0.5% plain prior to induction of general anaesthesia. The splanchnic uptake of glycerol was lower in the patients in the epidural group but the uptake of lactate and alanine were similar in both groups. Plasma catecholamines and serum cortisol levels were higher in the patients receiving only general anaesthesia while serum growth hormone was higher in the extradural group (Lund et al 1986).

Cardiac surgery

Hynynen et al (1986a) compared the use of continuous infusions of fentanyl or alfentanil for coronary artery bypass surgery (total dose ratio of fentanyl to alfentanil = 1:13) and found that cardiovascular stability was maintained with either drug postoperatively. Plasma cortisol levels decreased in both groups of patients before cardiopulmonary bypass after which levels rose significantly. Beta endorphin immunoreactivity increased with both fentanyl and alfentanil immediately after the onset of cardiopulmonary bypass and remained elevated. There were no significant changes in plasma AVP concentrations during anaesthesia and surgery. When the opiate infusions were discontinued there was an increase in AVP concentration which commenced earlier in the alfentanil group (Hynynen et al 1986b). Hynynen et al (1986a) also concluded that alfentanil no longer had a short duration of action when given in large doses and that the AVP response to coronary artery bypass surgery could be prevented by continuous infusion of fentanyl or alfentanil (Hynynen et al 1986b). In another study plasma renin activity (PRA) and AVP levels were measured during coronary artery surgery and PRA levels were increased but this followed no particular pattern. The AVP concentrations were all increased but the changes were not related to the postoperative arterial hypertension that occurred (Hawkins et al 1986). The AVP response to surgery was also compared in patients having coronary artery surgery with those undergoing thymectomy and levels rose in both groups during splitting of the sternum. There was a second more marked increase in AVP levels in those patients who had cardiopulmonary bypass (Knight et al 1986).

Depth of anaesthesia

It has been postulated that the endocrine response to surgery may depend on the depth of anaesthesia. Lacoumenta et al (1986) studied the effects of two different concentrations of halothane, in patients undergoing hysterectomy and found that there was no significant difference in the changes of blood glucose, lactate, plasma glycerol, insulin and catecholamines.

Spinal opioids

Intrathecal morphine (0.8 mg) administered prior to operation for cholecystectomy was compared with patients given intravenous papaveretum during operation. Although intrathecal morphine had no effect upon the hyperglycaemic response to surgery it did reduce the expected rise in serum cortisol concentration (Downing et al 1986). A similar effect was obtained by Child & Kaufman (1985) using intrathecal heroin.

In patients also undergoing cholecystectomy Normandale et al (1985) compared epidural diamorphine (10 mg) with intravenous papaveretum. They found little difference in the parameters measured during operation which included blood glucose, lactate, pyruvate and non-esterified fatty acids but the plasma cortisol levels were much lower in the epidural diamorphine group postoperatively when there was also better pain relief than in the control group. They concluded that epidural diamorphine does not influence the endocrine response to surgery but does so in the postoperative period, this being secondary to better pain relief. This is in contrast to the studies of Child & Kaufman (1985) who administered the diamorphine intrathecally.

The metabolic effects of intrathecal morphine have been evaluated in patients undergoing coronary artery surgery. 4 mg of morphine in 6 ml saline was administered prior to surgery and although it provided better postoperative analgesia than a control group it was ineffectual in modifying the response to surgery as assessed by plasma catecholamines and glucose. Cortisol suppression was noted in the postoperative period and lasted for 5 hours suggesting possibly a delayed effect of morphine (Sebel et al 1985).

Splanchnic nerves

Shirasaka et al (1986) discussed the role of the splanchnic nerves on the endocrine response to surgery. They measured plasma cortisol, glucose, free fatty acids and urinary adrenaline in patients having partial gastrectomy under general anaesthesia with splanchnic nerve blockade or under epidural analgesia. The inhibitory effect of the splanchnic blockade was only slightly less than that of the high epidural but in both these groups the parameters measured were depressed compared with the results under general anaesthesia alone. Urinary noradrenaline excretion was highest on the first postoperative day in the patients having general anaesthesia. Thus splanchnic nerve stimulation appears to account for the endocrine response to surgery although the results also suggested that pain stimulation was responsible for catecholamine release. The main stimulus for AVP release appears to be peritoneal stimulation (Melville et al 1985).

Other studies have compared the role of catabolic hormones with fasting. An infusion of cortisol, glucagon and adrenaline results in hypermetabolism, hyperglycaemia and hyperinsulinaemia but marked suppression of the ketosis of fasting (Watters & Wilmore 1986). The metabolic rate can be stimulated in man when the plasma adrenaline level is increased two to three times the basal rate but the physiological significance of this has still to be established (MacDonald et al 1985).

Respiratory depression

Most of the reports of respiratory depression have occurred after epidural morphine, but this complication has been noted to occur following diamorphine and appears to have occurred after inadvertent dural puncture (Corke & Wheatley 1985).

Stability of diamorphine

The stability of diamorphine in saline has been questioned and it is unlikely to be of importance when diamorphine is reconstituted in saline immediately prior to intrathecal or epidural injection. Hain & Kirk (1985) have shown that diamorphine in sodium chloride solution, at pH 4.9 and stored at a temperature of 23°C for 24 hours was quite stable. Macrae (1987) also confirmed that there was no significant degradation of diamorphine in saline for the same period.

Temperature

A fact which may affect some of the studies on the endocrine response to surgery may also be change in mean body temperature, especially in elderly patients undergoing large bowel surgery. An attempt was made to maintain the patients at normal temperatures during and after surgery by warming the fresh gases, the intravenous fluids, by padding exposed parts of the body at operation and covering patients with the equivalent of a space blanket in the postoperative period. In these patients the excretion of 3-methylhistidine (3-MeH), a marker of muscle protein breakdown and also urea nitrogen loss were measured in the urine and it was found that prevention of heat loss during and after surgery resulted in a significant decrease in the loss of muscle protein and nitrogen (Carli & Itiaba 1986). A novel technique involving the use of an oesophageal tube through which warm water circulates has been described by Kristensen et al 1986. They recommend the use of this apparatus which maintained body temperature satisfactorily. They considered this to be of great importance in patients with a limited cardiopulmonary reserve. The possible dangers of the apparatus are leakage of water and thermal injury to the oesophagus.

Fatigue and anxiety

Attempts have been made to correlate postoperative fatigue with preoperative anxiety but Christensen et al (1986) have been unable to confirm any correlation between the two. They suggested that nutritional status, neuromuscular function and the state of the cardiovascular system are more likely to be involved in the aetiology of fatigue than psychological factors. In fact Brough et al (1986) confirmed that muscle function was not influenced by long term steroids, trauma or surgery but by poor nutritional intake and muscle function could be restored with total parenteral nutrition in patients with insufficient dietary intake. Chan et al (1986) have adopted a regime of glucose-potassium prior to surgery as this has been shown to improve muscle power in undernourished patients. Brooks et al (1986) found that there was a correlation between cortisol growth hormone and anxiety but there was no correlation between anxiety and serum prolactin levels.

Atrial natriuretic peptide (atrial peptin)

Needleman & Greenwald (1986) have described atriopeptin as 'a cardiac hormone intimately involved in fluid, electrolyte and blood pressure homeo-stasis'. This peptide, recently discovered, is stored in granules in the atrium as a prohormone, atriopeptigen. The prohormone has 126 amino acids, is probably continuously released at low levels but the hormone detected in the plasma is a low molecular weight 28-amino-acid hormone, alpha atrial natriuretic peptide (alpha ANP). The hormone is released when the atrium is stretched in response to volume expansion, vasoconstrictors that elevate atrial pressure, atrial tachycardia and high intake of salt. The hormone increases glomerular filtration rate, renal blood flow, urine volume, sodium excretion and decreases plasma renin activity. There is inhibition of aldosterone secretion (irrespective of stimuli for its release such as angiotensin II, ACTH or potassium). The expected rise in AVP release in response to dehydration or haemorrhage is also suppressed. Blood vessels are relaxed by direct action. The main effects of alpha ANP therefore are to promote the loss of water and electrolytes and reduce vascular tone. If blood volume is reduced there is a negative feedback mechanism reducing plasma levels of alpha ANP. With radio-immunoassay techniques the normal resting level of alpha ANP ranges from 10 to 70 pg/ml. Needleman & Greenwald (1986) suggested the use of alpha ANP as a diuretic to produce water and sodium loss without a marked potassium loss and also in the treatment of cardiac failure. However ANP levels were elevated in patients with increased right and left atrial pressures. In heart failure sympathetic activity and the effects of the renin-angiotensin system may predominate over the relaxing property of ANP (Raine et al 1986). Richards et al (1986) found that the measurement of alpha ANP was a useful objec-tive indicator of the severity of cardiac disability (Leading Article Lancet 1986).

ANP concentrations are raised in patients following cardiac transplant surgery leading to the suggestion that the transplanted atria may secrete the hormone (Singer et al 1986). However Schwab et al (1986) found elevated levels in patients who had artificial hearts. Schwab et al (1986) concluded from their data that ANP is normally present in these patients and is released into the circulation as the right atrial pressure is increased.

Hyponatraemia

Hyponatraemia has been reported in mothers and infants at delivery especially when there has been maternal overload with non-electrolyte solution. Some of the infants had sodium concentrations of 125 mmol/l but no neurological damage resulted (Tarnow-Mordi et al 1981).

Arieff (1986) reported convulsions, respiratory arrest and permanent brain damage associated with hyponatraemia after elective surgery in healthy women. There were 15 healthy patients in the series whose pre-operative serum sodium level was 138 mmol/l and approximately 49 hours after surgery the serum sodium fell to 108 mmol/l. Grand mal seizures developed followed by respiratory arrest requiring intubation. Prior to the convulsion, symptoms included nausea, headache and vomiting. Half the patients were incontinent, some were disorientated, depressed or had hallucinations. A cerebrovascular accident was suspected and this delayed the diagnosis and treatment. Seven of the patients recovered from the comatose state after serum sodium had reached 131 mmol/l, but they became comatose again a few days later and either died or suffered permanent brain damage. In this series 60% were left with permanent brain damage, 27% died and 13% had limb paralysis.

On reviewing the postoperative fluid balance it transpired that the average intake was 8.8 ± 0.7 litres of 2.5 mmol/l glucose (containing less than 5 mmol of sodium chloride per litre). The mean urinary output was 1.3 ± 0.4 litres with an osmolality of 501 ± mosm/kg and a sodium level of 68 ± 10 mmol/l. Arieff (1986) concluded that with this level of elevated urinary sodium and osmolality in the presence of water intoxication and hyponatraemia there was inappropriate secretion of AVP. Response to therapy with sodium chloride often combined with frusemide was variable with some of the patients regaining consciousness only to relapse into coma later. One patient had permanent double vision and partial paralysis of one leg while the other had partial paralysis of one arm and one leg. Contributive factors were sought and some of the patients had been taking thiazide diuretics, phenothiazines, while one patient had idiopathic diabetes insipidus. One patient was on prednisone while another two were on propranolol. Seven of the patients were comatose while the serum sodium level was being increased from 105 to 131 mmol/l over a period of 41 hours, while 51 hours after awakening from the comatose state and being able to talk, eat and even walk they had convulsions, became comatose and did not recover. There have been suggestions that this may be due to the rapid correction of serum sodium although increasing the serum at the rate of 2 mmol/l appears to be an acceptable regime from a consensus of experts (Narins 1986).

Sterns et al (1986) have also described neurological damage associated with the rapid correction of hyponatraemia (greater than 12 mmol/l/day). Neurological damage that resulted was pontine myelinolysis. The symptoms may vary from failure to recover, generalised seizures, dysarthria, difficulty in walking, spastic quadriplegia, bulbar paralysis and hallucinations.

Although hyponatraemia may cause cerebral oedema there is less brain swelling as a result of loss of cell solute if the condition becomes chronic. Sterns et al (1986) concluded that it was dangerous to attempt to correct hyponatraemia rapidly as otherwise osmotic demyelination would ensue. Ayus (1986) has suggested that serum sodium concentration should not be corrected by more than 20 mmol/l in the first 24 hours.

These case reports underline the dangers of administering non-electrolyte solutions during surgical procedures and the need for monitoring the serum sodium at regular intervals in the postoperative period. Loss of sodium may occur prior to operation and fail to be detected as electrolyte levels are usually measured on admission and e.g. not after patients have had purgatives to empty the bowel prior to abdominal surgery. Diuretics prior to surgery and during surgery to maintain urinary output may further reduce the serum sodium.

ARGININE VASOPRESSIN (AVP)

Although the antidiuretic effects of vasopressin have been known for more than 50 years it is only recently that its other actions have been discovered prompting this extensive review.

AVP is synthesised in cells in the supra-optic and paraventricular nuclei and passes down the axon of these neurones to be stored in the posterior pituitary. It is rapidly destroyed in the liver and kidneys and has a half-life of 18 minutes. Its main action has always been considered to conserve water in response to haemorrhage when there was a decreased extracellular fluid volume and increased plasma osmotic pressure. Stimulation of portal osmo receptors releases vasopressin (Baertschi et al 1985). Pain and drugs such as morphine and barbiturates increase the secretion. Alterations in intravascular volume also affect AVP secretion (Epstein et al 1975), while intermittent positive pressure ventilation with positive end expiratory pressure (PEEP) can impair renal function and lead to increased AVP release (Priebe et al 1981, Annat et al 1983).

Recent studies have shown that AVP has an effect on blood pressure as well as possible other central effects. Johnston (1985) has reviewed the role of the hormone in circulatory control in the pathogenesis of hypertension. There is also the suggestion that AVP is involved in the release of ACTH, having at one time thought to have been the corticotrophin-releasing factor (CRF). It is now believed that it increases the activities of other CRFs (see Buckingham 1985). Peripheral plasma catecholamines at physiological concentrations have no effect on the CRF release of ACTH (Milsom et al 1986).

Mormede et al (1985) proposed that there were two mechanisms of action by which AVP could release ACTH — an indirect action via endogenous CRF release and a direct action on the pituitary. Gibbs (1986) while conceding that AVP and oxytocin (OT) attenuated the actions of CRF suggested they might also control the secretion of ACTH. Gibbs (1986) studied various species and found that AVP stimulated ACTH secretion in all species, whereas OT stimulated ACTH release in rats but inhibited the release in primates. AVP seemed to be important in ACTH release in response to physical stress whereas OT was more involved in neurogenic or emotional stress. In animal studies Young & Akil (1985) noted that both AVP and CRF acted synergistically for ACTH release. There may be blunted responses in ACTH and beta endorphin release which can be overcome by use of high doses of CRF and AVP. When animals are chronically stressed release of ACTH and beta endorphin is in the normal expected concentration. When animals are chronically stressed and then acutely stressed they do not exhibit the blunted release. This may indicate that there are adaptive mechanisms being developed for CRF receptor desensitisation. Redekopp et al (1986) found that plasma AVP levels not large enough to cause ACTH release were associated with an augmented response to CRF. They concluded that endogenous AVP was of physiological importance in increasing the ACTH response to stress.

The control of AVP secretion by dopamine mechanisms has been investigated by Chiodera et al (1986) who found that metoclopramide stimulated AVP secretion whereas domperidone was without effect. Metoclopramide has a central peripheral antagonistic action at dopamine receptors whereas domperidone does not cross the blood-brain barrier. Metoclopramide may also act through other neurotransmitters.

Cardiovascular system

Rossi & Schrier (1986) have drawn attention to the potential role of AVP in the maintenance of systemic blood pressure. It had been noted that large doses of AVP were necessary to produce small rises in mean arterial blood pressure, but following baroreceptor-denervation there was a marked increase in blood pressure following administration of the same dose of drug in dogs. Patients with autonomic neuropathy have a pressor response to small doses of AVP. AVP appears to play an important role in maintaining blood pressure in response to haemorrhage.

In animal studies Morris et al (1986) confirmed that there appears to be a central vasopressin receptor controlling blood pressure but the role of AVP in the pathogenesis of hypertension is less clear. In man infusion of AVP results in a decreased heart rate and cardiac output and a dose-dependent increase in total peripheral and forearm vascular resistance. There was no increase in blood pressure because of the fall in cardiac output (Ebert et al 1986). AVP augments the cardiopulmonary baroreflex-mediated increase of peripheral resistance and may play a vital role in the maintenance of blood pressure during haemorrhage. Chapman et al (1986) found that recovery of blood pressure following major haemorrhage was influenced by AVP especially in the first 20 minutes ascribing the effect to an increase in total peripheral resistance. This effect has been observed in clinical practice when AVP levels are suppressed following intrathecal heroin during major abdominal surgery and the blood pressure is sensitive to blood loss despite the fact that spinal opioids have no action on sympathetic nerves (personal study).

Bennett & Gardiner (1986) although confirming that AVP had an influence in cardiovascular regulation were not convinced of the evidence cited in many studies. Aylward et al (1986) noted that small doses of AVP resulted in mild bradycardia and a small increase in central venous pressure whereas large doses caused an increase in heart rate and central venous pressure, a fall in pulse pressure, no rise in blood pressure and vasodilatation in the forearm. The vasodilatation in the forearm was unexpected and it was concluded that it was the result of an increase of central venous pressure with facilitation of the baroreflex-mediated withdrawal of sympathetic tone.

l-Desamino-8-D-arginine vasopressin (DDAVP), the potent long acting synthetic analogue of AVP, caused facial flushing, fall in diastolic blood pressure and a rise in pulse rate. There was a rise in PRA and plasma cortisol concentration. Following hypotonic saline infusion the plasma AVP level rose to the same degree, both in the DDAVP-treated patients and the controls. It might have been expected that DDAVP might influence the secretion of AVP by negative feedback but in this study the DDAVP appears to exert its action by mechanisms other than antagonising circulating endogenous AVP (Williams et al 1986). Hiwatari et al (1986) also questioned the role of AVP in the maintenance of blood pressure.

Simpson et al (1986) have demonstrated that AVP is involved in the postural control of blood pressure. When subjects were tilted to 50° the fall in forearm blood flow was much greater with an infusion of AVP compared with controls. The cardiac output fell while diastolic pressure, mean arterial pressure and systemic vascular resistance rose. It was suggested that the increased effect of AVP when the subject is tilted is due to increased baroreceptor sensitivity or is a direct vascular action via vasopressin receptors.

There are other complex interactions of AVP with other agents. Angiotensin inhibits the cardio-inhibitory actions of AVP assisting in the maintenance of tissue perfusion when the circulating blood volume is reduced (Caine et al 1985). The renin-angiotensin-aldosterone system influences AVP release (Santucci et al 1985) while in congested cardiac failure the beneficial effect of captopril is not related to AVP suppression (Stanek et al 1985).

Diuretics

Baylis & De Beer (1981) investigated the AVP response to potent loop diuretics such as frusemide and piretanide. There was a large diuresis, a small increase in plasma osmolality but no change in mean arterial blood pressure. Despite a fall in blood volume of 7% within 1 hour of the administration of frusemide there was no significant rise in plasma AVP. Drieu et al (1986) measured AVP, plasma renin activity (PRA) and aldosterone (ALD) after the administration of frusemide in patients with cardiac denervation following heart transplant surgery. They found that the AVP response to the frusemide-induced plasma volume reduction was suppressed but that of PRA and ALD was maintained. Their studies showed that in man cardiac receptors and vagal activity are involved in the ADH response to reduced plasma volume but they are not essential for PRA or ALD secretion. In hypertensive patients intravenous frusemide lead to a significantly higher level of AVP compared with controls while the rate of increase of ALD was slower in the hypertensives. It is suggested that the higher levels of AVP after frusemide may be due to either a greater plasma volume reduction or reduced response of the renal tubules. They also found that serum potassium was reduced which would account for the slower increase in ALD (Pedersen et al 1986).

Thus the mechanisms controlling AVP secretion are complex, involving baroreceptors, volume depletion and cardiac receptors which may be ventricular as well as atrial. Imaizumi & Thames (1986) have even suggested that intravenous AVP acts on ganglionic transmission.

Volume expansion

There have been many studies on AVP release in response to hypovolaemia but little on the effects of volume expansion. Linne & Rundgren (1986) found that AVP excretion decreased in response to volume expansion in healthy individuals when related to glomerular filtration rate (GFR) and to body surface area. In patients with glomerulonephritis with normal blood pressure and normal GFR, AVP excretion tended to decrease but was not significantly different. Those with hypertension and normal GFR and those with hypertension and decreased GFR did not exhibit any change in renal excretion of AVP in response to volume expansion. However if these results are related to GFR those patients with hypertension and decreased GFR had a marked increased excretion of AVP. It is possible that in patients with a reduced GFR increased AVP secretion may stimulate renal prostaglandin synthesis which may maintain renal function.

Surgical operations

During abdominal operations requiring general anaesthesia it was found that plasma AVP levels rose from the normal of 0.5–5.0 fmol/ml to 25.2–100.8 fmol/ml (median level was 59.5 fmol/ml). These levels returned to below 5 fmol/ml within 24 hours. These values are well above that required to produce a maximal antidiuresis (5 fmol/ml). There is no clear relationship between plasma AVP concentrations and urinary volume (Fieldman et al 1985). Stimulus for the increased plasma levels of AVP appears to be peritoneal stimulation for within 3 minutes of peritoneal manipulation the response in AVP was noted (Melville et al 1985). This would explain the hyponatraemia and ADH secretion reported by Chung et al (1986) the former effect being due to the administration of hypotonic fluids and the latter response to painful stimulation. Surgical operations seem a potential cause of inappropriate secretion of ADH.

Anaesthesia

It is surprising that most of the agents in use for general anaesthesia have little effect in suppressing the endocrine response to surgical stimulation except for etomidate (see Ch. 5). On the other hand extradural techniques appear to be more successful. Bonnet et al (1982) showed that epidural analgesia almost completely suppressed the release of ADH during total hip replacement. Korinek et al (1985) found that ADH levels were unchanged during knee operations following the use of extradural bupivacaine. The addition of 0.1 mg/kg of morphine in 10 ml of saline led to a delayed and stepwise increase in plasma ADH. They suggested that this was due to morphine reaching the brain stem and thereby stimulating ADH secretion. During major and prolonged abdominal operations Bailey (1987) using intrathecal diamorphine (3–5 mg) was able to attenuate the level of ADH response to surgical stimulation. It was also noted that the blood pressure was significantly lower than the control group suggesting that the intrathecal diamorphine also antagonised the vasopressor effect of AVP. Another interesting observation noted in a similar group of patients was that the use of small doses of bumetanide (0.0075 mg/kg) given prior to surgical stimulation could also attenuate the AVP response and this was of longer duration than the diuretic effect and lasted for at least 5 hours in the post-operative period (Kaufman & Bailey 1987).

Metabolism

Insulin-induced hypoglycaemia is a stimulus for AVP release. Coiro et al (1986) designed a study to determine the nature of the pathway involved. In normal men, muscarinic receptors were blocked with pirenzepine while nicotine receptors were antagonised by trimetaphan which significantly reduced the AVP release of insulin by 50%. The study suggested that there was a cholinergic-nicotinic mechanism involved in the regulation of AVP response to hypoglycaemia. Infusion of AVP results in a small but significant rise in plasma glucose and this may be due to stimulation of glucagon release and possibly glycogen phosphorylase release which breaks down glycogen (Spruce et al 1985).

Zerbe et al (1985) have on the other hand shown that uncontrolled insulin diabetic patients have raised levels of plasma vasopressin. The exact mechanism of this is still obscure as studies have shown that the raised levels cannot be accounted for by osmotic or non-osmotic stimuli. They suggested that the osmo receptors for AVP secretion are reset at higher levels and this may also be related to serum sodium which is reduced in diabetic patients.

Selective deficiency in the osmo regulation of AVP secretion has been described by Smitz & Legros (1985) in a patient with chronic hypernatraemia. Another anomalous situation has been described by Kern et al

(1986). The syndrome of inappropriate antidiuresis is usually associated with hyperosmolar urine in the presence of dilutional hyponatraemia and elevated levels of AVP. They described a patient who had low levels of AVP and on investigation was found to have a chromophobe adenoma with hyperprolactinaemia. After prolonged treatment with bromocriptine plasma AVP was detected for the first time during hypertonic saline infusion. Kern et al (1986) suggested that there might be another antidiuretic substance distinct from AVP related to higher levels of prolactin.

Although the structure of oxytocin and AVP are similar, oxytocin is unlikely to have a significant place in the regulation of fluid balance in man. Studies of AVP and oxytocin in response to acute and chronic osmotic stimulation led to rises in AVP but not in oxytocin (Williams et al 1985). Under physiological conditions osmoregulation is the major stimulus controlling AVP release and other stimuli such as angiotensin II and dopamine are not significantly involved (Morton et al 1985).

Haemostasis

There is a possibility that AVP may be involved in haemostasis. Studies emulating stress such as seen during surgical operations show there is a highly significant correlation between the rise in AVP levels and factor VIII. The concentration of AVP appears to be important for at low levels, plasma fibrinolytic activities can be stimulated while higher doses induce a hyper-coagulable state (Grant et al 1985).

The central nervous system

Animal experiments (Greidanus et al 1985) suggest that endogenous AVP may have a role in relation to memory especially in the storage and retrieval of information.

There may also be a central role for AVP in restoring blood pressure following haemorrhage but this does not appear to be involved in limiting the fall in blood pressure. When an AVP antagonist is administered, naloxone improved the mean arterial pressure following haemorrhage suggesting that endogenous opioids oppose the restoration of mean arterial pressure (Bennett et al 1986).

Prostatic carcinoma

Treatment with stilboestrol results in expansion of plasma volume with activation of the renin-angiotensin-aldosterone system. Although there were no significant changes in blood pressure or changes in cardiac output these findings should be borne in mind if the patients develop cardiac failure or hypotension (Blyth et al 1985), and might also influence the management and the course of anaesthesia.

REFERENCES

Annat G, Viale J P, Bui Xuan B et al 1983 Effect of PEEP ventilation on renal function, plasma renin, aldosterone, neurophysins and urinary ADH and prostaglandins. Anesthesiology 58: 136–141

Arieff A I 1986 Hyponatremia, convulsions, respiratory arrest and permanent brain damage after elective surgery in healthy women. New England Journal of Medicine 314: 1529–1535

Aylward P E, Floras J S, Leimbach W N, Abboud F M 1986 Effects of vasopressin on the circulation and its baroreflex control in healthy men. Circulation 73: 1145–1154

Ayus J C 1986 Diuretic-induced hyponatremia. Archives of Internal Medicine 146: 1295–1296

Baertschi A J, Massy Y, Kwon S 1985 Vasopressin responses to peripheral and central osmotic pulse stimulation. Peptides 6: 1131–1135

Bailey P M 1988 British Journal of Anaesthesia (In press)

Baylis P H, De Beer F C 1981 Human plasma vasopressin response to potent loop-diuretic drugs. European Journal of Clinical Pharmacology 20: 343–346

Bennett T, Gardiner S M 1986 Influence of exogenous vasopressin on baroreflex mechanisms. Clinical Science 70: 307–315

Bennett G W, Hatton R, Johnson J V 1986 Effect of central and systemic administration of a vasopressin V1 antagonist on recovery of MAP after hypovolaemia in rats. British Journal of Clinical Pharmacology 88 (suppl): 310

Blyth B, McRae C U, Espiner E A, Nicholls M G, Conaglen J V, Gilchrist 1985 Effect of stilboestrol on sodium balance, cardiac state, and renin-angiotensin-aldosterone activity in prostatic carcinoma. British Medical Journal 291: 1461–1464

Bonnett F, Harari A, Thibonnier M, Viars P 1982 Suppression of antidiuretic hormone hypersecretion during surgery by extradural anaesthesia. British Journal of Anaesthesia 54: 29–35

Brooks J E, Herbert M, Walder C P, Selby C, Jeffcoate W J 1986 Prolactin and stress: some endocrine correlates of preoperative anxiety. Clinical Endocrinology 24: 653–656

Brough W, Horne G, Blount A, Irving M H, Jeejeebhoy K N 1986 Effects of nutrient intake, surgery, sepsis and long term administration of steroids on muscle function. British Medical Journal 293: 983–987

Buckingham J C 1985 Hypothalamo-pituitary responses to trauma. British Medical Bulletin 41: 203–211

Caine A C, Lumbers E R, Reid I A 1985 The effects and interactions of angiotensin and vasopressin on the heart of unanaesthetized sheep. Journal of Physiology 367: 1–11

Carli F, Itiaba K 1986 Effect of heat conservation during and after major abdominal surgery on muscle protein breakdown in elderly patients. British Journal of Anaesthesia 58: 502–507

Chan S T F, McLaughlin S J, Ponting G A, Biglin J, Dudley H A F 1986 Muscle power after glucose-potassium loading in undernourished patients. British Medical Journal 293: 1055–1056

Chapman J T, Hreash F, Laycock J F, Walter S J 1986 The cardiovascular effects of vasopressin after haemorrhage in anaesthetized rats. Journal of Physiology 375: 421–434

Child C S, Kaufman L 1985 Effect of intrathecal diamorphine on the adrenocortical, hyperglycaemic and cardiovascular responses to major colonic surgery. British Journal of Anaesthesia 57: 389–393

Chiodera P, Volpi R, Delsignore R et al 1986 Different effects of metoclopramide and domperidone on arginine-vasopressin secretion in man. British Journal of Clinical Pharmacology 22: 479–482

Christensen T, Hjortso N C, Mortensen E, Riis-Hansen M, Kehlet H 1986 Fatigue and anxiety in surgical patients. Acta Psychiatrica Scandinavica 73: 76–79

Chung H-M, Kluge R, Schrier R W, Anderson R J 1986 Postoperative hyponatremia. A prospective study. Archives of Internal Medicine 146: 333–336

Coiro V, Butturini U, Gnudi A, Delsignore R, Volpi R, Chiodera P 1986 Nicotinic-cholinergic involvement in arginine-vasopressin response to insulin-induced hypoglycemia in normal men. Metabolism 35: 577–579

Corke C F, Wheatley R G 1985 Respiratory depression complicating epidural diamorphine. Anaesthesia 40: 1203–1205

Downing R, Davis I, Black J, Windsor C W O 1986 Effect of intrathecal morphine on the adrenocortical and hyperglycaemic responses to upper abdominal surgery. British Journal of Anaesthesia 58: 858–861

Drieu L, Rainfray M, Cabrol C, Ardaillou R 1986 Vasopressin aldosterone and renin responses to volume depletion in heart-transplant recipients. Clinical Science 70: 233–241

Ebert T J, Cowley A W, Skelton M 1986 Vasopressin reduces cardiac function and augments cardiopulmonary baroreflex resistance increases in man. Journal of the American Society for Clinical Investigation 77: 1136–1142

Epstein M, Pins D S, Sancho J, Haber E 1975 Suppression of plasma renin and plasma aldosterone during water immersion in normal man. Journal of Clinical Endocrinology and Metabolism 41: 618–625

Fieldman N R, Forsling M L, Le Quesne L P 1985 The effect of vasopressin on solute and water excretion during and after surgical operations. Annals of Surgery 201: 383–390

Gibbs D M 1986 Vasopressin and oxytocin. Hypothalamic modulators of the stress response. A review. Psychoneuroendocrinology 11: 131–140

Grant P J, Davies J A, Tate G M, Boothby M, Prentice C R M 1985 Effects of physiological concentrations of vasopressin on haemostatic function in man. Clinical Science 69: 471–476

Greidanus T J, van Wiemersma B, Veldhuis H D 1985 Vasopressin: site of behavioral action and role in human mental performance. Peptides 6 (supple 2): 177–180

Hain W R, Kirk B 1985 Stability of diamorphine — sodium chloride solutions. Anaesthesia 40: 1241

Hawkins S, Forsling M, Treasure T, Aveling W 1986 Changes in pressor hormone concentrations in association with coronary artery surgery. Renin and vasopressin responses. British Journal of Anaesthesia 58: 1267–1272

Hiwatari M, Abrahams J M, Saito T, Johnston C I 1986 Contribution of vasopressin to the maintenance of blood pressure in deoxycorticosterone-salt induced malignant hypertension in spontaneously hypertensive rats. Clinical Science 70: 191–198

Hynynen M, Takkunen O, Salmenpera H, Haataja H, Heinonen J 1986a Continuous infusion of fentanyl or alfentanil for coronary artery surgery. Plasma opiate concentrations, haemodynamics and postoperative course. British Journal of Anaesthesia 58: 1252–1259

Hynynen M, Lehtinen A-M, Salmenpera M, Fyhrquist O, Takkunen O, Heinonen J 1986b Continuous infusion of fentanyl or alfentanil for coronary artery surgery. Effects on plasma cortisol concentration, beta-endorphin immunoreactivity and arginine vasopressin. British Journal of Anaesthesia 58: 1260–1266

Imaizumi T, Thames M D 1986 Influence of intravenous and intracerebroventricular vasopressin on baroreflex control of renal nerve traffic. Circulation Research 58: 17–25

Johnston C I 1985 Vasopressin in circulatory control and hypertension. Journal of Hypertension 3: 557–569

Kaufman L, Bailey P M 1987 Intravenous bumetanide attenuates the rise in plasma vasopressin levels during major surgical operations. British Journal of Clinical Pharmacology 23: 237–240

Kern P A, Robbins R J, Bichet D, Berl T, Verbalis J G 1986 Syndrome of inappropriate antidiuresis in the absence of arginine vasopressin. Journal of Clinical Endocrinology and Metabolism 62: 148–152

Knight A, Forsling M, Treasure T, Aveling W, Loh L, Sturridge M F 1986 Changes in plasma vasopressin concentration in association with coronary artery surgery or thymectomy. British Journal of Anaesthesia 58: 1273–1277

Korinek A M, Languille M, Bonnet F et al 1985 Effect of postoperative extradural morphine on ADH secretion. British Journal of Anaesthesia 57: 407–411

Kristensen G, Guldager H, Gravesen H 1986 Prevention of peroperative hypothermia in abdominal surgery. Acta Anaesthesiologica Scandinavica 30: 314–316

Lacoumenta S, Paterson J L, Burrin J, Causon R C, Brown M J, Hall G M 1986 Effects of two differing halothane concentrations on the metabolic and endocrine responses to surgery. British Journal of Anaesthesia 58: 844–850

Leading Article 1986 Atrial natriuretic peptide. Lancet 2: 371–372

Linne T, Rundgren M 1986 Arginine vasopressin excretion in response to volume expansion in the healthy human, and in patients with glomerulonephritis. Acta Physiologica Scandinavica 126: 45–49

Lund J, Stjernstrom H, Jorfeldt L, Wiklund L 1986 Effects of extradural analgesia on glucose metabolism and gluconeogenesis. British Journal of Anaesthesia 58: 851–857

Macrae D J 1987 Diamorphine in acqueous solution. Anaesthesia 42: 82–83

MacDonald I A, Bennett T, Fellows I W 1985 Catecholamines and the control of metabolism in man. Clinical Science 68: 613–619

Melville R J, Forsling M L, Frizis H I, Lequesne L P 1985 Stimulus for vasopressin release during elective intra-abdominal operations. British Journal of Surgery 72: 979–982

Milsom S R, Donald R A, Espiner E A, Nicholls M G, Livesey J H 1986 The effect of peripheral catecholamine concentrations on the pituitary-adrenal response to corticotrophin releasing factor in man. Clinical Endocrinology 25: 241–246

Mormede P, LeMoal M, Dantzer R 1985 Analysis of the dual mechanism of ACTH release by arginine vasopressin and its analogs in conscious rats. Regulatory Peptides 12: 175–184

Morris M, Sain L E, Schumacher S J 1986 Involvement of central vasopressin receptors in the control of blood pressure. Neuroendocrinology 43: 625–628

Morton J J, Connell J M C, Hughes M J, Inglis G C, Wallace E C H 1985 The role of plasma osmolality, angiotensin II and dopamine in vasopressin release in man. Clinical Endocrinology 23: 129–138

Narins R G 1986 Therapy of hyponatremia: does haste make waste? New England Journal of Medicine 314: 1573–1575

Needleman P, Greenwald J E 1986 Atriopeptin: a cardiac hormone intimately involved in fluid, electrolyte and blood pressure homeostasis. New England Journal of Medicine 314: 828–834

Normandale J P, Schmulian C, Paterson J L, Burrin J, Morgan M, Hall G M 1985 Epidural morphine and the metabolic response to upper abdominal surgery. Anaesthesia 40: 748–753

Pedersen E B, Danielsen H, Madsen M, Sorensen S S, Thomsen O O 1986 Abnormal vasopressin and aldosterone response to furosemide in essential hypertension. Acta Medica Scandinavica 219: 387–392

Priebe H J, Heinmann J C, Headley-White 1981 Mechanisms of renal dysfunction during positive end-expiratory pressure ventilation. Journal of Applied Physiology: Respiration, Environmental and Exercise Physiology 50: 643–649

Raine A E G, Erne P, Burgisser E et al 1986 Atrial natriuretic peptide and atrial pressure in patients with congestive heart failure. New England Journal of Medicine 315: 533–537

Redekopp C, Livesey J H, Sadler W, Donald R A 1986 The physiological significance of arginine vasopressin in potentiating the response to corticotrophin-releasing factor in sheep. Journal of Endocrinology 108: 309–312

Richards A M, Cleland J G F, Tonolo G et al 1986 Plasma alpha natriuretic peptide in cardiac impairment. British Medical Journal 293: 409–412

Rossi N F, Schrier R W 1986 Role of arginine vasopressin in regulation of systemic arterial pressure. Annual Review of Medicine 37: 13–20

Santucci A, Luparini R L, Ferri C, Ficara C, Giarrizzo C, Balsano F 1985 Relationship between vasopressin and the renin-angiotensin-aldosterone system in essential hypertension: effect of converting enzyme inhibitor on plasma vasopressin. Journal of Hypertension 3 (suppl 2): S133–S134

Schwab T R, Edwards B S, De Vries W C, Zimmerman R S, Burnett J C 1986 Atrial endocrine function in humans with artificial hearts. New England Journal of Medicine 315: 1398–1401

Sebel P S, Aun C, Fiolet J, Noonan K, Savege T M, Colvin M P 1985 Endocrinological effects of intrathecal morphine. European Journal of Anaesthesiology 2: 291–296

Seitz W, Leubbe N, Bechstein W, Fritz K, Kirchner E 1986 A comparison of two types of anaesthesia on the endocrine and metabolic responses to anaesthesia and surgery. European Journal of Anaesthesiology 3: 283–294

Shirasaka C, Tsuji H, Asoh T, Takeuchi Y 1986 Role of the splanchnic nerves in endocrine and metabolic response to abdominal surgery. British Journal of Surgery 73: 142–145

Simpson H C R, Zubillaga J E, Collier J G, Bennett E D, Mehta A N, Jenkins J S 1986 Haemodynamic effects of vasopressin in man are related to posture. Clinical Science 70: 177–184

Singer D R J, Buckley M G, MacGregor G A, Khaghani A, Banner N R, Yacoub M H

1986 Raised concentrations of plasma atrial natriuretic peptides in cardiac transplant recipients. British Medical Journal 293: 1391–1392

Smitz S, Legros J J 1985 Regulation of vasopressin secretion in a patient with chronic hypernatraemia. Acta Endocrinologica 110: 346–351

Spruce B A, McCulloch A J, Burd J et al 1985 The effect of vasopressin infusion on glucose metabolism in man. Clinical Endocrinology 22: 463–468

Stanek B, Bruckner U, Silberbauer K 1985 Plasma vasopressin as influenced by acute and chronic blockade of the renin-angiotensin system. Journal of Hypertension 3 (suppl 2): S129–S131

Sterns R H, Riggs J E, Schochet S S 1986 Osmotic demyelination syndrome following correction of hyponatremia. New England Journal of Medicine 314: 1535–1542

Tarnow-Mordi W O, Shaw J C L, Liu D, Gardner D A, Flynn F V 1981 Iatrogenic hyponatraemia of the newborn due to maternal fluid overload: a prospective study. British Medical Journal 283: 639–642

Watters J M, Wilmore D W 1986 Role of catabolic hormones in the hypoketonaemia of injury. British Journal of Surgery 73: 108–110

Williams T D M, Abel D C, King C M P, Yelley R Y, Lightman S L 1985 Vasopressin and oxytocin responses to acute and chronic osmotic stimuli in man. Journal of Endocrinology 108: 163–168

Williams T D M, Lightman S L, Leadbeater M J 1986 Hormonal and cardiovascular responses to DDAVP in man. Clinical Endocrinology 24: 89–96

Young E A, Akil H 1985 Corticotrophin-releasing factor stimulation of adrenocorticotrophin and beta endorphin release. Effects of acute and chronic stress. Endocrinology 117: 23–30

Zerbe R L, Vinicor F, Robertson G L 1985 Regulation of plasma vasopressin in insulin-dependent diabetes mellitus. American Journal of Physiology 249: E317–E325

Colloid-crystalloid controversy

INTRODUCTION

There can be few areas of critical care management where the clinician has been subject to such apparently conflicting advice as in the field of fluid therapy for the traumatized patient. Opinion has become polarized between the supporters of a crystalloid based regime on the one hand, and those recommending colloid therapy on the other. Each faction has published extensively, and come to apparently irreconcilable conclusions. Indeed over the last 2 years different authors have published such opposing opinions as 'the end of the crystalloid era?' (Twigley & Hillman 1985), and 'one wonders how their (colloids) further employment in clinical medicine can be justified' (Tranbaugh & Lewis 1986).

In this review the historical background to the present debate will be presented. The central question of the debate concerns the effects of the selected fluid regime on respiratory and cardiovascular function. To understand the published literature in this field it is necessary to re-examine the pathophysiology of the hypovolaemic state and the effects of fluid resuscitation on pulmonary function. Much of the data presented and reviewed relate to hypovolaemic shock as this has been most extensively researched, but the conclusions drawn will be discussed in the wider context of clinical fluid management policies.

THE HISTORICAL BACKGROUND

Intravenous fluid administration was first used in the 1830s when saline was used for the treatment of cholera. The first treatment of haemorrhage by intravenous fluid was described in *The Lancet* in 1891 in a tribute to a Dr Wooldridge (Lane 1891) who administered $3\frac{1}{2}$ pints of saline to a girl who had suffered prolonged bleeding, with remarkable effect. However up until the 1930s and 1940s it was still generally believed that the development of shock after severe trauma was due to the release of a toxin from damaged tissues, rather than being the result of hypovolaemia. A classic publication by Blalock (1930) demonstrated that shock was due to blood loss, rather than any humoral factor or histamine release, and recommended treatment by replacement of body fluids. Remarkably it was not until still later, during World War II, that the treatment of blood loss by giving intravenous fluids became widely accepted, with both blood and plasma being used with clearly beneficial results (Blalock 1943).

In the 1940s and 1950s publications by Coller et al (1944) and Moore & Ball (1952) described the sodium and water retention that occurred after surgery and trauma. Their warnings that the use of electrolyte solutions might produce salt poisoning supposedly produced widespread reluctance amongst surgeons and anaesthetists to administer crystalloids to their patients. Then in the 1960s several workers showed that survival after experimental haemorrhagic shock in animals was greatly increased if blood and crystalloids, rather than blood alone, were administered (Wolfman et al 1963, Shires et al 1964, Dillon et al 1966). A swing then occurred towards liberal administration of crystalloids. Indeed they came to be administered so generously that two leading authorities had to publish a joint editorial urging 'moderation' (Moore & Shires 1967). Over the next few years many articles were published which discussed the choice of fluids during resuscitation — the crystalloid versus colloid debate had begun.

THE PATHOPHYSIOLOGY OF HYPOVOLAEMIC SHOCK

Progressive haemorrhage produces a well known sequence of clinical events. In man, losses of 10–25% of blood volume produce a variable but usually small drop in arterial pressure, while cardiac output is reduced by 20–40%. In invasively monitored animals (Carey et al 1970) rapid removal of 25% of the blood volume causes a 20% fall in systemic and pulmonary arterial pressures and a 50% reduction in left and right atrial pressures and cardiac output. The systemic and pulmonary vascular resistance both rise by 100%. The initial compensatory responses to hypovolaemia include contraction of venous capacitance vessels, arteriolar vasoconstriction in muscle, skin, and splanchnic viscera, and increased myocardial contractility. Longer term compensatory mechanisms include refilling of the intravascular space, reduced urine output, and increased thirst. In addition numerous neuro-endocrine changes take place, some contributing to, and some resulting from, the above effects. There is immediate activation of the sympatho-adrenal system with massive release of catecholamines and angiotensin, with later increases in the release of ACTH, cortisol, growth hormone, glucagon, aldosterone, and antidiuretic hormone. Prostaglandins, leukotrienes, and other plasma kinins may all also be involved in the microvascular disturbances occurring during hypovolaemic shock (Ledingham & Ramsay 1986). When approximately 50% of the blood volume has been lost the phase of 'irreversible shock' is entered, and mortality approaches 100%, regardless of how rapidly and efficiently fluid replacement is carried out.

Commonly used clinical measurements in shock, such as arterial and venous pressures, give information about the intravascular space. However this is the smallest of the fluid compartments, containing only 12.5% of the total body fluids. Loss of fluid from this space not surprisingly causes disturbances of the fluid content of both the intracellular and interstitial spaces.

Interstitial fluid changes during shock

It is important to realize that it is the tissue cells which ultimately suffer from the effects of inadequate perfusion, and that these are separated from the bloodstream by the interstitial fluid. The interstitial fluid functions both as a transport medium for nutrients and metabolites, and also in maintaining a constant *milieu interieur* for cells by resisting changes in the local environment. The composition of interstitial fluid and the changes that occur in hypovolaemic shock have been reviewed by Haljamae (1984). The interstitial fluid has a volume three to four times that of the plasma, with over 90% being located in the skeletal muscle, skin, and viscera. The concentration of protein in interstitial fluid in skin and muscle is 20–40% of that of plasma, whereas in the lung it is much higher, at about 70% of that of plasma.

In early hypovolaemic shock fluid is transferred from the interstitial compartment into the intravascular space, producing haemodilution. This intravascular refilling is thought to be due to the sympatho-adrenal activation increasing the pre- to postcapillary resistance ratio. As a result of the loss of fluid from the interstitial space, capillary surface area is reduced and interstitial space osmotic pressure rises. These changes result in impairment of both flow- and diffusion-dependent exchanges between the bloodstream and the tissue cells.

Evidence of the reduction in volume of the interstitial space during haemorrhagic shock was first produced in the early 1960s (Wolfman et al 1963, Shires et al 1964). Shires' group used dogs subjected to controlled haemorrhage and fluid replacement. Their experiments showed that the reduction in 'functional' extracellular fluid volume (i.e. the sum of plasma and interstitial fluid volumes) after blood loss was far greater than the actual volume of blood removed. In addition if the removed blood was re-infused, then red cell mass and plasma volumes returned to normal but there was still a large deficit in the 'functional' extracellular fluid volume. Shire's group also claimed that 'functional' extracellular fluid losses occur during surgery with tissue trauma (Shires et al 1961). Not all workers have been able to demonstrate these reductions in interstitial fluid volume, and the extent of these losses is still a matter of some controversy. Tissue biopsies from hypovolaemic animals certainly show marked reductions in extracellular water content (Trunkey et al 1973). Generally it can be assumed that during hypovolaemia or traumatic surgery the interstitial fluid space becomes contracted, with fluid being lost to various possible sites: the intravascular space, 'non-functional' extracellular space (the so called 'third' space), and the intracellular space.

In prolonged severe shock there is a reversal in the direction of fluid transfer, with fluid leaving the intravascular space, resulting in haemoconcentration. This reversal of fluid migration is thought to be the result of dilatation of the precapillary resistance vessels (thus decreasing the pre- to postcapillary resistance ratio) secondary to local metabolic changes. It has been suggested that this development of precapillary vessel dilatation, with loss of response to sympathetic influences, marks the onset of 'irreversible shock', when no form of treatment can improve the outcome.

Cellular changes in shock

Studies on primate skeletal muscle using intracellular electrodes and concomitant tissue biopsies (Trunkey et al 1973) have shown that during shock there is a reduction in the cell membrane potential, and that muscle cells gain water, sodium, and chloride, while losing potassium. Essentially an isotonic swelling of the cells takes place. Similar studies on action potentials in skeletal muscle cells during shock have shown a decrease in resting membrane potential, decrease in amplitude of the action potential, and prolongation of both repolarization and depolarization times. Resuscitation rapidly reverses these changes, except for repolarization times which remain prolonged for several days.

Implications for the treatment of hypovolaemic shock

It is thus clear that during hypovolaemic shock profound changes take place in the constitution of both the interstitial and intracellular fluid spaces, and that intracellular metabolic disturbances are increasingly buffered from the bloodstream by the altered behaviour of the interstitial fluid. Though some regimens for fluid resuscitation may rapidly restore cardiovascular indices and blood volume, they may not necessarily be effective at returning interstitial space and cellular function to normal. For good longer term survival assumedly all the fluid compartments of the body require treatment.

EFFECTS OF FLUID RESUSCITATION UPON PULMONARY FUNCTION

Much of the early objection to crystalloid resuscitation was based on the assumption that dilution of the plasma proteins, with subsequent lowering of the plasma colloid oncotic pressure (PCOP), would inevitably cause pulmonary oedema. It was claimed that if the gradient between the PCOP and intravascular pressure became reduced, then fluid would accumulate in the pulmonary interstitial space. However there is actually little theoretical basis, or experimental evidence, to support this assumption.

The physiology of pulmonary fluid exchange

Fluid flow across capillary membranes is governed by the Starling equation, which states that the net fluid flux (Q_f) across a membrane is related to its permeability and to the relative hydrostatic and colloid osmotic pressures on each side. The full equation is —

$$Q_f = K_f[(Pmv - Ppmv) - \sigma(\pi mv - \pi pmv)]$$

in which —

K_f is the conductance of the capillary membrane, indicating its permeability to fluids

Pmv is the hydrostatic pressure inside the microvascular lumen, which in the lung is most commonly approximated to by using the left atrial pressure or pulmonary artery wedge pressure (PAWP). A more precise estimate is given by Gaar's equation: PAWP + 0.4 (pulmonary artery wedge pressure − PAWP).

$Ppmv$ is the hydrostatic pressure of the perimicrovascular (i.e. interstitial) space, probably zero or slightly negative

σ is the solute reflection coefficient, reflecting the permeability of the capillary membrane to protein relative to water, with a value normally of 0.8

πmv and πpmv are the colloid osmotic pressures of the intravascular and interstitial spaces respectively, thus πmv = PCOP

As described earlier the interstitial fluid in the lung has a much higher protein content than elsewhere, giving it a colloid oncotic pressure of 70% of that of plasma, thus the difference between intravascular and interstitial fluid colloid osmotic pressure in the lung is small. The earlier equation can now be simplified to —

$$Q_f = K_f [(PAWP - 0) - 0.8(PCOP - 0.7PCOP)]$$
$$= K_f [PAWP - 0.24PCOP]$$

Thus changes in PCOP have a far smaller effect on pulmonary fluid flux than changes of a similar magnitude in PAWP. Additional mechanisms counteracting any tendency to gain interstitial fluid include enormous increases in the rate of pulmonary lymph drainage, and dilution and washout of interstitial fluid proteins (thereby lowering the interstitial fluid colloid oncotic pressure). In tissues outside the lung the interstitial fluid colloid oncotic pressure is much lower and thus the gradient between plasma and tissue colloid oncotic pressures has greater influence on fluid flux. Unfortunately there are uncertainties about the estimation of almost all the variables used in the Starling equation, particularly assumptions that PAWP can be used for intravascular pressure, and that interstitial fluid pressure remains constant (Civetta 1979, Gabel & Drake 1979). It is fairly certain however that hypovolaemia and fluid resuscitation do not alter pulmonary vascular permeability.

The results of research aimed at determining the relative pulmonary effects of crystalloids and colloids, in both animals and man, are discussed below. Many techniques of assessment of pulmonary function have been used, including measurement of: radiological pulmonary oedema, lung volumes and compliance, physiological deadspace, blood gas tensions, alveolar to arterial oxygen tension gradients (P(A-a)O$_2$), intrapulmonary shunt, and extravascular lung water (EVLW). Additional techniques in animals include measurement of pulmonary lymph flow and protein content, and gravimetric and histological assessment of lungs post-mortem. However the validity of some of these is uncertain during major fluid loss and replacement, due to alterations in cardiac output and regional distribution of lung perfusion. It would appear that both radiological pulmonary oedema and impaired lung compliance can occur well before gas exchange becomes impaired. Large rises in EVLW also appear to have surprisingly little correlation with impairment of gas exchange (Brigham et al 1983). The effects upon pulmonary function in man in the presence of lung disease, cardiac disease, and sepsis are discussed separately.

Effects of fluid resuscitation on pulmonary function in animals

Demling et al (1979) compared the effects of crystalloid and colloid resuscitation on pulmonary lymph flow in sheep with chronic lung lymph fistulae. Pulmonary lymph is assumed to have a composition nearly identical to that of pulmonary interstitial fluid, and the flow rate is closely related to the transcapillary fluid flow. Giving crystalloid in two and a half times the volume of colloid, they found that lung lymph flow and protein flux increased transiently and equally. With crystalloid the drop in PCOP was mirrored by an equal drop in pulmonary interstitial fluid colloid oncotic pressure, thus the gradient between the two remained unaltered. They stated that fluid flux in the lung was dependent only on intravascular pressure. Zarins et al (1978) made similar measurements on baboons, which underwent plasmapheresis to reduce the PCOP by over 75%, whilst maintaining PAWP with crystalloid. As in Demling et al's experiments the drop in PCOP was paralleled by a similar change in the pulmonary lymph oncotic pressure, with the gradient between the two remaining unaltered. Pulmonary lymph flow was found to increase sevenfold. The PCOP-PAWP gradient dropped from a mean of 15.3 mmHg to −0.3 mmHg, but intrapulmonary shunt did not increase (see Fig. 7.1), nor did lung water, despite the development of peripheral oedema and ascites.

Holcroft & Trunkey (1974) measured EVLW in baboons using thermaldye methods, showing that at 1 hour after resuscitation there was a 60% increase in EVLW in those given colloids, while EVLW dropped slightly in those given crystalloid. At 24 hours the crystalloid group had a very small increase in EVLW and all the colloid group had died. A similar study by the same authors (Holcroft & Trunkey 1975) using only crystalloid showed

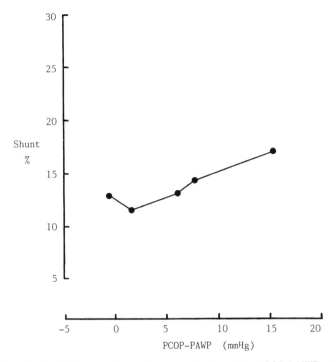

Fig. 7.1 The relationship between intrapulmonary shunt and the PCOP-PAWP gradient in baboons which underwent plasmapheresis to reduce their PCOP (from the data of Zarins et al 1978))

a small increase in EVLW at $2\frac{1}{2}$ hours, with return to normal by 24 hours. Other workers demonstrating no detrimental effect of crystalloid on EVLW include Moss et al (1971), Risberg et al (1981), Merrill et al (1981), Brinkmeyer et al (1981) and Gallagher et al (1985). The only study in animals which has shown a higher EVLW after crystalloid than colloid administration was by Magilligan et al (1972). However their study also showed a large rise in EVLW (using double isotope dilution) after return of the removed blood alone, and gravimetric measurement did not confirm raised lung weight in the crystalloid group. Using histological assessment of interstitial pulmonary oedema, Gaisford et al (1972) found interstitial oedema only in crystalloid-treated animals, while Moss et al (1979) only observed it in colloid-treated animals.

Measurements of pulmonary mechanics and gas exchange have given more varied results. Studies by Proctor et al (1969), Moss et al (1971), Gaisford et al (1972), Nees et al (1978), Risberg et al (1981), and Merrill et al (1981) have all found little difference in lung mechanics or gas exchange between colloid and crystalloid treatment groups. Brinkmeyer et al (1981) using severe haemodilution (down to a haematocrit of 10%) in dogs found little difference in shunt, but pulmonary compliance and airway resistance were worse in the crystalloid-treated group.

Effects of fluid resuscitation on pulmonary function in man

Shah et al (1977) studied 20 patients with multiple trauma, giving blood to replace estimated losses, and additional Ringer Lactate (RL), or RL with albumin, to maintain left ventricular stroke work index. The RL group required 16 litres of fluid during resuscitation, and the albumin group 11.5 litres. They found no difference in intrapulmonary shunt over the first 3 days. Tranbaugh et al (1982) studied EVLW in 16 patients with severe trauma. All patients received blood and crystalloid only, the average fluid requirement in the first 48 hours being 33 litres. The EVLW only rose in six patients, five of whom had severe lung contusion or sepsis, and the sixth having cardiac failure. In those without chest injury or sepsis there was no rise in EVLW. They concluded that EVLW only became increased after massive crystalloid resuscitation if lung contusion, sepsis, or fluid overload were present. Virgilio et al (1979) studied 29 patients undergoing abdominal aortic surgery. They gave blood and RL, or blood and RL with albumin, to maintain PAWP and cardiac ouput, ten patients requiring over 20 litres of fluid. The PCOP-PAWP gradient decreased from a mean of 11 mmHg to 2 mmHg in the RL group, and actually became negative in seven

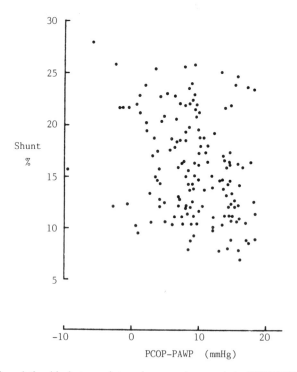

Fig. 7.2 The relationship between intrapulmonary shunt and the PCOP-PAWP gradient in patients undergoing abdominal aortic surgery, with crystalloid or colloid fluid replacement (from Virgilio et al (1979) with permission of the publishers)

patients, but there was no difference in intrapulmonary shunt between the two groups (see Fig. 7.2).

Similarly Shires et al (1983) studied 18 patients undergoing aortic surgery, giving either blood and RL, or blood and RL with albumin, to maintain PAWP, cardiac output, and urine output. They found no difference in EVLW or shunt between the two groups. Lowe et al (1979) studied 141 patients with abdominal trauma, randomly allocated to receive either RL, or RL with albumin, given to maintain blood pressure and urine flow. They found no significant differences between the two groups in shunt or physiological deadspace. Lucas et al (1980) studied 94 patients with severe trauma, allocated to receive blood and RL, or blood and RL with albumin supplements for 5 days. They found worse pulmonary function in the albumin-treated group, with markedly longer times required for postoperative ventilation (8 days for the albumin group versus 3 days for the crystalloid group). However the albumin group had a higher central venous pressure (CVP) postoperatively than the crystalloid group, and thus may have received excessive volumes of fluid. Carey et al (1971), in discussion of the management of severe haemorrhage during the Vietnam War, states that resuscitation using enormous quantities of crystalloids, with replacement of estimated blood loss, did not produce pulmonary problems (in those without thoracic injury), though most patients were not monitored in detail.

Four studies have claimed deleterious effects of crystalloids on lung function when compared to colloids. Skillman et al (1975) studied patients undergoing aortic surgery, allocated to receive blood and RL, or blood and albumin in saline. In addition both groups received albumin supplements postoperatively. The $P(A-a)O_2$ gradients were higher in the RL group in the early postoperative course. However no criteria for fluid administration was stated, and no cardiovascular measurements quoted, thus differences in cardiac output between the two groups may have been partly responsible for the differences in arterial oxygen tensions. Boutros et al (1979) studied similar patients, allocated to receive RL, dextrose/saline, or dextrose/saline with albumin. The $P(A-a)O_2$ gradients were greater in the non-albumin groups but intrapulmonary shunts were not significantly worse. Laks et al (1976) haemodiluted eight patients, half with RL, and half with RL and albumin, given to maintain CVP. EVLW and $P(A-a)O_2$ gradients were greater in the RL group but not significantly so. Modig (1983) assessed pulmonary function in patients with pelvic and femoral fractures, allocated to receive RL, or dextran 70, given to maintain blood pressure and CVP. Four out of 11 RL patients developed impaired pulmonary gas exchange in the RL group, but none out of 12 in the dextran group.

Summary

These animal and human studies support the theoretical prediction that the interstitium of the normal lung is able to resist the accumulation of excess fluid, even in the face of markedly reduced plasma oncotic pressure. The major determinant in fluid movement across the pulmonary capillary is not the plasma oncotic pressure, but is the intravascular hydrostatic force. These observations do not support the contention that colloid resuscitation has a specific advantage in protecting the lungs from oedema.

COMPARATIVE EFFICACY DURING RESUSCITATION

The effectiveness of either type of solution has usually been assessed by determining the comparative volumes that are needed to return cardiovascular variables such as arterial pressure, CVP, PAWP, and cardiac output to normal. Some authors have suggested that CVP and PAWP may not be accurate guides to volume replacement after major haemorrhage, due to gross alterations in vasomotor tone. Most of the studies have replaced measured or estimated blood loss with blood, using additional crystalloid or colloid to maintain cardiovascular function. The fact that large volumes of the chosen replacement fluid have been required in addition to the measured losses is evidence in support of the occurrence of fluid losses outside the intravascular space.

Using animals with induced haemorrhagic shock Moss et al (1969), Gaisford et al (1972), Proctor et al (1969), Holcroft & Trunkey (1974), and Smith & Norman (1982), all found that to return cardiovascular variables to normal crystalloid was required in between 1.5 and 2.9 times the volume of colloid. Other workers have given pre-set volumes of different fluids to animals after induced blood loss and compared the response, again finding similar ratios of volumes to be required for similar effect (Carey et al 1970, Nees et al 1978, Dawidson & Eriksson 1982). Carey et al (1970) estimated that 2 hours after the infusion of RL only 17.5% remained in the circulation, whereas 43% of dextran 40 was still present. Brinkmeyer et al (1981) as discussed earlier, and Takaori & Safar (1967) have performed experiments with severe haemodilution in dogs, removing blood and simultaneously replacing it with crystalloid or colloid. When haemodiluted down to a haematocrit of 10% of normal, crystalloids were required in much larger volumes than colloids (seven times more in the study of Brinkmeyer et al), and mortality was far greater in the crystalloid groups. Thus in the event of loss of 90% of the blood volume, administration of some colloid appears to be vital.

In man, studies are available using patients undergoing elective surgery with major blood loss, and from patients found to be hypovolaemic on admission or whilst in hospital. Three studies on patients undergoing aortic surgery have compared crystalloid and colloid treatment (Virgilio et al 1979, Shires et al 1983, Skillman et al 1975). After replacement of blood loss the fluid requirements were found to be between 1.5 and 1.8 times greater if crystalloid was used rather than colloid. Comparisons in patients already hypovolaemic are more difficult since different treatment groups may not have had similar blood loss. Several workers have given set volumes of different fluids to hypovolaemic patients and measured the responses. Rackow et al (1983) found that fluid challenges with saline needed to be 3.5 times larger than albumin, and 2.4 times larger than with hydroxyethyl starch (HES) to obtain the same cardiovascular effect. Hauser et al (1980) found that in hypovolaemic patients with respiratory failure 1 litre of RL expanded the plasma by less than 200 ml, while hyperoncotic albumin caused a greater plasma expansion than the volume given. Similar experiments by Shoemaker (1976) showed that RL produced plasma expansion of less than 25% of the volume given, while blood, dextran 70, and albumin all produced plasma expansion equal to or slightly greater than the volume given.

All these studies have shown that colloids cause a much greater expansion of the intravascular space than crystalloid — a fact that is not in dispute by the proponents of each type of solution. Several workers have noticed that if resuscitated to an identical CVP, colloid groups have a significantly greater cardiac output (Gaisford et al 1972, Laks et al 1976, Sturm et al 1979, Smith & Norman 1982). This has been attributed to the fact that colloids cause a greater reduction in systemic vascular resistance than crystalloids. Fears that the administration of large quantities of lactate in RL might exacerbate lactic acidosis have not been confirmed. This has been studied by Carey et al (1971) and Canizaro et al (1971) amongst others, and all have found a rapid drop in lactate levels during RL administration as tissue perfusion improves.

Summary

Thus in the case of resuscitation from hypovolaemic shock it can be shown that the major difference between crystalloid and colloid-based regimes is in the total volume required to refill the intravascular space. The end-point for such resuscitation is based on measurements of circulatory function. It should be emphasized that such observations shed no light on the adequacy of the restoration of interstitial fluid volume. Several of the studies suggest that high volumes of colloid may have detrimental effects on pulmonary function. On the other hand it has been shown that some colloid replacement is mandatory after massive blood loss.

The conclusion must be that neither fluid can be used in isolation, as each has its place in the complete resuscitation from the hypovolaemic state. The clinician should plan his therapy based on a sound understanding of the pathophysiology of fluid movement across the pulmonary vascular bed. Furthermore it is necessary to achieve some insight into the limitations of currently available measurement techniques in providing a full picture of fluid repletion in the three relevant spaces: intravascular, interstitial, and intracellular.

SPECIAL CLINICAL PROBLEMS IN FLUID REPLACEMENT

As was stated above, the hypovolaemic model provides an excellent basis to examine the controversy concerning the choice of resuscitative fluids. However there are a number of clinical circumstances that warrant special attention and these will be briefly reviewed in this final section.

The pulmonary effects of fluid administration in the presence of respiratory and cardiac disease

Patients with impaired pulmonary gas exchange have an increased barrier between the pulmonary capillaries and alveolar gas. In the absence of chronic pathological changes (e.g. emphysema or fibrosis) this is commonly due to interstitial or alveolar oedema or inflammatory exudate. In the absence of raised intravascular pressure, assumedly pulmonary capillary membrane permeability must have increased. Several workers have tried to assess whether alterations in PCOP have any greater influence on lung function under these circumstances.

Finch et al (1983) studied dogs with a dual insult of haemorrhage and chemically induced lung injury. The removed blood was returned, equal volumes of RL or various colloids given, then PAWP maintained using RL. EVLW (measured using thermal-dye dilution) was increased by 570% in the RL and dextran groups, and by 430% and 370% in the albumin and starch groups respectively. Despite this, $P(A-a)O_2$ gradients and physiological dead-space values were similar for all of the groups. They could not explain the lack of difference in gas exchange with such widely varying EVLW results. Rutili et al (1984) measured lymph flow and EVLW in dogs with chemically induced lung damage. They were then partly exchange transfused with dextran 70 or saline. Pulmonary lymph flow increased much more in the saline-treated group, but EVLW increases were identical in the two groups. They emphasized that EVLW is essentially related to microvascular hydrostatic pressure.

Studies in humans have usually used groups of intensive care unit patients with respiratory failure of varying aetiologies. Few have managed to maintain comparable CVP, PAWP, or cardiac output levels in different treatment groups. Hauser et al (1980) gave patients with adult respiratory distress syndrome (ARDS) either 1 litre of RL, or 100 ml of 25% albumin. Neither caused a significant change in shunt, though RL caused a small but not significant rise in $P(A-a)O_2$ gradients. Sibbald et al (1983) infused albumin solutions into patients with ARDS (administering diuretics to prevent rises in PAWP) and measured the transmicrovascular flux of macromolecules. They found that the flux of macromolecules was essentially related to intravascular pressure, that increasing PCOP did not reduce the flux, and that shunt increased significantly after the albumin infusion. Metildi et al (1984) treated patients with severe respiratory failure (due to sepsis in 50%) with RL, or RL and albumin, to maintain cardiac filling pressures. There were no differences between the two groups until the end of the second day, when the shunt was higher in the RL group, the authors claiming no overall difference in pulmonary function between the two groups.

Patients in cardiac failure also frequently have raised lung water content, assumedly due to the raised pulmonary intravascular pressure. If cardiac failure is severe, gross interstitial and alveolar oedema can develop. In cardiogenic pulmonary oedema fluid must collect in the interstitial space at a rate exceeding the maximal capacity of lymph drainage and other protective mechanisms. Imbalance in the contractility of the right and left sides of the heart can cause a greater output from the right than left heart, with inevitable fluid accumulation. Several studies of fluid administration in patients with cardiac failure have claimed that PCOP is important in determining the risk of pulmonary oedema, most using radiographic assessment only. Da Luz et al (1975) studying patients with acute myocardial infarction claimed a good relationship between PCOP-PAWP and pulmonary oedema, as did Rackow et al (1977) in a study of 128 patients, over half of whom had primary myocardial disease. Stein et al (1975) compared the development of pulmonary oedema with the PAWP and PCOP in 37 patients, some of whom had primary myocardial disease. They claimed that the administration of crystalloid predisposed to the development of pulmonary oedema by reducing the PCOP-PAWP gradient. However the diagnosis for most of the patients was not specified, some had excessively high PAWP values, and the reduction in PCOP-PAWP in those who developed pulmonary oedema was similar whether treated with colloid or crystalloid.

Certainly low PCOP values seem to be associated with a high mortality rate in ITU patients, and appear to be more common in patients with radiographic pulmonary oedema. However a cause and effect relationship has not been clearly demonstrated. Attempts to clear pulmonary oedema by administering hyperoncotic fluids have always provided very mixed and unsatisfactory results.

The pulmonary effects of fluid administration in the presence of sepsis

Impaired respiratory function is common in patients with trauma complicated by sepsis (Demling 1986). In the absence of fluid overload it must again be asked whether pulmonary capillary permeability has become increased. In septic shock the systemic vascular resistance drops due to increased arteriovenous shunting at the precapillary level. However in animals, and to a lesser extent in humans, a pronounced rise occurs in pulmonary vascular resistance and pulmonary artery pressure. Under these circumstances it may no longer be acceptable to use PAWP as an estimate of pulmonary capillary intravascular pressure. Also the end-points for resuscitation can be difficult to ascertain since subjects may have a low cardiac output in spite of a high CVP and PAWP.

Brigham et al (1979) studied sheep given intravenous *Escherichia coli* endotoxin. They found that with left atrial pressure kept fairly constant, lung lymph flow increased by a factor of five, and lung lymph protein concentration increased slightly. They stated that there was markedly increased permeability to water and proteins, and that this persisted for over 6 days. Sturm et al (1979) measured pulmonary lymph flow and protein content, and EVLW, in sheep after injecting *E. coli* intravenously. They administered RL or albumin to maintain CVP. They found that during the 4 hours of their study, pulmonary lymph flow increased with both fluids, with lymph albumin levels maintaining a constant ratio to those in the plasma. EVLW was raised only in the albumin-treated animals, due to a greater lung albumin content. Unlike Brigham's group they stated that during sepsis pulmonary capillary permeability was not increased, and that pulmonary fluid and albumin flux were proportional to intravascular pressure and plasma albumin concentration respectively. These opposing conclusions are due to different estimations of intravascular pressure in the pulmonary capillaries. Brigham's group used left atrial pressure (LAP), while Sturm's group used Gaar's formula, which during sepsis-induced pulmonary hypertension gives markedly different results. Esrig & Fulton (1975) subjected dogs to various combinations of haemorrhage, resuscitation, and intratracheal injections of *Pseudomonas aeruginosa*. Haemorrhage followed by resuscitation produced little change in arterial oxygenation, dead-space ratio, pulmonary compliance, or lung weight; however the combined insult of haemorrhage and intratracheal bacteria caused severe derangements of all these variables, with a greatly increased mortality.

Rackow et al (1983) compared the cardiorespiratory effects of saline, albumin, and HES in 26 hypovolaemic patients, 70% of whom had septicaemic shock. Fluid was given to maintain PAWP at 15 mmHg. At 24 hours radiological pulmonary oedema was present in 87.5% of those given saline, compared to 22% in those given albumin or starch. Arterial oxygen tensions were lower in those given saline but the reduction was not statistically significant. Tranbaugh et al (1980) in a study on EVLW in burns patients resuscitated with crystalloids found a significant rise in EVLW in patients with sepsis, but normal values in those without sepsis. Metildi et al's previously mentioned study (1984), in which over half the patients were suffering from septic shock, showed no differences in pulmonary function between crystalloid- and colloid-treated groups.

CONCLUSIONS

In the initial resuscitation from hypovolaemia the choice of fluid is less important than the rapidity and adequacy of fluid replacement. It has been suggested that preferences as to the type of fluid used 'centre mainly on issues relating to philosophy, side-effects, and economics' (Ledingham & Ramsay 1986). In the USA it has been estimated that treating hypovolaemia with colloids rather than crystalloids involves a difference in cost of 500 million dollars per year (Tranbaugh & Lewis 1986).

It is clear that colloids cause a greater expansion of the intravascular space than crystalloids, the latter being required in approximately two and a half times the volume for equivalent effect. Certain statements can also be made concerning the pulmonary effects of fluid administration in previously healthy patients.

1. Transudation of fluid in the lung is primarily controlled by the pulmonary intravascular pressure.
2. Changes in PCOP do not alter the oncotic pressure gradient between the plasma and the pulmonary interstitial fluid.
3. If any increase in fluid transudation does occur, it is normally compensated for by an increase in pulmonary lymph drainage.
4. Large increases in lung water content can occur before gas exchange becomes impaired.

Thus in many patients crystalloids can be administered in enormous quantities with very little harmful effect on the lung, even though peripheral oedema may occur during the recovery phase. The situation is less clear in the presence of lung injury, acute respiratory disease, and sepsis, when pulmonary oedema, raised EVLW, and impaired gas exchange are more common. If intravascular pressure is not raised assumedly capillary permeability must be increased, with the increased fluid flux overwhelming the protective mechanisms. It would seem that the intravascular pressure is still the most important factor in controlling fluid flux, but the question of whether in the critically ill patient the raising of PCOP is beneficial or detrimental cannot be confidently answered. In patients such as these, and those with cardiac failure, cardiac filling pressures must not be allowed to rise above normal and thus more intensive monitoring will be required during fluid resuscitation.

In practice minor blood loss is usually treated by crystalloid alone, and major blood loss by a combination of blood, crystalloid and varying proportions of colloid. One should aim to maintain haemoglobin levels at 8–10 g/dl or a haematocrit of 30–35%. In situations where virtually the entire red cell mass has been lost, the administration of at least some colloid would appear essential. Indeed a combination of both crystalloid and colloid appears to be required for the best results during treatment of major hypovolaemia (Smith & Norman 1982). In addition, in situations where blood loss is extremely rapid, or resuscitation is required very rapidly, colloids will have greater effect than equal volumes of crystalloids, and thus can be effectively administered faster.

REFERENCES

Blalock A 1930 Experimental shock: the cause of the low blood pressure produced by muscle injury. Archives of Surgery 20: 959–996

Blalock A 1943 A consideration of the present status of the shock problem. Surgery 14: 487–508

Boutros A R, Ruess R, Olson L, Hoyt J L, Baker W H 1979 Comparison of hemodynamic, pulmonary, and renal effects of use of three types of fluids after major surgical procedures on the abdominal aorta. Critical Care Medicine 7: 9–13

Brigham K L, Bowers R E, Haynes J 1979 Increased sheep lung vascular permeability caused by Escherichia coli endotoxin. Circulation Research 45: 292–297

Brigham K L, Kariman K, Harris T R, Snapper J R, Bernard G R, Young S L 1983 Correlation of oxygenation with vascular permeability-surface area but not with lung water in humans with acute respiratory failure and pulmonary edema. Journal of Clinical Investigation 72: 339–349

Brinkmeyer S, Safar P, Motoyama E, Stezoski W 1981 Superiority of colloid over electrolyte solution for fluid resuscitation (severe normovolemic hemodilution). Critical Care Medicine 9: 369–370

Canizaro P C, Prager M D, Shires G T 1971 The Infusion of Ringer's lactate solution during shock. American Journal of Surgery 122: 494–501

Carey J S, Scharsmidt B F, Culliford A T, Greenlee J E, Scott C R 1970 Hemodynamic effectiveness of colloid and electrolyte solutions for replacement of simulated operative blood loss. Surgery, Gynecology & Obstetrics 131: 679–686

Carey L C, Lowery B D, Cloutier C T 1971 Hemorrhagic shock. Current Problems in Surgery January: 1–48

Civetta J M 1979 A new look at the Starling equation. Critical Care Medicine 7: 84–89

Coller F A, Campbell K N, Vaughan H H, Iob L V, Moyer C R 1944 Postoperative salt intolerance. Annals of Surgery 119: 533–542

Da Luz P, Schubin H, Weil M H, Jacobson E J, Stein L 1975 Pulmonary edema related to changes in colloid osmotic and pulmonary artery wedge pressure in patients after acute myocardial infarction. Circulation 51: 350–357

Dawidson I, Eriksson B 1982 Statistical evaluation of plasma substitutes based on 10 variables. Critical Care Medicine 10: 653–657

Demling R H 1986 The cardiopulmonary effects of sepsis on the trauma patient. Critical Care Clinics 2: 853–867

Demling R H, Manohar M, Will J A 1979 Response of the pulmonary microcirculation to fluid loading after hemorrhagic shock and resuscitation. Surgery 87: 552–559

Dillon J, Lynch L J, Myers R, Butcher H R, Moyer C A 1966 A bioassay of treatment of hemorrhagic shock. Archives of Surgery 93: 537–555

Esrig B C, Fulton R L 1975 Sepsis, resuscitated hemorrhagic shock and "Shock Lung". Annals of Surgery 182: 218–227

Finch J S, Reid C, Bandy K, Fickle D 1983 Compared effects of selected colloids on extravascular lung water in dogs after oleic acid-induced lung injury and severe hemorrhage. Critical Care Medicine 11: 267–270

Gabel J C, Drake R E 1979 Pulmonary capillary pressure and permeability. Critical Care Medicine 7: 92–97

Gaisford W D, Pandey N, Jensen C G 1972 Pulmonary changes in treated hemorrhagic shock II. Ringer's lactate solution versus colloid infusion. American Journal of Surgery 124: 738–743

Gallagher T J, Banner M J, Barnes P A 1985 Large volume crystalloid resuscitation does not increase extravascular lung water. Anesthesia and Analgesia 64: 323–326

Haljamae J 1984 Interstitial fluid response. In: Shires G T (ed) Shock and related problems. Clinical Surgery International vol 9. Churchill Livingstone, Edinburgh, Ch 4, p 44–60

Hauser C J, Shoemaker W C, Turpin I, Goldberg S J 1980 Oxygen transport responses to colloids and crystalloids in critically ill surgical patients. Surgery, Gynecology & Obstetrics 150: 811–816

Holcroft J W, Trunkey D D 1974 Extravascular lung water following hemorrhagic shock in the baboon. Annals of Surgery 180: 408–417

Holcroft J W, Trunkey D D 1975 Pulmonary extravasation of albumin during and after hemorrhagic shock in baboons. Journal of Surgical Research 18: 91–97

Laks H, O'Connor N E, Anderson W, Pilon R N 1976 Crystalloid versus colloid hemodilution in man. Surgery, Gynecology & Obstetrics 142: 506–512

Lane W A 1891 A surgical tribute to the late Dr Wooldridge. Lancet ii: 626–627

Ledingham I McA, Ramsay G 1986 Hypovolaemic shock. British Journal of Anaesthesia 58: 169–189

Lowe R J, Moss G D, Jilek J, Levine H D 1979 Crystalloid versus colloid in the etiology of pulmonary failure after trauma — a randomized trial in man. Critical Care Medicine 7: 107–112

Lucas C E, Ledgerwood A M, Higgins R F, Weaver D W 1980 Impaired pulmonary function after albumin resuscitation from shock. Journal of Trauma 20: 446–451

Magilligan D J, Oledkyn T W, Schwartz S I, Yu P N 1972 Pulmonary intravascular and extravascular volumes in hemorrhagic shock and fluid replacement. Surgery 72: 780–788

Merrill D G, Rosenthal M H, Mihn F G, Feeley T W, Ashton J P A, Howse J J 1981 Fluid resuscitation and lung water accumulation. Anesthesiology 55: A78

Metildi L A, Shackford S R, Virgilio R W, Peters R M 1984 Crystalloid versus colloid in fluid resuscitation of patients with severe pulmonary insufficiency. Surgery, Gynecology & Obstetrics 158: 207–212

Modig J 1983 Advantages of dextran 70 over Ringer acetate solution in shock treatment and in prevention of adult respiratory distress syndrome. Resuscitation 10: 219–227

Moore F D, Ball M R 1952 The metabolic response to surgery. Charles C Thomas, Springfield, Illinois

Moore F D, Shires G T 1967 Moderation. Annals of Surgery 166: 300–301

Moss G S, Proctor H J, Homer L D, Herman C M, Litt B D 1969 A comparison of asanguinous fluids and whole blood in the treatment of hemorrhagic shock. Surgery, Gynecology & Obstetrics 129: 1247–1257

Moss G S, Siegel D C, Cochin A, Fresquez V 1971 Effects of saline and colloid solutions on pulmonary function in hemorrhagic shock. Surgery, Gynecology & Obstetrics 130: 53–58

Moss G S, Das Gupta T K, Brinkman R, Seghal L, Newsom B 1979 Changes in lung ultrastructure following heterologous and homologous serum albumin infusion in the treatment of hemorrhagic shock. Annals of Surgery 189: 236–242

Nees J E, Hauser C J, Shippy C, Shoemaker W C 1978 Comparison of cardiorespiratory effects of crystalline hemoglobin, whole blood, albumin, and Ringer's lactate in the resuscitation of hemorrhagic shock in dogs. Surgery 83: 639–647

Proctor H J, Moss G S, Homer L D 1969 Changes in lung compliance in experimental hemorrhagic shock and resuscitation. Annals of Surgery 169: 82–92

Rackow E C, Fein A F, Leppo J 1977 Colloid osmotic pressure as a prognostic indicator of pulmonary edema and mortality in the critically ill. Chest 72: 709–713

Rackow E C, Falk J L, Fein A et al 1983 Fluid resuscitation in circulatory shock: a comparison of the cardiorespiratory effects of albumin, hetastarch, and saline infusions in patients with hypovolemic and septic shock. Critical Care Medicine 11: 839–850

Risberg B, Miller E, Hughes J 1981 Comparison of the pulmonary effects of rapid infusion of a crystalloid and a colloid solution. Acta Chirurgica Scandinavica 147: 613–618

Rutili G, Parker J C, Taylor A E 1984 Fluid balance in ANTU-injured lungs during crystalloid and colloid infusions. Journal of Applied Physiology 56: 993–998

Shah D M, Browner B D, Dutton R E, Newell J C, Powers S R 1977 Cardiac output and pulmonary wedge pressure. Archives of Surgery 112: 1161–1164

Shires T, Williams J, Brown F 1961 Acute changes in extracellular fluids associated with major surgical procedures. Annals of Surgery 154: 803–810

Shires T, Coln D, Carrico J, Lightfoot S 1964 Fluid therapy in haemorrhagic shock. Archives of Surgery 88: 688–693

Shires G T, Peitzman A B, Albert S A, I Uner H, Silane M F, Perry M O 1983 Response of extravascular lung water to intraoperative fluids. Annals of surgery 197: 515–519

Shoemaker W C 1976 Comparison of the relative effectiveness of whole blood transfusions and various types of fluid therapy in resuscitation. Critical Care Medicine 4: 71–78

Sibbald W J, Driedger A A, Wells G A, Myers M L, Lefcoe M 1983 The short-term effects of increasing plasma colloid osmotic pressure in patients with noncardiac pulmonary edema. Surgery 93: 620–633

Skillman J J, Restall D S, Salzman E W 1975 Randomized trial of albumin vs electrolyte solutions during abdominal aortic operations. Surgery 78: 291–303

Smith J A R, Norman J N 1982 The fluid of choice for resuscitation of severe shock. British Journal of Surgery 69: 702–705

Stein L, Beraud J-J, Morissette M, da Luz P, Weil M H, Shubin H 1975 Pulmonary edema during volume infusion. Circulation 52: 483–489

Sturm J A, Carpenter M A, Lewis F R, Graziano C, Trunkey D D 1979 Water and protein movement in the sheep lung after septic shock: effect of colloid versus crystalloid resuscitation. Journal of Surgical Research 26: 233–248

Takaori M, Safar P 1967 Treatment of massive hemorrhage with colloid and crystalloid solutions: studies in dogs. Journal of the American Medical Association 199: 297–302

Tranbaugh R F, Lewis F R 1986 Crystalloid vs colloid in the initial fluid resuscitation of the acutely injured patient. In: Askanazi J, Starker P M, Weissman C (eds) Fluid and electrolyte management in critical care. Butterworths, Boston, pp 189–202

Tranbaugh R F, Lewis F R, Christensen J M, Elings V B 1980 Lung water changes after thermal injury. The effects of crystalloid resuscitation and sepsis. Annals of Surgery 192: 479–490

Tranbaugh R F, Elings V B, Christensen J, Lewis F R 1982 Determinants of pulmonary interstitial fluid accumulation after trauma. Journal of Trauma 22: 820–826

Trunkey D D, Illner H, Wagner I Y, Shires C T 1973 The effect of hemorrhagic shock on intracellular muscle action potentials in the primate. Surgery 74: 241–250

Twigley A J, Hillman K M 1985 The end of the crystalloid era? Anaesthesia 40: 860–871

Virgilio R W, Rice C L, Smith D E et al 1979 Crystalloid vs colloid resuscitation: is one better? Surgery 85: 129–139

Wolfman E F, Neill S A, Heaps D K, Zuidema G D 1963 Donor blood and isotonic salt solution. Archives of Surgery 86: 869–873

Zarins C K, Rice C L, Peters R M, Virgilio R W 1978 Lymph and pulmonary response to isobaric reduction in plasma oncotic pressure in baboons. Circulation Research 43: 925–930

Hyperglycaemia and ischaemic brain damage

INTRODUCTION

The brain does no mechanical work: nevertheless, its consumption of energy is substantial. Energy is required to sustain ionic pumps, to preserve the ion fluxes that accompany the transfer of information between the cells of the brain, to maintain the integrity of barriers such as the blood-brain and blood-CSF barriers, and to support the synthesis of a variety of neurotransmitters (both excitatory and inhibitory). Indeed, such is the requirement for energy by the brain that it utilises one quarter of the glucose (31 μmol/100 g/min) consumed by the entire body (as well as around 20% of oxygen required by the body at rest).

The cells of the brain, in particular the neurones, are continually active and, not surprisingly, consume substantial amounts of energy. However, since the brain cannot store oxygen, and since its content of energy-generating substances is small, the normal functioning of the central nervous system is dependent upon the continuous supply of appropriate energy substrates, in particular oxygen and glucose, and the adequate removal of the waste products of metabolism. Fortunately, most evidence indicates that, in conscious man under physiological conditions, the blood flow to the brain parallels the demand for energy by the brain and, consequently, the level of oxygen consumption and glucose utilisation. When cerebral function is depressed, as in coma, and the requirement for energy decreased, total cerebral blood flow, oxygen consumption and glucose utilisation are much lower than in the normal fully conscious state. In contrast, during seizures the demand for oxygen and glucose increases markedly and this must be met from a concomitant increase in supply.

The peculiar vulnerability of the cells of the brain (particularly the neurones) has been ascribed to their sensitivity to an imbalance between supply and demand. As will be appreciated, any inadequacy of supply will lead to the rapid depletion of available substrate — be this oxygen or glucose (or both). Not surprisingly, therefore, in times past it was assumed that any increase in the 'stores' of energy-generating substances before, or any decrease in the consumption of such substances during, an episode of

119

ischaemia (or hypoxia) would improve the tolerance of the brain to the insult. Nevertheless, although energy stores in the brain have been shown to increase following the administration of glucose (and decrease after the injection of insulin) (Hansen 1978) there is more recent, substantial, evidence to suggest that the administration of glucose before an episode of ischaemia (or hypoxia) will exacerbate the subsequent brain damage.

In this chapter data will be presented (from studies in laboratory animals and man) supportive of the above and we then attempt to highlight the clinical relevance of the relationship between hyperglycaemia and ischaemic brain damage.

ISCHAEMIA

Intuitively, one would anticipate that complete global ischaemia (the total cessation of the supply of oxygen and glucose) would be infinitely worse, as far as the brain is concerned, than incomplete global, or focal, ischaemia. One could be forgiven for assuming that the continuing supply of substrate — albeit in substantially decreased concentration — would delay the onset of cell damage, and the infarction of brain tissue. Although this latter view has been supported by the studies of Marshall et al (1975), Steen et al (1979) and Schurr et al (1986), the conclusions drawn by other groups were different. For example, Hossmann & Olsson (1970) flushed the cerebral vascular system (of the cat) with non-oxygenated Ringer's solution during 30 minutes of ischaemia and were able to demonstrate a greater degree of neurological recovery in these animals than in other animals in which the blood flow had been stopped for an equivalent period. Three years later, this same group (Hossmann & Kleihues 1973) noted *en passant* that the brains of animals, subjected to 60 minutes of ischaemia, appeared to fare worse in the presence of persisting (although low) blood flow. This particular question was studied in more detail by Nordstrom et al (1978a,b) using models of complete ischaemia (no blood flow) or incomplete ischaemia (blood flow 5–10% of control). These workers observed that the recovery of the cerebral (cortical) energy state was significantly less in those animals subjected to incomplete ischaemia. Ultimately, this disparity between the findings in different laboratories was largely resolved when it was noted that in some studies the animals were fed ad libitum (Nordstrom et al 1978b) whereas in others (Steen et al 1979) the animals had been fasted prior to the period of ischaemia. Although difficult to reconcile initially, these disparate views and the ensuing controversy highlighted significantly the whole question of the exacerbation of ischaemic brain damage in association with hyperglycaemia.

Complete ischaemia

Myers & Yamaguchi (1976, 1977) provided the first direct in vivo evidence that glucose, and in particular hyperglycaemia, was detrimental to the recovery of cerebral function following a defined ischaemic insult. Two monkeys receiving glucose (35 and 70 ml/kg i.v.) before experimentally-induced complete global ischaemia (14 minutes of cardiac arrest) suffered substantially more brain damage than did four saline-pretreated animals. Likewise, fasted monkeys given glucose (2.5 or 5.0 g/kg i.v.) fared worse neurologically than similar animals receiving physiological saline (Myers 1976). Siemkowicz & Hansen (1978) induced complete ischaemia (10 minutes' duration) in rats pretreated to produce different blood glucose concentrations (1.9 mmol/l: 7.8 mmol/l: 24 mmol/l) and assessed survival and neurological damage at 21 days. All of the rats in the normoglycaemic group were alive at the end of the period of observation: some had recovered completely, others had persistent minor neurological deficits. In contrast, all of the rats in the hyperglycaemic group died within 12 hours of the insult. Recovery in the hypoglycaemic group of animals was significantly inferior to that in the normoglycaemic group (three out of eight animals died): nevertheless, it was substantially better than in the group of hyperglycaemic animals. More recently, Lanier et al (1987) induced complete ischaemia in monkeys and demonstrated that the administration of clinically relevant doses of 5% dextrose solution (that is, in the absence of frank hyperglycaemia (blood glucose concentration pre-insult 11 ($\pm$ 1SE) mmol/l)) resulted in a significantly poorer neurological state following resuscitation than that obtained in similar animals pretreated with lactated Ringer's solution (blood glucose concentration pre-insult 8.5 ($\pm$ 0.4SE) mmol/l). In addition, these workers were able to show that the degree of brain damage was proportional to the blood glucose concentration.

Incomplete ischaemia

In general terms, studies based on models of *incomplete* ischaemia have drawn conclusions similar to those described above. In a rat model of incomplete ischaemia (bilateral carotid ligation: arterial hypotension to a mean of 50 mmHg for 30 minutes followed by restoration of arterial pressure and blood flow for 90 minutes) Rehncrona et al (1981) and Kalimo et al (1981) demonstrated that the recovery of the cortical energy state was impaired significantly in hyperglycaemic animals (blood glucose concentrations between 10.9 and 25.3 mmol/l). In addition, these workers demonstrated increased morphological damage following the period of ischaemia, and lower values of cerebral blood flow in the recovery period when compared with the findings in animals given an equivalent volume of physiological saline. Pulsinelli et al (1982) examined the effect of hyperglycaemia in an animal model (rat) that simultaneously produces severe (virtually complete) ischaemia of the forebrain with moderate ischaemia of the hindbrain — in which there is a continued but lower delivery of substrate. Morphological damage in the animals pretreated with physiological saline (blood glucose concentration 10 ± 1 mmol/l) was characterised by ischaemic cell damage limited to selectively vulnerable neurones. There was no evidence of infarction of brain tissues (vide infra). In the animals pretreated with glucose (blood glucose concentration 18 ± 2 mmol/l) there was significant morphological damage throughout the forebrain, and more ischaemic cell damage in the hindbrain than in the saline-treated control animals. Moreover, evidence of severe cerebral oedema, and of infarction of brain tissue (in three out of nine animals) were present in the group of animals which received glucose pre-insult. Further evidence was provided by Ginsberg et al (1980) who reported that, in a model of incomplete ischaemia, animals pretreated with glucose developed evidence of brain damage (post-ischaemic heterogeneity of perfusion in the cerebral cortex and deep grey structures) after a 15-minute period of ischaemia. In animals not so pretreated 30 minutes of ischaemia was required to induce a similar degree of damage.

Thus the events associated with incomplete ischaemia are particularly complex and we will return to these later. At this point in our discussion it is sufficient to note that, in general terms, the brain damage following a period of incomplete ischaemia is greater than that associated with an episode of complete ischaemia of similar duration (Nordstrom et al 1978b, Siesjo 1981). The only caveat to the above is that *fasted* animals subjected to a period of incomplete ischaemia recover more completely than those exposed to complete ischaemia — as evidenced by the return of electrical activity in the brain (EEG and evoked potentials) (Kalimo et al 1981).

Studies in man

Evidence that the phenomenon described above pertains also to man is less clear. Nevertheless, detrimental effects of increases in blood glucose concentration, on neurological outcome after ischaemia, have been reported.

Epidemiological studies have indicated that the incidence of ischaemic stroke is greater in diabetic, than in non-diabetic, patients. Although this difference has been attributed to the frequency of hypertension, cardiac disease and proliferative cerebral angiopathy, in the patients with diabetes it has been shown that, even when these risk factors were taken into account (Wolf & Kannell 1982), diabetes per se increases the incidence of stroke. Similar conclusions were drawn by Pulsinelli et al (1983). In a retrospective study these workers noted that recovery of neurological function in diabetic patients with a stroke was significantly worse than in non-diabetic patients, and that the incidence of stroke-related deaths was greater in the diabetic patients. In a prospective study, this same group (Pulsinelli et al 1983) reported that, among a group of non-diabetic patients with an ischaemic stroke, 76% of those with a blood glucose concentration (on admission) of less than 7.3 mmol/l returned to 'full or partial work-related activities' whereas only 43% with values greater than 7.3 mmol/l regained a similar status. These observations are corroborated by those of Melamed (1976) and Longstreth & Inui (1984). Melamed, for example, noted that the severity of an acute stroke could be related to the increase in blood glucose concentration induced by the cerebrovascular accident. Longstreth & Inui (1984) carried out a retrospective review of the neurological outcome of 430 patients resuscitated from a cardiac arrest occurring outside hospital. All of the patients had received varying amounts of 5% dextrose solution i.v. They reported that the blood glucose concentrations (on admission to hospital) of those patients who did not regain consciousness after the arrest were significantly greater than the values obtained in the patients who regained consciousness. Moreover, they found that, of the patients regaining consciousness, the blood glucose concentration was greater in those patients with persisting neurological deficits than in those patients surviving without deficit.

Although certain of the studies cited above could be criticised on a number of counts the overwhelming impression from the data presented is that, in an energy-depleted state, hyperglycaemia, even of modest degree, can aggravate the damage produced by an ischaemic insult of defined density and duration. For some reason, the concentration of glucose in the brain immediately prior to an episode of cerebral ischaemia appears to determine whether the period of ischaemia causes infarction of brain tissue and, consequently, more extensive tissue damage, or whether it results in a more limited degree of injury — localised ischaemic cell damage (Plum 1983). Why?

Lactate in brain tissue

Lactate is a normal constituent of brain tissue (resting concentration around 1.5 μmol/g). Following the sudden acute onset of complete ischaemia the tissue content of lactate will increase from around 1.5 to 12–14 μmol/g as a result of the continued metabolism of the normal (pre-ischaemic) stores of glucose and glycogen (Ljunggren et al 1974). However, the ultimate lactate concentration depends on the pre-ischaemic nutritional state: in particular, on the pre-ischaemic blood glucose concentration (Ljunggren et al 1974). For example, lactate concentrations in ischaemic tissue of 4.8, 12.1 and 20.7 μmol/g have been associated, respectively, with blood glucose concentrations of 2.4, 7.8 and 28 mmol/l. Since starved animals do not become hyperglycaemic during a period of ischaemia the lactate concentration in such animals does not exceed the values obtained in normoglycaemic animals. In contrast, the administration of food, or the infusion of glucose, increases the blood, and hence the brain, glucose concentration and, under these circumstances, cerebral tissue lactate concentration may exceed 30 μmol/g (Siesjo & Wieloch 1985).

Numerous attempts have been made to define a tissue concentration above which lactic acid becomes toxic. Myers (1979) suggested that a value of around 20 μmol/g may be critical, and Siesjo (1981) observed that animals in which the lactate concentration exceeded 20–25 μmol/g failed 'to recover a "normal" cerebral energy state'. In general terms, therefore, the available data would suggest that there is a critical threshold somewhere between 16 and 25 μmol/g.

With this as background it is not surprising that the increase in brain damage associated with hyperglycaemia has been ascribed to the anaerobic production of 'critical' concentrations of lactic acid (Myers 1979, Welsh et al 1980, Siemkowicz & Gjedde 1980, Plum 1983). Since an exogenous, or even an endogenous, increase in blood glucose concentration is associated with a parallel increase in brain tissue glucose concentration it follows that, during an ischaemic event, there would be a proportionally greater production of lactate and, hence, more extensive brain damage. However, although this argument appears reasonable, it is unclear whether it is, indeed, the absolute lactate concentration per se which produces the damage. Any increase in lactate concentration decreases tissue pH and increases the osmolality of the tissue. Although most investigators suspect that the decrease in pH is the primary determinant of the damage, either mechanism could be harmful. Although attractive in its simplicity this scenario may lack precision. Certainly, Welsh et al (1983) argue strongly against the increase in tissue lactate concentration being the fundamental mechanism underlying the poorer outcome. They point out that the actual increase in lactate concentration is relatively small in absolute terms, and that, although the accumulation of lactate in the cortex was regionally homogeneous, the changes in blood flow and energy metabolites observed post-insult were obviously heterogeneous in distribution. Not surprisingly, a number of groups, including Siemkowicz & Gjedde (1980), Ginsberg et al (1980) and Welsh et al (1983) have considered the possibility that the poorer outcome was due to regional impairment of perfusion following the period of ischaemia. However, the evidence is inconclusive: it is difficult to determine whether the observed changes in flow are the primary event or whether they are secondary to other factors such as an increase in extracellular brain water (vide infra).

The amount of lactic acid which can accumulate during *complete* ischaemia is determined by, and limited by, the pre-ischaemic stores of substrate: the supply of oxygen and glucose is zero and the diffusion of lactate out of the brain negligible. In *incomplete* ischaemia, on the other hand, the presence of some residual blood flow (the 'trickle of flow') provides a continuing supply of exogenous glucose. In addition, during incomplete ischaemia, the final tissue concentration of lactate will depend on the blood glucose concentration and the duration of the period of incomplete ischaemia. It is possible that these facts could explain the apparent paradox discussed earlier: namely, of a poorer outcome following incomplete than after complete ischaemia. Interestingly, Nordstrom & Siesjo

(1978) and Nordstrom et al (1978a,b) demonstrated that the increases in brain tissue lactate concentration associated with incomplete ischaemia were twice those resulting from a period of complete ischaemia.

Be that as it may, we have, as yet, not addressed the second, and more fundamental, part of the question posed earlier: why should the damage to brain tissue resulting from a defined ischaemic insult be more extensive when associated with hyperglycaemia? Is the degree of damage merely a reflection of the higher tissue lactate concentration (or the greater increase in osmolality, or the more marked decrease in pH) per se, or is there more to it than that?

Lactate and cell death

Ischaemia leads to swelling of the astrocytes due, most probably, to a trans-location of water from the extracellular to the intracellular space. If the ischaemia is of short duration the net increase in brain tissue water content may be zero or very small. In the presence of more prolonged ischaemia, and especially if hyperglycaemia is present, the swelling of the astrocytes becomes much more pronounced, and there is a net increase in brain tissue water content (cerebral oedema). Such oedema, which may be augmented substantially during the period of recirculation which follows the ischaemic insult, can be sufficient to cause infarction of tissue. However, as alluded to above, the water content of the *intracellular* space (of the astrocyte) may be increased also.

Astrocytes contain more glycogen than other cells in the adult brain. Therefore, it is conceivable that, during a period of ischaemia, the osmolality and the hydrogen ion concentration should increase to a greater extent in the astrocyte than in other cells (for example, neurones). As a result Plum (1983) has postulated that, when the lactate concentration is low, ischaemia damages 'nerve cells by a process that is independent of pH or osmolal change and presumably relates directly to oxygen lack and the associated energy failure'. In this hypothesis astrocytes and endothelial cells are not damaged until the brain tissue lactate concentration exceeds a threshold value (approximately 16 μmol/g). At concentrations above this value the accumulation of lactate (or the sequelae of the accumulation of lactate) causes the already anoxic (and swollen) astrocytes to rupture and the endothelial cells to necrose. The neurones now bereft of mechanical, nutritional and metabolic support die: an infarct becomes established (Fig. 8.1). As both neuronal and supporting elements have been affected regionally it is not really surprising that neurological outcome is poorer under such circumstances. For more detailed information on the precise biochemical mechanisms which are thought to subserve the swelling of the astrocytes, and the development of the oedema (both intracellular and extracellular) the interested reader is referred to reviews by Siesjo (1981), Siesjo & Wieloch (1985) and Plum (1983).

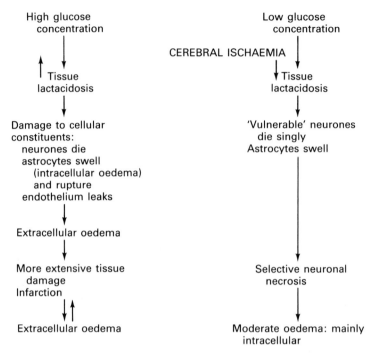

Fig. 8.1 A hypothesis for the adverse effects of hyperglycaemia in association with cerebral ischaemia (adapted from Plum (1983) with permission)

CLINICAL IMPLICATIONS

In this section of the chapter it is apposite that we consider the clinical implications, if indeed there are any, of the points discussed previously. However, before doing so, there is some merit in highlighting two additional points, from the various experimental studies, which could have a direct bearing on clinical practice. First, it must be stressed that the deleterious effects of hyperglycaemia relate to those situations in which the glucose concentration has been above its physiological value *before* and, in the case of incomplete ischaemia, during the period of ischaemia. At the present time, the effects of the administration of glucose during complete ischaemia, or following the ischaemic insult, are unclear. However, the balance of the evidence appears to suggest that such manoeuvres of themselves neither augment, nor diminish, post-ischaemic neurological damage.

In the second place, it is relevant to note that the glucose concentration in brain need not always reflect the blood glucose concentration. For example, there is some evidence which suggests that the brain will not release excess glucose to the blood in response to a decreasing blood glucose concentration. Instead, free water will be absorbed by the brain until an equilibrium is established between the concentrations in blood and brain (Welsh et al 1980). Thus, in circumstances in which the blood glucose values were decreasing — as, for example, following the discontinuation of an infusion of glucose — it is conceivable that the glucose concentration in the brain could lag behind that in the blood. Thus, theoretically at least, the risk of hyperglycaemia-induced neurological damage could be present, following an infusion of glucose, despite acceptable blood glucose concentrations immediately prior to the ischaemic insult.

As far as the clinical anaesthetist is concerned the relevance of this topic centres around, first, the definition of those patients, and clinical situations, associated with a risk of cerebral ischaemia and, second, an assessment of the advisability of withholding glucose-containing solutions in such patients. If we take the second point first it is evident that a number of workers now advise against the use of such solutions and/or the development of hyperglycaemia in such patients (Newberg 1985, Lanier et al 1987). One potential problem with such a recommendation, however, is the possibility that the fasted patient could become hypoglycaemic during the surgical procedure. It has, of course, been acknowledged for some time that hypoglycaemia can, of itself, cause brain damage. Recently, Sieber et al (1985) addressed this particular aspect in patients with supratentorial tumours. They obtained blood glucose concentrations of around 14 ($\pm$ 0.7) mmol/l in patients receiving approximately 1 litre of 5% dextrose solution over 4 hours. In a similar group of patients given physiological saline the mean blood glucose concentration was 10 ($\pm$ 0.4) mmol/l. In other words the patients receiving physiological saline solution did not become hypoglycaemic. In addition, they showed that the intra-operative administration of glucose (over the period of their study) exerted no beneficial effect on protein catabolism. They recommended that, since the blood glucose concentrations obtained by the administration of glucose were within the range thought to augment brain damage, 'glucose-containing solutions be avoided in patients undergoing operations that may have a significant risk of intraoperative ischaemia'. There are situations in which the need for intra-operative glucose does exist: for example, the unstable diabetic, the stable but insulin-dependent diabetic, the patient in receipt of parenteral nutrition involving the use of concentrated solutions of dextrose. However, in all probability, the average patient does not require the intra-operative administration of glucose — at least as long as the duration of surgery is not greater than 4 hours. During more protracted procedures there may be merit in monitoring the blood glucose concentration more closely than is customary at present, and tailoring the administration of glucose to the patient's actual requirements.

It behoves us to consider those clinical situations in which there is defined risk of ischaemia. The most common are presented in Table 8.1. It is to

Table 8.1 Clinical situations in which there is a significant risk of cerebral ischaemia

---

Cardiovascular
    Cardiac arrest
    Arterial hypotension
    Cardiopulmonary bypass
    Severe arrhythmia

Neurological
    Cerebrovascular/intracranial surgery
    Subarachnoid haemorrhage: 'spasm'
    Stroke
    Carotid endarterectomy

Endocrine
    Diabetic with cerebrovascular disease
    Severe hyperglycaemia in diabetic

---

be hoped that none of the patients in our care sustain an episode of complete global cerebral ischaemia (cardiac arrest). However, many may require the deliberate clipping of an intracerebral artery (complete focal ischaemia) during the surgical management of an intracranial aneurysm or during an intracranial-extracranial bypass. Likewise, incomplete global ischaemia may be associated with cardiopulmonary bypass and the deliberate, or inadvertent, induction of systemic arterial hypotension. One would include patients undergoing carotid endarterectomy as being at risk of developing ischaemia during the period of carotid clamping. Likewise, it would be possible to argue that patients requiring excision of a brain tumour are also at risk since the pressure exerted by the brain retractor(s) may compromise cerebral perfusion (Albin et al 1980).

Incidents such as cardiac arrest, stroke, and cardiopulmonary bypass, for example, are stressful events and are associated with a physiological response which includes an increase in blood glucose concentration. Conceivably, this endogenous release of glucose could be a means of augmenting brain damage should it be superimposed on an ischaemic background.

The patient with a head injury must also be considered to be at risk. The clinician has no control over the pre-insult blood glucose concentration: nevertheless, more frequent measurements, than heretofore, of blood glucose concentrations may be advisable. An interesting aside was highlighted by the results of a study by Dearden et al (1986) in which they showed that outcome was poorer in head-injured patients in whom the intracranial pressure was greater than 20 mmHg following the administration of dexamethasone. Subsequent correspondence (Reynolds & Flint 1986) highlighted the fact that the glucose concentrations in the group receiving the dexamethasone were higher than in the control group. Would it be too far-fetched to speculate whether any of the discrepancies in the literature in regard to the efficacy of various cerebral resuscitation regimens could be ascribed to differences (possibly quite small) in pre-insult blood (or brain) glucose concentrations?

CONCLUSION

The vulnerability of the brain to ischaemia is well known: the case for the augmentation of ischaemic damage by hyperglycaemia, even of moderate degree, has been presented. The anaesthetist must consider the whole patient but I submit that there are situations in which the use of glucose-containing solutions may be more harmful than beneficial.

REFERENCES

Albin M S, Bunegin B S, Martin A, Helsel B S, Phillips W, Babinski M F 1980 Brain retraction pressure and cerebral perfusion (abstract). Anesthesiology 53: S117

Dearden N M, Gibson J S, McDowall D G, Gibson R M, Cameron M M 1986 Effect of high-dose dexamethasone on outcome from severe head injury. Journal of Neurosurgery 64: 81–88

Ginsberg M D, Welsh F A, Budd W W 1980 Deleterious effect of glucose pretreatment on recovery from diffuse cerebral ischaemia in the cat: 1. Local cerebral blood flow and glucose utilisation. Stroke 11: 347–354

Hansen A J 1978 The extracellular potassium concentration in brain cortex following ischaemia in hypo- and hyperglycaemic rats. Acta Physiologica Scandinavica 102: 324–329

Hossmann K-A, Kleihues P 1973 Reversibility of ischaemic brain damage. Archives of Neurology 29: 375–382

Hossmann K-A, Olsson Y 1970 Suppression and recovery of normal function in transient cerebral ischaemia. Brain Research 22: 313–325

Kalimo H, Rehncrona S, Soderfeldt B, Olsson Y, Siesjo B K 1981 Brain lactic acidosis and ischaemic cell damage: 2. Histopathology. Journal of Cerebral Blood Flow and Metabolism 1: 313–327

Lanier W L, Strangland K J, Scheithauer B W, Mude J H, Michenfelder J D 1987 The effects of dextrose infusion and head position on neurologic outcome after complete cerebral ischemia in primates: examination of a model. Anesthesiology 66: 39–48

Longstreth W T, Inui T S 1984 High blood glucose level on hospital admission and poor neurological recovery after cardiac arrest. Annals of Neurology 15: 59–63

Ljunggren B, Norberg K, Siesjo B K 1974 Influence of tissue acidosis upon restitution of brain energy metabolism following total ischaemia. Brain Research 77: 173–186

Marshall L F, Durity F, Lounsbury R, Graham D I, Welsh F, Langfitt T W 1975 Experimental cerebral oligemia and ischemia produced by intracranial hypertension. Part 1: pathophysiology, electroencephalography, cerebral blood flow, blood-brain barrier, and neurological function. Journal of Neurosurgery 43: 308–317

Melamed E 1976 Reactive hyperglycaemia in patients with acute stroke. Journal of Neurological Science 29: 275–276

Myers R E 1976 Anoxic brain pathology and blood glucose (abstract). Neurology 26:345

Myers R E 1979 Lactic acid accumulation as cause of brain edema and cerebral necrosis resulting from oxygen deprivation. In: Horobkin R, Guilleminault C (eds) Advances in perinatal neurology. Spectrum, New York, pp 85–114

Myers R E, Yamaguchi S 1976 Effects of serum glucose concentration on brain response to circulatory arrest (abstract). Journal of Neuropathology and Experimental Neurology 33:301

Myers R E, Yamaguchi S 1977 Nervous system effects of cardiac arrest in monkeys. Archives of Neurology 34: 65–74

Newberg L A 1985 Use of intravenous glucose solutions in surgical patients (Correspondence). Anesthesiology and Analgesia 64: 558

Nordstrom C H, Rehncrona S, Siesjo B K 1978a Restitution of cerebral energy state, as well as of glycolytic metabolites, citric acid cycle intermediates and associated amino acids after 30 minutes of complete ischaemia in rats anaesthetised with nitrous oxide or phenobarbital. Journal of Neurochemistry 30: 479–486

Nordstrom C H, Rehncrona S, Siesjo B K 1978b Effects of pentobarbital in cerebral ischaemia. Part II: restitution of cerebral energy state, as well as of glycolytic metabolites, citric acid intermediates and associated amino acids after pronounced incomplete ischaemia. Stroke 9: 335–343

Nordstrom C H, Siesjo B K 1978 Effects of phenobarbital in cerebral ischemia. I: cerebral energy metabolism during pronounced, incomplete ischemia. Stroke 9: 327–335

Plum F 1983 What causes infarction in ischaemic brain? The Robert Wartenberg Lecture. Neurology 33: 222–233

Pulsinelli W A, Waldman S, Rawlinson D, Plum F 1982 Moderate hyperglycaemia augments ischaemic brain damage: A neuropathologic study in the rat. Neurology 32: 1239–1246

Pulsinelli W A, Levy D E, Sigsbee B, Scherer P, Plum F 1983 Increased damage after ischemic stroke in patients with hyperglycemia with or without established diabetes mellitus. American Journal of Medicine 74: 540–544

Rehncrona S, Rosen I, Siesjo B K 1981 Brain lactic acidosis and ischaemic cell damage. I: biochemistry and neurophysiology. Journal of Cerebral Blood Flow and Metabolism 1: 287–311

Reynolds G A, Flint G A 1986 Dexamethasone in severe head injury (Correspondence). Journal of Neurosurgery 65: 427

Schurr A, West C A, Reid K H, Tseng M T, Rigor B M 1986 Hyperglycemia improves recovery from cerebral hypoxia: an in vitro study. Anesthesiology 65: A314

Sieber F E, Smith D S, Crosby L et al 1985 The effects of intraoperative glucose on protein catabolism and serum glucose levels in patients with supratentorial tumours (abstract). Anesthesiology 63: A261

Siemkowicz E, Gjedde A 1980 Post-ischemic coma in rat: effect of different pre-ischemic blood glucose levels on cerebral metabolic recovery after ischaemia. Acta Physiologica Scandinavica 110: 225–232

Siemkowicz E, Hansen A J 1978 Clinical restitution following cerebral ischaemia in hypo-, normo- and hyperglycemic rats. Acta Neurologica Scandinavica 38: 1–8

Siesjo B K 1981 Cell damage in the brain: a speculative synthesis. Journal of Cerebral Blood Flow and Metabolism 1: 155–185

Siesjo B K, Wieloch T 1985 Cerebral metabolism in ischaemia: neurochemical basis for therapy. British Journal of Anaesthesia 57: 47–62

Steen P A, Michenfelder J D, Milde J H 1979 Incomplete versus complete cerebral ischaemia: improved outcome with a minimal blood flow. Annals of Neurology 6: 389–398

Welsh F A, Ginsberg M D, Rieder W, Budd W W 1980 Deleterious effect of glucose pretreatment on recovery from diffuse cerebral ischaemia in the cat. II: regional metabolite levels. Stroke 11: 355–363

Welsh F A, Sims R E, McKee A E 1983 Effect of glucose on recovery of energy metabolism following hypoxia–oligemia in mouse brain: dose-dependence and carbohydrate specificity. Journal of Cerebral Blood Flow and Metabolism 3: 486–492

Wolf P, Kannell W B 1982 Controllable risk factors for stroke: preventative implications of trends in stroke mortality. In: Meyer J S, Shaw T (eds) Diagnosis and management of stroke and TIAs. Addison-Wesley, Menic Park, California, pp 25–61

Cerebral ischaemia: pathophysiology and treatment

INTRODUCTION

Ischaemia is an important cause of brain damage following cardiac arrest, haemorrhagic hypotension and head injury. Cerebral ischaemia may also complicate the management of patients with raised intracranial pressure (as a result of tumour, intracranial haematoma or hydrocephalus), anomalies of the cerebral vascular system and, increasingly, those undergoing craniotomy only days following a subarachnoid haemorrhage (Ljunggren et al 1985). The anaesthetist is uniquely skilled in managing cerebral ischaemia in most of these conditions and the therapies employed for preventing or treating it, such as the use of cerebral metabolic depressant drugs, manipulation of fluid balance, induced alterations of blood pressure, and induced hypothermia, must be familiar to the trained anaesthetist. The purpose of this chapter is to outline normal cerebral perfusion, describe the effects of cerebral ischaemia and discuss methods of treatment.

CEREBRAL PERFUSION

The function of the normal brain depends on a supply of oxygen and glucose adequate to maintain the aerobic metabolism of the cerebral neurones. In health, overall cerebral blood flow is 50 ml.100 g^{-1}.min^{-1} (Lassen 1985) and cerebral metabolic rate for oxygen ($CMRO_2$) is 3.8 ml.100 g^{-1}.min^{-1} (Graham 1985). Within these global figures there are wide regional variations and it appears that there normally exists a close coupling of regional metabolic rate and blood flow in the unanaesthetised subject (Jones et al 1985).

Perfusion of the normal brain depends on an adequate cerebral perfusion pressure (CPP) which is the difference between mean arterial pressure (MAP) and intracranial pressure (ICP), i.e.,

CPP = MAP − ICP

A CPP of more than 40 mmHg ensures a normal perfusion in the normal brain.

The cerebral circulation exhibits *autoregulation* i.e., the cerebral blood flow remains constant over a range of mean arterial blood pressures. In normal patients this pressure range is 60–130 mmHg (Lassen & Christensen 1979) but both the upper and lower limits of this range are increased in chronic hypertension.

The range is decreased (i.e., the lower limit is raised) by severe haemorrhage or raised intracranial pressure. The lower limit may be decreased (i.e., the range extended) by drug-induced hypotension (Fitch et al 1976) and sodium nitroprusside (of the commonly available intravenous agents) preserves perfusion best (McDowall 1985a).

CEREBRAL ISCHAEMIA

Cerebral ischaemia results when the blood supply to the brain is less than is required for normal function (Siesjo 1978). Ischaemia combines the effects of anoxia and hypoglycaemia, depriving the brain of both oxygen and glucose (Siesjo 1981). Ischaemia may be global or focal depending on whether the whole brain or only part of it is affected and may be complete or incomplete depending on whether the blood flow is arrested or merely reduced. Table 9.1 illustrates the categories of ischaemia and some situations in which they may arise.

Many experimental models of the various types of cerebral ischaemia have been reported. It is now possible to define threshold values of cerebral blood flow below which electrical and metabolic indices of cerebral function are perturbed (Heuser & Guggenberger 1985, Symon 1985). The indices of cerebral function used include: spontaneous and evoked cerebral electrical activity (Heiss et al 1976, Prior 1985); cerebral extracellular fluid ionic activities (as an index of the integrity of cellular membranes and metabolism) (Harris et al 1981); and direct tissue analyses of such biochemical intermediates as lactate, pyruvate, creatine phosphate and adenosine triphosphate (Siesjo & Nilsson 1971, Siesjo 1978).

Table 9.2 illustrates threshold cerebral blood flows and the effects produced. In addition to direct biochemical measurements on tissue samples, the derived indices of the lactate:pyruvate ratio (Siesjo & Nilsson 1971) and the adenylate energy charge are commonly used. The adenylate energy charge is the most useful expression of the availability of high energy

Table 9.1 Categories and causes of cerebral ischaemia

Category of ischaemia		Potential Cause
Global	Complete	Cardiac arrest
	Incomplete	Cerebral perfusion pressure <40 mmHg (hypotension; raised ICP)
Focal	Complete	Cerebrovascular occlusion
	Incomplete	Cerebrovascular stenosis (with hypotension)

Table 9.2 Effects of reduced cerebral blood flow

CBF (ml.100 g^{-1}.min^{-1})	Index		
	Electrical	ECF ion activity	Metabolites
15–20	EEG silent SEP present but altered	–	–
15	EEG silent SEP absent	pH $\downarrow$	Lactate $\uparrow$ Creatine phosphate $\downarrow$
10–15	EEG silent	pH $\downarrow$ K$_e$$\uparrow$ Na$_e$ $\downarrow$ Cl$_e$ $\downarrow$	Lactate $\uparrow$ ATP and adenylate energy charge $\downarrow$
10	EEG silent	pH $\downarrow\downarrow$ K$_e$ $\uparrow\uparrow$ Ca$_e^{2+}$$\downarrow$	Lactate $\uparrow\uparrow$ ATP and adenylate energy charge $\downarrow\downarrow$

phosphates in the presence of a reduced adenine nucleotide pool size (Siesjo 1981) and is defined as

$$([ATP] + 0.5\ [ADP]) / ([ATP] + [ADP] + [AMP])$$

The consequences of cerebral ischaemia outlined in Table 9.2 are:

1. Loss of spontaneous electrical activity at a blood flow of 15–20 ml.100g^{-1}.min^{-1} (Heiss et al 1976, Astrup et al 1977, Prior 1985, Symon 1985). There is no indication of metabolic disturbance at the threshold of electrical silence (Siesjo & Wieloch 1985). Evoked potentials are still present but with reduced amplitudes and increased latencies (Prior 1985).
2. With a further reduction in flow to around 15 ml.100 g^{-1}.min^{-1} there is increased production of lactic acid resulting in a fall in intracellular and extracellular pH (Siesjo & Wieloch 1985, Heuser & Guggenberger 1985). Cellular metabolism begins to be anaerobic but high energy phosphate availability is still normal (Siesjo & Nilsson 1971). Somatosensory evoked potentials are lost (Astrup et al 1977).
3. At a flow of 10–15 ml.100 g^{-1}.min^{-1} there is a rise in extracellular K$^+$ activity and a fall in Na$^+$ and Cl$^-$ activities (Ljunggren et al 1974, Astrup et al 1980, Heuser & Guggenberger 1985, Siesjo & Wieloch 1985). Lactate production continues and intracellular and extracellular pH fall progressively. High energy phosphate availability is reduced resulting in a failure of ionic pumps to maintain transmembrane concentration gradients and producing a net efflux of K$^+$ from cells (Morris et al 1983) and uptake of Na$^+$ and Cl$^-$ predominantly into astrocytes (Hertz 1981). The obligatory movement of water with these ion shifts results in a

decrease in extracellular fluid volume detectable experimentally as a rise in tissue impedance (Siesjo & Wieloch 1985) and a swelling of astrocytic processes, evident histologically (Siesjo 1981).

4. As cerebral blood flow falls to less than 10 ml.100g^{-1}.min^{-1}, the extra-cellular potassium, K_e^+, which has been slowly increasing from baseline values of around 3 mmol.l^{-1} to 10–15 mmol.l^{-1}, suddenly increases to values in excess of 30–40 mmol.l^{-1} (Heuser & Guggenberger 1985, Siesjo & Wieloch 1985). This marks the onset of so-called 'anoxic depolarisation'. At this point there may be a small and temporary reversal in the decline of extracellular pH before it resumes its fall (Heuser & Guggenberger 1985). Of more importance at this stage is the fall in extracellular fluid Ca^{2+} activity (Harris et al 1981) reflecting the uptake of Ca^{2+} ions into cells. Neuronal depolarisation and the influx of calcium result in the release of neurotransmitters, amongst which the excitatory amino acids, glutamate and aspartate, cause epileptiform burst discharging in selec-tively vulnerable cells in the hippocampus (Schwartzkroin & Wyler 1980).

MECHANISMS OF TISSUE INJURY

Several mechanisms are involved in the process of tissue injury following ischaemia. These will be outlined below.

Intracellular calcium

In all normal cells intracellular calcium activity is tightly controlled and within neurones it is maintained within the range of 10^{-6}–10^{-8} mol.l^{-1} by various processes all of which ultimately depend on the availability of high energy phosphates (Siesjo & Wieloch 1985). In severe cerebral ischaemia these mechanisms are either inoperative or rapidly saturated because of the markedly reduced availability of high energy phosphates and the gross disturbances of intracellular ionic homeostasis. As a result intracellular Ca^{2+} activity rises rapidly and catabolic reactions are triggered by this rise. A raised intracellular calcium activity causes activation of phospholipase A_2 resulting in the generation of arachidonic acid from the phospholipids of the plasma membrane and intracellular organelle membranes (Farber et al 1981). The arachidonic acid thus generated becomes the substrate for the formation of prostaglandins and leukotrienes which may also be cell damaging (Wolfe 1982).

Proteases are also activated by a rise in intracellular free Ca^{2+}. There is a resultant degradation of neurofilaments (Schlaepfer & Zimmerman 1981) and neurotubules are depolymerised in the presence of increased Ca^{2+} activity. These elements make up the cytoskeleton of the cell which is disrupted by these processes (Siesjo & Wieloch 1985). Proteolysis may also increase the affinity of post-synaptic membranes for excitatory transmitters, particularly in the hippocampus (Lynch et al 1982) resulting in post-ischaemic hyperactivity of these neurones.

Phosphorylation of proteins by kinases, also stimulated by increased Ca^{2+} activity, may also enhance post-ischaemic neuronal discharge by both pre- and post-synaptic effects on neurotransmission (Siesjo & Wieloch 1985).

Free radical production

The excessive production of free radicals in injured tissues may lead to further extension of tissue damage. Free radicals are molecules or ions which have a lone electron in an outer orbital and as a result they are highly reactive. The generation of free radicals is a by-product of normal aerobic metabolism in the mitochondrial electron transport chain, forming O_2^-, H_2O_2 and $OH\cdot$. The cell is normally guarded against free radical damage by: the presence of enzymes (superoxide dismutase, catalase and peroxidase); endogenous free radical scavengers (vitamin E (alpha tocopherol), vitamin C (ascorbic acid), and thiol-containing amino acids and peptides); and by the containment of free radical production within mitochondria (Siesjo 1981).

Paradoxically the re-introduction of O_2 following complete cerebral ischaemia or the continued inadequate supply of O_2 during incomplete ischaemia enhances free radical production by at least three mechanisms. Firstly, mitochondrial electron transfer is abnormal, resulting in a 'damming up' of electrons and increased generation of O_2^-, H_2O_2 and $OH\cdot$ (Kogure et al 1985). Secondly the enzyme xanthine oxidase which is formed in ischaemic tissue from xanthine dehydrogenase, metabolises hypoxanthine to uric acid and produces O_2^- as a by-product (McCord 1985). Thirdly metabolism of arachidonic acid generates O_2^- as a by-product. The most important effect of free radicals is peroxidation of membrane phospholipids. This is postulated to be an important part of the mechanism in 'reperfusion injury'.

Arachidonic acid metabolism

Arachidonic acid generated by the action of phospholipases on cellular membranes is the precursor of prostaglandins (PGs) thromboxane ($TBXA_2$) prostacyclin (PGI_2) and leukotrienes (LTs) (Wolfe 1982). In normal cerebral tissue the administration of PGE_2 and $PGF_{2\alpha}$ causes a reduction in $CMRO_2$ and in cerebral blood flow (CBF).

Thromboxane ($TBXA_2$) causes cerebral vasoconstriction and platelet aggregation. It is itself mostly formed by platelets (Pickard 1981). PGI_2 (prostacyclin) is derived predominantly from vascular endothelium. PGI_2 is a platelet anti-aggregatory factor and vasodilator, in a wide variety of situations (Wolfe 1982). It causes relaxation of isolated previously constricted human pial arteries in vitro but this may be a species and site dependent phenomenon as PGI_2 causes vasoconstriction in isolated feline cerebral and basilar arteries (Uski et al 1983). These compounds are all derived from arachidonic acid from a metabolic pathway catalysed by the enzyme cyclo-oxygenase (prostaglandin synthetase) the action of which generates oxygen free radicals (O_2^-) in addition to the other products.

Arachidonic acid may also be metabolised by 15-lipoxygenase, 12-lipoxygenase or 5-lipoxygenase. The action of the last of these results in generation of the precursor of the leukotriene, LTA_4, which itself is the precursor of LTB_4 and LTC_4. LTC_4 is metabolised to form LTD_4 (Pickard 1981). LTC_4 and LTD_4 are, with another agent (LTE_4) responsible for the effects of 'slow reacting substance of anaphylaxis' (SRS-A) in immune and allergic reactions, causing powerful and prolonged smooth muscle contraction and increased microvascular permeability (Wolfe 1982). Topically applied LTB_4, LTC_4 and LTD_4 cause constriction of cerebral arterioles (Rosenblum 1985). Reperfusion following complete cerebral ischaemia in gerbils results in the generation of PGE_2 and $TBXB_2$ (a stable metabolite of thromboxane A_2), LTB_4, LTC_4 and LTD_4 (Kiwak et al 1985, Dempsey et al 1986). The leukotriene content does not return to normal until almost 24 hours after the period of reperfusion begins (Kiwak et al 1985).

It therefore seems likely that arachidonic acid metabolites play a major role in ischaemic injury in brain: directly by causing vasoconstriction and platelet aggregation, and indirectly by the production of free radical species during their generation.

Lactic acidosis

It is possible to show that the severity of neuropathological changes induced by complete cerebral ischaemia is related to the degree of lactic acidosis caused by the ischaemia (Kalimo et al 1981). In turn the higher the pre-ischaemic blood glucose concentration the more severe is the acidosis resulting from complete ischaemia (Ljunggren et al 1974). In incomplete cerebral ischaemia the continued supply of glucose, with inadequate oxygen, fuels the progressive production of lactic acid and results in more severe cerebral acidosis, with extracellular pH perhaps falling to values less than 6 (Heuser & Guggenberger 1985).

Ischaemic brain oedema

Cerebral ischaemia results in cerebral oedema via two major mechanisms (Klatzo 1985). Firstly, the catabolic processes triggered by ischaemia result in the generation of many small (osmotically active) molecules and a rise in tissue osmolality (Symon 1985), which draws water across an intact blood-brain barrier, resulting in *cytotoxic oedema*. Secondly, *vasogenic oedema* occurs in situations in which the blood-brain barrier is open. The barrier opens following complete ischaemia if the initial reperfusion pressure is excessive. There may also be a later opening of the barrier some hours following the re-introduction of cerebral perfusion (Klatzo 1985).

TREATMENT

Treatment of cerebral ischaemia encompasses brain protection in which the treatment is given before the ischaemic episode and brain resuscitation in which treatment is given after the insult.

Interest has centred on: (a) reduction of cerebral metabolic rate; (b) reduction of calcium entry and its effects; (c) modulation of arachidonic acid metabolism; (d) treatment of ischaemic brain oedema; (e) treatment of post-ischaemic seizure activity; (f) reduction of free radical damage; and (g) improvement of microcirculation.

Reduction of cerebral metabolic rate

Cerebral metabolic rate for oxygen ($CMRO_2$) is reduced by some anaesthetic agents in an approximately dose-related manner until the EEG becomes isoelectric (Siesjo 1978, Newberg et al 1983). Thiopentone (Steen & Michenfelder 1978), isoflurane (Newberg & Michenfelder 1983), etomidate (Milde & Milde 1986) and midazolam (Nugent et al 1982) all offer a degree of preservation of high energy metabolites when given prior to and during a period of incomplete ischaemia.

However, halothane at high concentrations (above 4.5%) obtunds aerobic metabolism and results in cerebral lactacidosis in non-ischaemic tissue (Michenfelder & Theye 1975).

Preliminary results of a comparison of thiopentone, isoflurane and the recently introduced intravenous agent, propofol, in a model of global incomplete cerebral ischaemia suggest that pretreatment with thiopentone or propofol results in better recovery of ionic homeostasis in the post-ischaemic period than in the isoflurane-treated or control groups of animals (Weir & Goodchild 1987).

Hypothermia also reduces $CMRO_2$ having an additive effect with pharmacological depression of cerebral metabolism. Mild hypothermia to 33–36°C may be a clinically appropriate mode of cerebral protection (McDowall 1985b).

Clinical evidence of the benefit of cerebral protection in patients undergoing cardiopulmonary bypass is now established for thiopentone pretreatment (Nussmeier et al 1986, Michenfelder, 1986). Patients given thiopentone by infusion sufficient to produce a burst suppression pattern on the EEG from 10 minutes before aortic cannulation, during cardiopulmonary bypass and weaning from bypass suffered significantly less long term neurological damage than a control group to whom thiopentone was not given. Ten days postoperatively no thiopentone-treated patient (in a group of 89) had any detectable neurological or psychiatric disability whereas seven of the control group of 93 had neuropsychiatric disability not present pre-operatively.

Conversely there appears to be no benefit to be gained from the administration of high dose thiopentone for cerebral resuscitation following cardiac arrest (Abramson et al 1986). This is not perhaps unexpected if thiopentone exerts a beneficial effect by suppressing cerebral metabolism to the point of isoelectricity of the EEG but has no effect on cerebral metabolism if ischaemia has already rendered the EEG flat (Michenfelder 1986).

In focal cerebral ischaemia (stroke) occurring either clinically or experimentally the administration of barbiturates is of benefit, presumably by causing a reversed steal effect. As a result of the reduced $CMRO_2$ and CBF in normal brain surrounding the ischaemic area, blood flow is diverted towards it and the volume of tissue ultimately undergoing irreversible ischaemia and necrosis is reduced. Hypotension which may occur due to the administration of barbiturates must be avoided (Shapiro 1985).

Reduction of the effect of calcium

Many calcium entry blocking drugs have now been described including nifedipine, verapamil, nimodipine, lidoflazine, diltiazem, cinnarizine, flunarizine and nicardipine. Modulation of calcium metabolism in ischaemia may be of benefit in three ways: by reducing Ca^{2+} influx into ischaemic neurones; reducing vasospasm (particularly in association with subarachnoid haemorrhage) by reducing the entry of Ca^{2+} into cerebrovascular smooth muscle; and improving the flow properties of blood.

Nimodipine is the most promising calcium channel blocker in cerebral ischaemia. When given post-ischaemia in a canine model of complete global cerebral ischaemia, neurological outcome was improved and post-ischaemic blood flow was increased (Steen et al 1984). In the same model lidoflazine failed to produce any improvement in outcome or to ameliorate post-ischaemic hypoperfusion (Fleisher et al 1987). In a similar model nicardipine increased post-ischaemic blood flow but failed to improve outcome (Sakabe et al 1986). Vasodilatation caused by nimodipine may result in raised intracranial pressure and a steal effect and make its use inappropriate in focal cerebral ischaemia (Young et al 1986) but it has also been suggested that nimodipine does not increase cerebral blood flow to non-ischaemic areas of the brain (Forsman et al 1986). Nimodipine does not completely prevent Ca^{2+} uptake by ischaemic neurones in focal ischaemia (Symon 1985) but delays it resulting in better preservation of the adenylate energy charge in the first minute of complete ischaemia (Heffez & Passonneau 1985).

Cinnarizine and flunarizine may reduce red blood cell stiffness in response to high Ca^{2+} concentrations with a consequent improvement in blood flow in ischaemic or post-ischaemic tissue (Gisvold & Steen 1985).

Vasospasm associated with subarachnoid haemorrhage (SAH) both clinical and experimental, may be lessened by the topical application of several calcium antagonists (Gisvold & Steen 1985). Subarachnoid haemorrhage-induced vasospasm is relaxed by the *systemic* administration of nimodipine, an effect enhanced by disruption of the blood-brain barrier (Harper et al 1981).

Calcium antagonism may therefore be of benefit in global cerebral ischaemia, particularly in the post-ischaemic period and perhaps in focal ischaemia if a rise in intracranial pressure is avoided. Vasospasm associated with subarachnoid haemorrhage is a specific indication for the use of a calcium antagonist.

Ischaemic brain oedema

Osmotic diuretics such as mannitol and dimethylsulphoxide (DMSO) are effective in cytotoxic brain oedema (Gisvold & Steen 1985, Hoff 1986,). Vasogenic brain oedema may be treated by promoting diuresis and reducing cerebrospinal fluid production with such agents as frusemide and acetazolamide (Klatzo 1985). It would be helpful to have a clinically applicable index of blood-brain barrier permeability such as is available for the alveolar-capillary membrane (Barrowcliffe & Jones 1987).

Post-ischaemic seizure activity

Hyperexcitability is likely following cerebral ischaemia in certain vulnerable neurones (Siesjo 1985, Meldrum et al 1985). The resulting increase in metabolic demand for oxygen occurs at a time when oxygen delivery to the brain may be critical and result in hypoxia. Seizure activity must be treated as soon as it is diagnosed. This may be achieved either with the cerebral function monitor (CFM) or the cerebral function analysing monitor (CFAM) (Prior 1985). Drugs which depress cerebral metabolic rate (thiopentone, etomidate, midazolam (Gisvold & Steen 1985)) will suppress seizure activity.

Phenytoin (Artru & Michenfelder 1981) and lignocaine (Astrup et al 1981) additionally have stabilising effects on cell membranes, delaying the dissipative ion fluxes associated with cerebral ischaemia. These effects are valuable adjuncts in the treatment of post-ischaemic seizures.

Modulation of arachidonic acid metabolism

Prostaglandin synthesis may be inhibited by a variety of agents including aspirin, indomethacin, phenylpropionates and fenamates (Wolfe 1982).

Pretreatment with indomethacin and ibuprofen has been shown to result in improved post-ischaemic blood flow (Symon 1985, Grice et al, 1986). This probably results from greater inhibition of thromboxane synthesis than of prostacyclin synthesis by these agents, thus promoting higher post-ischaemic tissue flow (Symon 1985). The clinical value of this finding is reduced (Hoff 1986) by the fact that indomethacin increases post-ischaemic oedema formation and *increases* the cerebral blood flow threshold at which transmembrane ion shifts occur in response to ischaemia (Symon 1985).

Inhibition of prostaglandin synthesis may increase the production of leukotrienes in ischaemic tissue (Pickard 1981, Dempsey et al 1986). It may be possible to antagonise their actions with specific leukotriene receptor blocking drugs (Rosenblum 1984). The development of such agents promises the ability to prevent the adverse effects of prostaglandin synthesis (by indomethacin for example) and also of leukotrienes. At present, however, modulation of arachidonic acid metabolism is inappropriate in the treatment of cerebral ischaemia.

The prophylactic use of low dose aspirin in patients at risk of ischaemic vascular diseases may however be recommended as it appears to be 'better than nothing and may not be harmful' (Marcus 1983).

Reduction of free radical damage

Administration of vitamins C and E is beneficial in in vivo and in vitro models of cerebral ischaemia and hypoxia (Hoff 1986, Acosta et al 1986) presumably because of their actions as free radical scavengers. Free radical scavenging may contribute to the effectiveness of thiopentone, mannitol and dimethylsulphoxide (DMSO) in the treatment of cerebral ischaemia (Flamm et al 1977, Smith et al 1980, Gisvold & Steen 1985).

Improved microcirculation

Following a short period of cerebral ischaemia, if there is a prompt and adequate return of cerebral perfusion pressure, cerebral blood flow rises to levels above normal for perhaps 10–15 minutes. After this hyperaemic phase cerebral blood flow falls below normal (despite an adequate perfusion pressure) in a phase of delayed hypoperfusion (Sundt & Waltz 1971). During this period capillary blood flow may be adversely affected by platelet activation, increased red blood cell 'stiffness' (Gisvold & Steen 1985), and oedema and astrocytic swelling in the perivascular space (Siesjo & Wieloch 1985).

Flow in the microcirculation may be promoted by a variety of therapies. Some calcium entry blocking drugs may improve flow by effects on red blood cells, platelets and cerebrovascular smooth muscle (Gisvold & Steen 1985, Heuser & Guggenberger 1985). Manipulation of haematocrit by administration of albumin or low molecular weight dextran to result in hypervolaemic haemodilution may be beneficial (Hoff 1986). A combination of heparin, indomethacin and prostacyclin administered after ischaemia has been shown to improve post-ischaemic cerebral blood flow (Hallenbeck & Furlow 1979).

Reduction of blood viscosity by the administration of perfluorocarbons (perfluorochemicals) may also be beneficial in ischaemia. Solutions of perfluorochemicals such as Fluosol-DA have a lower viscosity than blood and unlike blood do not increase their viscosity at low flow rates (Faithfull 1987). The outcome of experimental focal ischaemia is improved by giving Fluosol-DA before and after the period of ischaemia (Peerless et al 1985), particularly when combined with mannitol (Faithfull 1987). However, current perfluorochemical preparations have long-lasting inhibitory effects on the reticulo-endothelial system and leukocyte function which caused the American Food and Drug Administration to refuse their use in humans (Kahn et al 1985).

Finally, the induction of hypertension has been shown to improve outcome in experimental models of focal cerebral ischaemia. It is inappropriate following global cerebral ischaemia, subarachnoid haemorrhage or cerebral trauma (Hoff 1986).

CONCLUSION

A unified account of the pathophysiology of cerebral ischaemia has been given but attempts to prevent or treat it must take account of the type of ischaemia in question. No one therapy or combination of therapies is invariably successful.

In the future there is likely to be an increasing range of drugs available to manipulate the biochemical processes initiated by ischaemia. Such drugs may interact significantly with anaesthetic agents, as is already evident with calcium entry blocking drugs, and present the anaesthetist with even more challenging pharmacological and physiological problems than now.

REFERENCES

Abramson N S, Safar P, Detre K M et al 1986 Randomized clinical study of thiopental loading in comatose survivors of cardiac arrest. New England Journal of Medicine 314: 397–403
Acosta D, Kass I, Cottrell J E 1986 Vitamin E protects against anoxic brain damage in the hippocampal slice. Anesthesiology 65 (suppl): A317
Artru A A, Michenfelder J D 1981 Anoxic cerebral potassium accumulation reduced by phenytoin: mechanism of cerebral protection? Anesthesia & Analgesia 60: 41–45
Astrup J, Symon L, Branston N M, Lassen N A 1977 Cortical evoked potential and extracellular K^+ and H^+ at critical levels of brain ischaemia. Stroke 8: 51–57
Astrup J, Rehncrona S, Siesjo B K 1980 The increase in the extracellular potassium concentration in the ischaemic brain in relation to the pre-ischaemic functional activity and cerebral metabolic rate. Brain Research 199: 161–174
Astrup J, Sorensen P M, Sorensen H R 1981 Inhibition of cerebral oxygen and glucose consumption in the dog by hypothermia, pentobarbital and lidocaine. Anesthesiology 55: 263–268
Barrowcliffe M P, Jones J G 1987 Solute permeability of the alveolar capillary barrier. Thorax 42: 1–10
Dempsey R J, Roy M W, Meyer K, Cowen D E, Tai H 1986 Development of cyclo-oxygenase and lipoxygenase metabolites of arachidonic acid after transient cerebral ischaemia. Journal of Neurosurgery 64: 118–124

Faithfull N S 1987 Fluorocarbons: Current status and future applications. Anaesthesia 42: 234–242

Farber J L, Chien K R, Mittnacht S 1981 The pathogenesis of irreversible cell damage in ischemia. American Journal of Pathology 102: 271–281

Fitch W, Ferguson G C, Sengupta D, Garibi J, Harper A M 1976 Autoregulation of cerebral blood flow during controlled hypotension in baboons. Journal of Neurology, Neurosurgery and Psychiatry 39: 1014–1022

Flamm E S, Demopoulos H B, Seligman M L, Ranshoff J 1977 Possible molecular mechanisms of barbiturate-mediated protection in regional cerebral ischaemia. Acta Neurologica Scandinavica 56 (suppl 64): 150–151

Fleischer J E, Lanier W L, Milde J H, Michenfelder J D 1987 Effect of lidoflazine on cerebral blood flow and neurological outcome when administered after complete cerebral ischemia in dogs. Anesthesiology 66: 304–311

Forsman M, Fleischer J E, Milde J H, Steen P A, Michenfelder J D 1986 The effects of nimodipine on cerebral blood flow and metabolism. Journal of Cerebral Blood Flow and Metabolism 6: 763–767

Gisvold S E, Steen P A 1985 Drug therapy in brain ischaemia. British Journal of Anaesthesia 57: 96–109

Graham D I 1985 The pathology of brain ischaemia and possibilities for therapeutic intervention. British Journal of Anaesthesia 57: 3–17

Grice S C, Chappell E T, Prough D S, Watkins W D, Whitley J M 1986 Ibuprofen improves cerebral blood flow after global cerebral ischaemia in dogs. Anesthesiology 65 (suppl): A312

Hallenbeck J M, Furlow T W 1979 Prostaglandin I_2 and indomethacin prevent impairment of post-ischemic brain perfusion in the dog. Stroke 10: 629–637

Harper A M, Craigen L, Kazda S 1981 Effect of the calcium antagonist, nimodipine, on cerebral blood flow and metabolism in the primate. Journal of Cerebral Blood Flow and Metabolism 1: 349–356

Harris R S, Symon L, Branston N M, Bayhan M 1981 Changes in extracellular calcium activity in cerebral ischaemia. Journal of Cerebral Blood Flow and Metabolism 1: 203–209

Heffez D S, Passonneau J V 1985 Effect of nimodipine on cerebral metabolism during ischemia and recirculation in the Mongolian gerbil. Journal of Cerebral Blood Flow and Metabolism 5: 523–528

Heiss W D, Hayakawa T, Waltz A G 1976 Cortical neuronal function during ischaemia: effects of occlusion of one middle cerebral artery on single-unit activity in cats. Archives of Neurology 33: 813–820

Hertz L 1981 Features of astrocytic function apparently involved in the response of central nervous tissue to ischemia- hypoxia. Journal of Cerebral Blood Flow and Metabolism 1: 143–153

Heuser D, Guggenberger H 1985 Ionic changes in brain ischaemia and laterations produced by drugs. British Journal of Anaesthesia 57: 23–33

Hoff J T 1986 Cerebral protection. Journal of Neurosurgery 65: 579–591

Jones J G, Heneghan C P H, Thornton C 1985 Functional assessment of the normal brain during general anaesthesia. In: Kaufman L (ed) Anaesthesia Review-3 Churchill Livingstone, Edinburgh, ch 8, pp 83–98

Kahn R A, Allen R W, Baldassare J 1985 Alternate sources and substitutes for therapeutic blood components. Blood 66: 1–12

Kalimo H, Rehncrona S, Soderfeldt B, Olsson Y, Siesjo B K 1981 Brain lactic acidosis and ischemic cell damage: 2 histopathology. Journal of Cerebral Blood Flow and Metabolism 1: 313–327

Kiwak K H, Moskowitz M A, Levine L 1985 Leukotriene production in gerbil brain after ischemic insult, subarachnoid hemorrhage and concussive head injury. Journal of Neurosurgery 62: 865–869

Klatzo I 1985 Brain oedema following brain ischaemia and the influence of therapy. British Journal of Anaesthesia 57: 18–22

Kogure H, Arai H, Abe K, Nakano M 1985 Free radical damage of the brain following ischaemia. Progress in Brain Research 63: 237–259

Lassen N A 1985 Normal average value of cerebral blood flow in younger adults is 50 ml/100 g/min. Journal of Cerebral Blood Flow and Metabolism 5: 347–349

Lassen N A, Christensen M S 1979 Physiology of cerebral blood flow. British Journal of Anaesthesia 48: 719

Ljunggren B, Norberg K, Siesjo B K 1974 Influence of tissue acidosis upon restitution of brain energy metabolism following total ischemia. Brain Research 77: 173–186

Ljunggren B, Schutz H, Siesjo B K 1974 Changes in energy state and acid-base parameters of the rat brain during complete compression ischemia. Brain Research 73: 277–289

Ljunggren B, Saveland H, Brandt L, Zygmunt S 1985 Early operation and overall outcome in aneurysmal sub-arachnoid haemorrhage. Journal of Neurosurgery 62: 547–551

Lynch G, Halpain S, Bandry M 1982 Effects of high-frequency synaptic stimulation on glutamate receptor binding studied with a modified in vitro hippocampal slice preparation. Brain Research 244: 101–111

McCord J M 1985 Oxygen derived free radicals in postischemic tissue injury. New England Journal of Medicine 312: 159–163

McDowall D G 1985a Induced hypotension and brain ischaemia. British Journal of Anaesthesia 57: 110–119

McDowall D G 1985b Brain ischaemia — its prevention and treatment (editorial). British Journal of Anaesthesia 57: 1–2

Marcus A J 1983 Recent progress in the role of platelets in occlusive vascular disease. Stroke 14: 475–479

Meldrum B, Evans M, Griffiths T, Simon R 1985 Ischaemic brain damage: the role of excitatory activity and of calcium entry. British Journal of Anaesthesia 57: 44–46

Michenfelder J D 1986 A valid demonstration of barbiturate-induced brain protection in man — at last. Anesthesiology 64: 140–142

Michenfelder J D, Theye R A 1975 In vivo toxic effects of halothane on canine cerebral metabolic pathways. American Journal of Physiology 229: 1050–1055

Milde L N, Milde J H 1986 Preservation of cerebral metabolites by etomidate during incomplete cerebral ischemia in dogs. Anesthesiology 65: 272–277

Morris P J, Heuser D, McDowall D G, Hashiba M, Myers D 1983 Cerebral cortical extracellular fluid H^+ and K^+ activities during hypotension in cats. Anesthesiology 59: 10–18

Newberg L A, Michenfelder J D 1983 Cerebral protection by isoflurane during hypoxemia or ischemia. Anesthesiology 59: 29–35

Newberg L A, Milde J H, Michenfelder J D 1983 The cerebral metabolic effects of isoflurane at and above concentrations that suppress cortical electrical activity. Anesthesiology 59: 23–28

Nugent M, Artru A A, Michenfelder J D 1982 Cerebral metabolic, vascular and protective effects of midazolam maleate. Comparison to diazepam. Anesthesiology 56: 172–176

Nussmeier N A, Ralund C, Slogoff S 1986 Neuropsychiatric complications after cardiopulmonary bypass: cerebral protection by a barbiturate. Anesthesiology 64: 165–170

Peerless S J, Nakamura R, Rodriguez-Salazar A, Hunter I G 1985 Modification of cerebral ischemia with Fluosol. Stroke 16: 38–43

Pickard J D 1981 Role of prostaglandins and arachidonic acid derivatives in the coupling of cerebral blood flow to cerebral metabolism. Journal of Cerebral Blood Flow and Metabolism 1: 361–384

Prior P F 1985 EEG monitoring and evoked potentials in brain ischaemia. British Journal of Anaesthesia 57: 63–81

Rosenblum W I 1985 Constricting effect of leukotrienes on cerebral arterioles of mice. Stroke 16: 262–263

Sakabe T, Nagai I, Ishikawa T et al 1986 Nicardipine increases cerebral blood flow but does not improve neurologic recovery in a canine model of complete cerebral ischaemia. Journal of Cerebral Blood Flow Metabolism 6: 763–767

Schlaepfer W W, Zimmerman U-J P 1981 Calcium mediated breakdown of glial filaments and neurofilaments in rat optic nerve and spinal cord. Neurochemical Research, 6: 243–255.

Schwartzkroin P A, Wyler A R 1980 Mechanisms underlying epileptiform burst discharge. Annals of Neurology 7: 96–107

Shapiro H M 1985 Barbiturates in brain ischaemia. British Journal of Anaesthesia 57: 82–95

Siesjo B K 1978 Brain energy metabolism. John Wiley, Chichester

Siesjo B K 1981 Cell damage in the brain: a speculative synthesis. Journal of Cerebral Blood Flow and Metabolism. 1: 155–185

Siesjo B K, Nilsson L 1971 The influence of arterial hypoxaemia upon labile phosphates and upon extracellular and intracellular lactate and pyruvate concentration in the rat brain. Scandinavian Journal of Clinical and Laboratory Investigation 27: 83–96

Siesjo B K, Wieloch T 1985 Cerebral metabolism in ischaemia: neurochemical basis for therapy. British Journal of Anaesthesia 57: 47–62

Smith D S, Rehncrona S, Siesjo B K 1980 Inhibitory effects of different barbiturates on lipid peroxidation in brain tissue in vitro: comparison with the effects of promethazine and chlorpromazine. Anesthesiology 53: 186–194

Steen P A, Michenfelder J D 1978 Cerebral protection with barbiturates: relation to anesthetic effect. Stroke 9: 140–142

Steen P A, Newberg L A, Milde J H, Michenfelder J D 1984 Cerebral blood flow and neurologic outcome when nimodipine is given after complete cerebral ischemia in the dog. Journal of Cerebral Blood Flow and Metabolism 4: 82–87

Sundt T M, Waltz A G 1971 Cerebral ischemia and reactive hyperemia. Studies of cortical blood flow and microcirculation before, during and after temporary occlusion of middle cerebral artery of squirrel monkeys. Circulation Research 28: 426–433

Symon L 1985 Flow threshold in brain ischaemia and the effects of drugs. British Journal of Anaesthesia 57: 34–43

Uski T, Anderson K-E, Brandt L, Edvinsson L, Ljunggren B 1983 Responses of isolated feline and human cerebral arteries to prostacyclin and some of its metabolites. Journal of Cerebral Blood Flow and Metabolism 3: 238–245

Weir D L, Goodchild C S 1987 Cortical extracellular fluid activities of K^+, Ca^{++} and pH in severe hypotension: effects of thiopentone, isoflurane and propofol. Journal of Cerebral Blood Flow and Metabolism 7 (suppl 1): S119

Wieloch T, Siesjo B K 1982 Ischaemic brain injury: the importance of calcium lipolytic activities, and free fatty acids. Pathological Biology 5: 269–277

Wolfe L S 1982 Eicosanoids: prostaglandins, thromboxanes, leukotrienes, and other derivatives of carbon-20 unsaturated fatty acids. Journal of Neurochemistry 38: 1–14

Young W L, Josevitz K, Morales O, Chien S 1986 The effect of nimodipine on post-ischemic cerebral glucose utilization and blood flow. Anesthesiology 65 (suppl): A309

The influence of absorption on analgesic therapy

INTRODUCTION

Drugs are selected for use on the basis of their pharmacodynamic properties, i.e. their ability to produce a desired effect with minimal side effects. Nevertheless, the pharmacokinetics of drugs may be important in optimizing therapy, i.e. maximizing efficacy while minimizing toxicity.

It is usually assumed that drug effects (therapeutic or adverse) are proportional to the concentration of the free drug at the receptor site. It is rarely possible to measure this concentration and studies of pharmacokinetics usually involve plasma concentrations of drugs which may have an inconstant relationship with receptor concentrations except at steady state. Plasma concentration is affected by the processes of absorption, distribution, metabolism and excretion. Drug absorption is particularly important for a first administration of a drug because it is axiomatic that a drug will

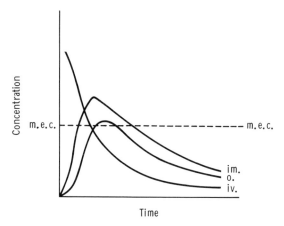

Fig. 10.1 The changes in plasma concentration of a drug with time after intravenous (i.v), intramuscular (i.m.) and oral (o.) administration. The minimum effective concentration (m.e.c.) is indicated. The initial high concentration achieved by the i.v. route declines rapidly, while the concentrations by i.m. and oral routes rise more slowly, peak later and at a lower value than the i.v. The initial rate of fall of plasma concentrations may be slower after i.m. or oral than after i.v.

exert no therapeutic effect or a delayed effect if it is not absorbed or if its absorption is delayed. If distribution and elimination remain constant, the rate of drug absorption will influence the rate of onset of action of a drug.

If a drug is administered directly into the bloodstream by intravenous injection its concentration in the systemic circulation will reach a peak almost immediately and will decline because of the processes of distribution and elimination. In this way the total amount of the administered drug is 'absorbed' almost instantaneously. However, if the same drug is administered by another route, e.g. intramuscularly, it may take some time before plasma concentration reaches a peak (Fig. 10.1). As soon as the drug starts to appear in the plasma the processes of distribution and elimination will start to operate. The total amount of administered drug may be absorbed but the peak blood concentrations (and the peak drug effect) will be delayed as there is no initial large peak and consequent concentration gradient. If the route of administration is such that the metabolic processes can start before the drug reaches the systemic circulation, e.g. orally, all the drug administered may not be absorbed (Fig. 10.1).

Plasma concentration/effect relationship

Changes in pharmacokinetic values may alter the drug concentration at the receptor sites at any particular time and so may alter the duration or intensity of the effect. However, other factors can alter the effect also, e.g. changes in receptor sensitivity. This is more difficult to measure. It is often assumed that the concentration of drug in the blood correlates with that at the receptors, but this may not be true. In a study of dogs the concentration of morphine in brain did not parallel that in plasma (Nishitateno et al 1979) and in a study of intramuscular methadone in postoperative cancer patients peak analgesic effect lagged behind the peak plasma concentration (Kaiko 1982).

There is also a delay between peak plasma pentazocine concentration and analgesia following intravenous administration (Berkowitz et al 1969). This delay is less with drugs which are more lipid soluble. Pethidine and fentanyl are both more lipid soluble than morphine and, as a result, they are taken up into the brain more rapidly than morphine (Hertz & Teschemacher 1971). It is clear, therefore, that caution must be exercised when considering the relationship between blood concentrations of drugs and analgesic effect.

FACTORS INFLUENCING DRUG ABSORPTION: A. ENTERAL ADMINISTRATION

1. Sublingual and buccal administration

The mouth has been investigated as a route of administration of drugs in an attempt to avoid the effects of drug degradation or metabolism in the gut and liver which occur for some drugs after they are swallowed. Although the surface area available for absorption is considerably less than in the small intestine (200 cm^2 compared with 2 000 000 cm^2), the mucosa of the mouth has a very rich supply of blood and lymphatic vessels. These drain into the systemic circulation and so any absorbed drug avoids the effects of first-pass metabolism. This route also has an in-built safety feature, in that if adequate response or intolerable side effects occur, the tablet may be removed and thus stop or at least minimize absorption. In addition, if the drug undergoes a large degree of first-pass metabolism, swallowing it should not cause any harm.

Tablets are used almost exclusively for both sublingual and buccal drug administration. The drug used must be potent or else the size of the tablet would be too great to achieve reasonable patient acceptance. The taste must not be too unpleasant or cause irritation to the mucosa in order to prevent removal or swallowing of the tablet. The tablet must dissolve in saliva to release free drug which must be moderately lipophilic to cross the mucosal membrane. On the other hand, drugs which have very high partition coefficients may be too water-insoluble to gain a sufficiently high concentration in saliva (Gibaldi & Kanig 1965, De Boer et al 1984). An overproduction of saliva may lead to excessive swallowing so reducing drug absorption while too little saliva may result in poor dissolution of the tablet.

The opioid drug buprenorphine, a partial agonist with high affinity for the μ receptor, has been found to be well absorbed by the sublingual route. Its systemic availability is in the region of 58% (Bullingham et al 1982), and peak plasma concentrations occur at 2 to 3 hours after administration (Bullingham et al 1981). In a study of 20 patients undergoing cholecystectomy, sublingual buprenorphine (0.2 mg) on patient demand produced good postoperative analgesia (Shah et al 1986). Similar results were found in 74 patients undergoing elective total hip replacement who received sublingual buprenorphine (0.4 mg), 8 hourly (Bullingham et al 1984). A comparison of mandatory sublingual buprenorphine, mandatory intramuscular morphine and self-administered intravenous pethidine postoperatively showed that sublingual buprenorphine was as effective as the other two methods (Ellis et al 1982).

A buccal preparation of morphine is undergoing clinical trial. In volunteers who received 13.3 mg of buccal morphine, plasma concentrations of 16 ng.ml^{-1} at 10 minutes and peak plasma concentrations of 36–47 ng.ml^{-1} within 1 hour were found (Bardgett et al 1984). A comparison of buccal morphine (13.3 mg) and intramuscular morphine (13.3 mg) in 40 patients experiencing pain after elective orthopaedic operations was carried out in a double blind, double-dummy, prospective fashion (Bell et al 1985). Plasma morphine concentrations were similar after buccal and intramuscular administration. The mean plasma concentration was greater than 10 ng.ml^{-1} after 5 minutes with intramuscular morphine and after 10 minutes with buccal morphine. Peak plasma concentrations were higher after intramuscular administration but declined more rapidly than did those after buccal administration.

The use of the sublingual and buccal routes of drug administration in analgesic therapy may have considerable potential. Attention must be paid to the presentation of the drug to achieve good patient co-operation and some degree of patient training may be required to ensure that the drug will have the opportunity to be absorbed. These routes may be more effective in maintenance of pain control once analgesia has been achieved by another route, e.g. intravenous.

2. Oral administration

Most drugs are given orally. It is the most convenient route and usually the least unpalatable for the patient. However, it may present the greatest number of problems for the drug to achieve its therapeutic effects.

Pharmaceutical formulation

After oral administration, drugs are absorbed from solution in the small intestine. If the drug is given as a tablet it must disintegrate into smaller particles and subsequently dissolve in the gastrointestinal contents to release free drug before absorption can occur. Apart from active drug in a tablet there are various other ingredients with varying functions (Orme 1984) (Table 10.1)

Differences in tablet formulation can lead to different bioavailabilities and different rates of absorption. The rate at which a tablet dissolves may be the rate-limiting step in its absorption. In a study in man it was shown that the absorption of aspirin varied depending upon whether it was in solution, in tablets with alkaline additives or in 'plain' tablets (Levy et al 1965). Absorption was far faster in solution than in alkaline conditions which was faster than with 'plain' tablets. Effervescent tablets allow quicker dissolution and so quicker absorption.

In vivo results can also differ from in vitro results as shown by two different brands of paracetamol tablet with similar in-vitro disintegration rates (Rawlins 1981). Peak plasma concentrations were higher and occurred

Table 10.1 Composition of a 'typical tablet' (adapted from Rowland & Tozer (1980) with permission)

Ingredient	Amount	Function
Drug	x mg	Therapy
Lactose	30 mg	Diluent
Starch	20 mg	Binder and disintegrant
Talc and magnesium	30 mg	Lubricants
Colouring	1 mg	Aesthetic and identification

earlier with one brand than with the other brand (30 minutes compared with 2 hours).

pH partition

The absorption of a drug from the gastrointestinal tract is dependent upon its ability to cross the lipid cell membrane. Consequently, ionization, lipid solubility and molecular weight may determine the rate and extent of the drug's absorption. The non-ionized form of an acidic or basic drug is preferentially absorbed by passive diffusion. Therefore, the more non-ionized drug available at the site of absorption, the greater will be the rate of absorption. The fraction of non-ionized drug is determined by the pH at the site of absorption and the pK_a of the drug according to the Henderson-Hasselbalch equation.

For acids: $pH = pK_a + \log ([\text{ionized}]/[\text{non-ionized}])$
For bases: $pH = pK_a + \log ([\text{non-ionized}]/[\text{ionized}])$

where pK_a is defined as the pH at which half of the drug is non-ionized.

So, for a weakly acidic drug the conditions in the stomach favour an increase in the concentration of the non-ionized form and so it should be absorbed more rapidly. A weak base (e.g. opioid analgesics) will have a much greater fraction in the non-ionized form in the alkaline conditions of the small intestine. A quaternary ammonium compound, which is always ionized, is not readily absorbed from the gastrointestinal tract. Non-ionized drugs (e.g. ethanol) and compounds of low molecular weight (e.g. urea) are rapidly absorbed but few drugs are of this form so it has very little clinical significance.

Gastric emptying

Although the pH partition theory of drug absorption indicates that weak acids are absorbed better in the stomach than weak bases, the much greater surface area of the intestinal mucosa relative to that of the gastric mucosa more than compensates for the potentially reduced rate of absorption per unit area of intestinal mucosa. All drugs are absorbed much more readily from the small intestine than from the stomach.

It seems likely that the rate of drug absorption and, in turn, the onset of pharmacological response is related directly to the rate at which drugs pass from the stomach to the small intestine. It follows that any factor that influences the rate of gastric emptying will influence the rate of absorption and the onset of action of an orally administered agent. Paracetamol has been used as a model drug for absorption studies since it is a weak acid (pK_a 9.5) that is largely non-ionized in both gastric and intestinal fluids. Its rate of absorption is largely independent of pH changes and is directly related to the rate of gastric emptying (Heading et al 1973, Prescott et al

1977). When gastric emptying is inhibited by diamorphine, the absorption of paracetamol is similarly inhibited (Nimmo et al 1975a,b, Prescott et al 1977).

Physiological factors. The presence of food in the stomach delays gastric emptying, solids more so than liquids, as does sleep and the recumbent position. Paracetamol is absorbed more rapidly in subjects who are ambulant than in those who swallow their tablets while they are lying down (Nimmo & Prescott 1978). Gastric dilatation is the only known physiological cause of increased rate of gastric emptying. Drugs may be absorbed more rapidly when given in a large volume of liquid.

Pathological factors. It is part of classical teaching that trauma and pain delay gastric emptying but pre-operative anxiety and pain themselves may not cause a delay in gastric emptying (Marsh et al 1984). Any observed delay in gastric emptying or drug absorption may be related to personality trait (Simpson & Stakes 1987). Increasing pain and distress during labour prolongs gastric emptying time slightly but is insignificant compared to that which occurs in patients who have received pethidine (Nimmo et al 1975b) (Fig. 10.2).

Pharmacological factors. Anticholinergics, antihistamines, tricyclic antidepressants, phenothiazines, opioid analgesics and aluminium hydroxide-containing antacids all delay gastric emptying and slow the rate of absorption of any drug given orally. Metoclopramide, domperidone, anticholinesterases, sodium bicarbonate and cigarette smoking all increase the rate of gastric emptying. When metoclopramide (10 mg i.m.) is given at the same time as an opioid analgesic, it fails to reverse the opioid-induced delay in

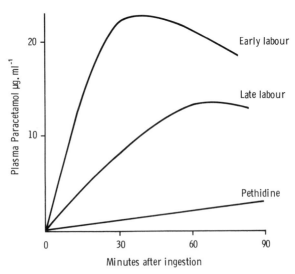

Fig. 10.2 The effect of increasing pain and distress in women during labour on the absorption of paracetamol compared with the effect of pethidine (150 mg intramuscularly). Redrawn, with permission, using data from Nimmo (1981).

paracetamol absorption and gastric emptying (Nimmo et al 1975a). Naloxone largely reverses this inhibition (Nimmo et al 1979), as does cisapride, a new gastric prokinetic drug undergoing clinical trial (Rowbotham & Nimmo 1987).

Biotransformation

Drugs can be metabolized by bacteria present in the gut and can take part in enterohepatic circulation. A drug excreted as a conjugate in the bile can be released by the action of glucuronidase and sulphatase enzymes contained in the bacteria in the colon so that free drug is available for re-absorption. Indomethacin is a drug for which this occurs. Alterations in the gut flora by the use of broad-spectrum antibiotics may, at least in theory, reduce the amount of available drug and consequently influence plasma concentrations.

During absorption, the drug must pass through the cells of the intestinal mucosa where it faces a variety of enzymes. These include the enzymes of phase 1 drug metabolism (oxidases, reductases, hydrolases and a small amount of cytochrome P-450 related enzymes). The phase 2 reaction enzymes (glucuronyl transferase, sulphokinase, methyl transferase, acety-lase and amino acid conjugase) are also active.

After passing through the gut wall the drug is carried to the liver in the blood of the portal vein to face the same metabolizing enzymes but in a greater concentration. Some drugs have a high hepatic extraction ratio (concentration of drug in hepatic vein/concentration of drug in portal vein is very low) and therefore are subject to extensive first-pass metabolism.

Acetylsalicylic acid is hydrolyzed in the gut wall and in the liver. Evidence in dogs indicates that there is no intestinal wall metabolism of paracetamol and that the liver is the only site.

In rats, 55% of orally administered morphine is extracted across the gut wall and the liver then extracts 60% of the morphine that is presented to it via the portal vein (Iwamoto & Klassen 1977). This means that the bioavailability of orally administered morphine is in the region of 18%. MST is a slow release formulation of morphine which is orally administered and it has been shown that during the first 7 hours after administration the bioavailability of its contained morphine is also 18% in volunteers (Vater et al 1984).

Studies of oral dextropropoxyphene in dogs have shown a bioavailability of 25% but this can be increased to 54% by the construction of a porto-caval shunt indicating that both gut wall and liver take part in dextropropoxy-phene metabolism (Levy & Giacomini 1981). In the same paper, the authors studied the effects of oral dextropropoxyphene in normal, cirrhotic and anephric patients and concluded that the much higher plasma concentrations that they found in the cirrhotic and anephric patients was largely due to decreased presystemic biotransformation of dextropropoxyphene.

In a study of oral dihydrocodeine in normal subjects and patients with end-stage renal failure plasma concentrations were significantly higher at 4 and 6 hours in the patients than in the normal subjects (Barnes et al 1985). The area under the curve was also significantly higher in the patients than in the normal subjects. These data are compatible with reduced first-pass metabolism in patients with renal failure.

Pethidine is absorbed better than morphine having a bioavailability in the region of 50%. The side effects of pethidine are mainly depressant but those of its metabolite norpethidine are excitatory to the central nervous system. An oral overdose of pethidine may be more dangerous than a parenteral overdose and may cause convulsions due to a relative excess of norpethidine produced by first-pass metabolism.

It can be seen that despite the convenience that the oral route provides there are disadvantages in its use. In order to promote good absorption of an orally administered drug it should be presented as a large volume of a dilute solution to a starved, pain-free patient who is sitting up (or preferably ambulant), and who has had no drugs which could delay gastric emptying, especially the opioids.

3. Rectal administration

The rectum has been used as a route of administration of drugs since the times of the pharaohs. Its surface area is slightly greater than that of the oral cavity, 200–400 cm^2, but still considerably less than the surface area available in the small intestine. Venous drainage is by three pairs of rectal veins, superior, middle and inferior. The superior ones drain into the portal system while the others drain directly into the systemic circulation. However, there are extensive anastamoses between the veins so that there is great variability in the proportion of blood entering the portal system. In general, if the drug is deposited high up in the rectum more of it will be absorbed via the superior rectal veins and pass into the portal circulation. This provides the possibility of a route of drug administration by which some of the effects of first-pass metabolism may be avoided (De Boer & Breimer 1981). The advantages and disadvantages of rectal administration are shown in Table 10.2.

Drugs for rectal administration can be formulated as suppositories, in gelatin capsules or enemas. Suppositories are suspensions of drug in a fatty base which melts at body temperature. Gelatin capsules dissolve to release active drug and enemas are solutions of drug. Due to the small volume of the rectum and the presence of fecal material dissolution and absorption may be impaired. Loss of sphincter control will result in loss of drug and, therefore, loss of therapeutic effect, as will also occur in the presence of diarrhoea.

When acetylsalicylic acid is administered as a suppository it is absorbed slowly, but if given as an aqueous enema of 20 ml at pH 4 its absorption

Table 10.2 Advantages and disadvantages of rectal administration of drugs (from Hanning (1985) with permission)

Advantages

Independent of gastric emptying
Unaffected by nausea and vomiting
Some bypass of first-pass metabolism
Administration easily stopped
Suitable for sustained-release formulations

Disadvantages

Patient acceptability
Variable interindividual absorption
Slow onset

is as rapid as by oral administration. Similar plasma concentrations of salicylate can be obtained when sodium salicylate is administered in suppository form (De Boer et al 1982). Paracetamol is absorbed in suppository form as well as from enemas, absorption being more rapid in the latter but still slower than by the oral route (Moolenaar et al 1979). Indomethacin can be given as a suppository and its absorption has been found to be more rapid by this route than by mouth (Holt & Hawkins 1965). In a study of patients who had undergone major abdominal surgery, indomethacin suppositories improved analgesia (Reasbeck et al 1982).

Opioids undergo a large degree of first-pass metabolism (see above) so the rectal route has been used in an attempt to avoid at least some of this. Very little is known about the use of rectal opioids in acute pain but there is a definite place for them in the management of chronic pain, especially in cancer. The bioavailability of morphine by the rectal route is approximately 30% in man (compared with 18% by the oral route) but shows great interindividual variability (Westerling et al 1982). Studies have been done using inert hydrophilic gels (hydrogels) as vehicles for morphine by the rectal route (Hanning et al 1983). These showed that analgesic plasma concentrations of morphine could be achieved using a specially developed device which delivered a bolus followed by a constant release of drug. This could provide a background level of analgesia which could be supplemented by boluses of parenteral drug as necessary.

It is clear that the rectal route offers some opportunities for drug administration that other routes may not. In patients who are unco-operative, relatively unskilled attendants can administer the drug. If nausea or vomiting prevents oral administration then the rectal route will allow access to an absorptive area. Drugs which are irritant to gastric mucosa can be given rectally, so avoiding, or at least reducing, the risk of gastrointestinal haemorrhage. Unpleasant tasting agents can be given in this way and this may be of particular use in children. The delay in onset of drug effect probably precludes the rectal route in the management of acute pain but it could be of great benefit in chronic pain.

B. PARENTERAL ADMINISTRATION

1. Intramuscular and subcutaneous administration

The most common route for postoperative analgesia is the intramuscular route. This involves the deposition of a quantity of drug within an area of muscle by a relatively blind injection. The drug must then be absorbed from the site of injection into the bloodstream before it can be distributed to its site of action. Several factors affect the rate of absorption and these will influence the analgesic effect.

Site

When 10 mg of methadone hydrochloride was administered into the deltoid muscle or the gluteal muscle and the plasma concentration of methadone measured, a significant difference was found (Kaiko 1982). Deltoid injection resulted in significantly higher concentrations of methadone at 15, 30 and 60 minutes after administration, compared with gluteal injection. This difference in absorption rate may be related to differences in deltoid and gluteal blood flow (Evans et al 1974). If the blood flow in the region of drug deposition is altered, for example, by shock, changes in temperature or vaso-active agents, then the rate of drug absorption would be similarly altered. Similar results were found when lignocaine was administered intramuscularly at different sites in order to produce anti-arrhythmic effects (Schwartz et al 1974). Injections into the deltoid gave greater plasma concentrations than did injections into the lateral thigh. Both of these sites produced higher plasma concentrations than did injection into the buttocks.

Sex

Plasma methadone concentrations after gluteal administration of 10 mg were consistently higher in males than in females despite the fact that the females received a greater amount of drug on a mg/kg basis (Kaiko 1982). This is probably due to variation in the distribution of adipose and lean tissue between the sexes in the gluteal region and the perfusion of these tissues. When administration was into the deltoid muscle the plasma concentrations were similar in males and females. When analgesia scores were compared with plasma concentrations it was found that females had a higher analgesia score for the same plasma concentration than males (produced by deltoid administration). After gluteal administration analgesia scores were similar when considered at fixed times after administration, indicating that females were achieving similar degrees of analgesia at lower plasma concentrations.

Age

The same author compared the effects of methadone in patients who were less than 40 years old and those who were more than 40 years old when the drug was given into the deltoid muscle. Plasma concentrations were consistently higher in the younger patients, and this may reflect their greater cardiac output and muscle perfusion.

In a study of nine patients to determine the relationship between blood pethidine concentration and analgesic response it was found that the concentration/effect curves were steep (Austin et al 1980). There was a difference of 0.05 μg.ml^{-1} between the mean concentration associated with severe pain (MCP) and the minimum effective analgesic concentration (MEAC) (0.41 and 0.46 μg.ml^{-1} respectively). There was no tendency for the MEACs to be dependent on the type of surgical procedure. Simple variabilities such as personality inventory scores correlated with MCPs.

The same factors which influence drug absorption from intramuscular sites influence absorption from subcutaneous tissue. Generally speaking, the blood supply to subcutaneous tissue is less than that to the muscles so that absorption may be slower from the subcutaneous site. However, in volunteers, plasma concentrations of unchanged morphine were similar after administration of 5.75 mg.m^{-2} of morphine (10 mg approx.) by intramuscular or subcutaneous routes (Brunk & Delle 1974). Care should be taken in extrapolating the results of studies in volunteers to patients. Factors such as pain, hypotension, hypothermia and the use of vasoconstrictor or vasodilator drugs may alter the perfusion of the depot site and so the rate of drug absorption.

2. Inhalational administration

Drugs given by inhalation may be absorbed from the nasal and bronchial mucosa but this has little significance when compared with the absorption from the vast surface area of the alveoli of the lungs. The principles of the uptake of volatile agents by inhalation are well described in standard texts (Nimmo 1985). The major factors are alveolar ventilation, drug solubility, the concentration gradient of drug between the alveoli and the blood in the pulmonary capillaries and the cardiac output. Increasing ventilation will increase alveolar concentration more with soluble agents (e.g. methoxyflurane) than with insoluble agents (e.g. nitrous oxide). Increasing cardiac output will increase the rate of uptake of the agent from the alveoli and reduce the rate of onset of its effect. Decreasing cardiac output will decrease the rate of uptake of agent from the alveoli so that the rate of onset of drug effect will be increased, especially with the more soluble agents.

The analgesic properties of nitrous oxide were first noted by Davy in 1799 and its use as an analgesic has become widespread in anaesthesia, labour and after trauma. It is a gas at room temperature and is delivered to the patient at a fixed rate with oxygen, either from separate sources or as a pre-mixed 50% mixture known as Entonox by way of a patient demand valve.

Although nitrous oxide is a weak anaesthetic agent (MAC of 105) it is a potent analgesic, 30–50% being equivalent to 10 mg of morphine intramuscularly (Hanning 1985). However, patient response is extremely variable. Nitrous oxide has a very low blood/gas solubility coefficient (0.47) which allows a rapid rate of onset of analgesia and also a very rapid rate of decline once administration is stopped. This makes it a suitable agent for use in conditions where pain is intermittent such as labour or for physiotherapy but not for constant pain. However, its use in postoperative pain as a continuous inhalation has been shown to abolish the usual reduction in functional residual capacity (Kripke et al 1983). Bone marrow depression, pollution and the effects on staff of exposure to trace amounts, limits its use for prolonged periods.

Trichloroethylene is a potent analgesic used in obstetric practice at a concentration of 0.35–0.5% from fixed concentration, temperature-compensated vaporizers such as the Emotril and the Tecota. Many patients found the smell unpleasant and the incidence of nausea and vomiting was quite high. Its relatively high blood/gas solubility (9.0) causes a slow onset of action and a prolonged recovery. This permits analgesia to continue even if administration is stopped for a short period so that, although its use in intermittent pain is limited, it is of use where more prolonged analgesia is required.

Methoxyflurane has physical properties similar to those of trichloroethylene. It produces analgesia in labour in concentrations of 0.35–0.5% in air. Its high blood/gas solubility (13.0) ensures an extremely slow onset of analgesia but a relatively prolonged duration of action.

3. Transdermal administration

Some drugs can penetrate the skin in sufficient quantities to achieve effective blood concentrations. One of these is the synthetic opioid fentanyl which has been formulated into a transdermal therapeutic system (TTS). A quantity of the drug is enclosed between an occlusive backing and a rate controlling membrane. This is applied to the skin, usually on the chest, as an adhesive patch.

In a study of 23 patients who had undergone upper abdominal surgery plasma fentanyl concentrations were compared after intravenous infusion or TTS administration of fentanyl for 24 hours as postoperative analgesia (Nimmo & Duthie 1986). Fentanyl TTS produced plasma fentanyl concentrations similar to those after constant rate intravenous infusion from 8 hours to 24 hours after the start of the infusion. A study comparing different rates of intravenous fentanyl infusion with fentanyl TTS in patients who had undergone major surgery found serum fentanyl concentrations somewhat higher in the TTS group than in the 100 μg.h^{-1} intravenous infusion group (Holley & van Steennis 1986).

Another study of 10 patients undergoing elective shoulder surgery under regional anaesthesia found good postoperative analgesia with the use of fentanyl TTS. No respiratory depression (< 8 breaths min^{-1}) was observed but nausea and vomiting did occur in some patients (Caplan et al 1986). A study of eight orthopaedic patients found similarly good analgesia with some nausea and sedation (Plezia et al 1986).

CONCLUSIONS

The route of administration of a drug may affect the total amount of the drug which is available to exert its therapeutic activity. More importantly, it may influence the rate at which the drug reaches an effective concentration at its receptor site. This will determine the length of time between drug administration and therapeutic effect.

Factors which influence absorption should be considered for each patient before a drug is prescribed. For example, it may be useless to prescribe a drug orally to a patient who is vomiting or one rectally to a patient with diarrhoea. Intramuscular or subcutaneous injections vary with blood flow and may be ineffective in shocked patients.

Although drugs are selected on the basis of their pharmacodynamic properties, their pharmacokinetics may have a profound effect on their ability to produce their effects. The route by which they are administered and the frequency at which they are repeated may be as important as drug selection in analgesic therapy.

REFERENCES

Austin K L, Stapleton J V, Mather L E 1980 Relationship between blood meperidine concentration and analgesic response. Anesthesiology 53: 460–466
Bardgett D, Howard C, Murray G R, Calvey T N, Williams N E 1984 Plasma concentration and bioavailability of a buccal preparation of morphine sulphate (proceedings of the BPS 7–9 September 1983). British Journal of Clinical Pharmacology 17: 198P–199P
Barnes J N, Williams A J, Tomson M J F, Toseland P A, Goodwin F J 1985 Dihydrocodeine in renal failure: further evidence for an important role of the kidney in the handling of opioid drugs. British Medical Journal 290: 740–742
Bell M D D, Mishra P, Weldon B D, Murray G R, Calvey T N, Williams N E 1985 Buccal morphine — a new route for analgesia? Lancet 1: 71–73
Berkowitz B A, Asling J H, Shnider S M, Way E L 1969 Relationship of pentazocine plasma levels to pharmacological activity in man. Clinical Pharmacology and Therapeutics 10: 320–328
Brunk S F, Delle M 1974 Morphine metabolism in man. Clinical Pharmacology and Therapeutics 16: 51–57
Bullingham R E S, McQuay H J, Dwyer D, Allen M C, Moore R A 1981 Sublingual buprenorphine used postoperatively: clinical observations and preliminary pharmacokinetic analysis. British Journal of Clinical Pharmacology 12: 117–122
Bulllingham R E S, McQuay H J, Porter E J B, Allen M C, Moore R A 1982 Sublingual buprenorphine used postoperatively: ten hour plasma drug concentration analysis. British Journal of Clinical Pharmacology 13: 665–673
Bullingham R E S, O'Sullivan G, McQuay H J et al 1984 Mandatory sublingual buprenorphine for postoperative pain. Anaesthesia 39: 329–334

Caplan R A, Ready L B, Olsson G L, Nessly M L 1986 Transdermal delivery of fentanyl for postoperative pain control. ASA abstracts. Anesthesiology 65: A196

De Boer A G, Breimer D D 1981 Rectal absorption: portal or systemic? In: Prescott L F, Nimmo W S (eds) Drug absorption (proceedings of the Edinburgh International Conference). Adis Press, Auckland, pp 61–71

De Boer A G, Moolenaar F, De Leede L G J, Breimer D D 1982 Rectal Drug administration; clinical pharmacokinetic considerations. Clinical Pharmacokinetics 7: 285–311

De Boer A G, De Leede L G J, Breimer D D 1984 Drug absorption by sublingual and rectal routes. British Journal of Anaesthesia 56: 69–82

Ellis R, Haines D, Shah R, Cotton B R, Smith G 1982 Pain relief after abdominal surgery — a comparison of i.m. morphine, sublingual buprenorphine and self-administered i.v. pethidine. British Journal of Anaesthesia 54: 421–427

Evans E F, Proctor J D, Fratkin M J, Velandia J, Wasserman A J 1974 Blood flow in muscle groups and drug absorption. Clinical Pharmacology and Therapeutics 17: 44–47

Gibaldi M, Kanig J L 1965 Absorption of drugs through the oral mucosa. Journal of Oral Therapeutics and Pharmacology 1: 440–450

Hanning C D 1985 Non-parenteral techniques. In: Smith G and Covino B G (eds) Acute pain. Butterworths, London, pp 180–204

Hanning C D, Smith G, McNeill M, Graham N B 1983 Rectal administration of morphine from a sustained release hydrogel suppository. British Journal of Anaesthesia 55: 236–237

Heading R C, Nimmo W S, Prescott L F, Tothill P 1973 The dependence of paracetamol absorption on the rate of gastric emptying. British Journal of Pharmacology 47: 415–421

Hertz A, Teschemacher H J 1971 Activities and sites of antinociceptive action of morphine-like analgesics. In: Harper N J, Simmonds A B (eds) Advances in drug research. Academic Press, New York, pp 79–119

Holley F O, van Steennis C 1986 Transdermal administration of fentanyl for postoperative analgesia. ASA abstracts. Anesthesiology 65: A548

Holt L P J, Hawkins C F 1965 Indomethacin: studies of absorption and of the use of indomethacin suppositories. British Medical Journal 1: 1354–1356

Iwamoto K, Klassen C D 1977 First-pass effect of morphine in rats. Journal of Pharmacology and Experimental Therapeutics 200: 365–376

Kaiko R F 1982 Methadone plasma levels and analgesia in postoperative cancer patients. In: Walker C A, Tterlikkis L P (eds) Application of pharmacokinetics to patient care. Praeger Scientific, New York, pp 119–134

Kripke B J, Justice R E, Hechtman H B 1983 Postoperative nitrous oxide analgesia and the functional residual capacity. Critical Care Medicine 11: 105–109

Levy G, Giacomini K M 1981 First-pass effects in health and disease: pharmacokinetic studies on dextropropoxyphene. In: Prescott L F, Nimmo W S (eds) Drug absorption (proceedings of the Edinburgh International Conference). Adis Press, Auckland, pp 115–122

Levy G, Leonards J R, Procknal J A 1965 Development of in vitro dissolution tests which correlate quantitatively with dissolution-rate limited absorption. Journal of Pharmaceutical Sciences 54: 1719

Marsh R H K, Spencer R, Nimmo W S 1984 Gastric emptying and drug absorption before surgery. British Journal of Anaesthesia 56: 161–164

Moolenaar F, Schoonen A J M, Evers A, Huizinga T 1979 Absorption rate and bioavailability of paracetamol from fatty suppositories. Pharmaceutisch Weekblad Scientific Edition 1: 89

Nimmo W S 1981 Gastric emptying and drug absorption. In: Prestcott L F, Nimmo W S (eds) Drug absorption (Proceedings of the Edinburgh International Conference). Adis Press, Auckland, p 16

Nimmo W S 1985 Principles of general pharmacology and pharmacokinetics. In: Smith G, Aitkenhead A R (eds) Textbook of anaesthesia. Churchill Livingstone, Edinburgh, pp 113–124

Nimmo W S, Duthie D J R 1986 Plasma fentanyl concentrations after transdermal or intravenous infusion of fentanyl. ASA abstracts. Anesthesiology 65: A559

Nimmo W S, Prescott L F 1978 The influence of posture on paracetamol absorption. British Journal of Clinical Pharmacology 5: 348–349

Nimmo W S, Heading R C, Wilson J, Tothill P, Prescott L F 1975a Inhibition of gastric emptying and drug absorption by narcotic analgesics. British Journal of Clinical Pharmacology 2: 509–513

Nimmo W S, Wilson J, Prescott L F 1975b Narcotic analgesics and delayed gastric emptying during labour. Lancet 1: 890–893

Nimmo W S, Heading R C, Wilson J, Prescott L F 1979 The reversal of narcotic induced delay in gastric emptying and drug absorption by naloxone. British Medical Journal 2: 1189–1190

Nishitateno K, Ngai S H, Fink A D, Berkowitz B A 1979 Pharmacokinetics of morphine: concentrations in the serum and brain of the dog during hyperventilation. Anesthesiology 50: 520–523

Orme M 1984 Drug absorption in the gut. British Journal of Anaesthesia 56: 59–67

Plezia P M, Linford J, Kramer T H, Iacona R P, Hameroff S R 1986 Transdermal therapeutic system (fentanyl) for postoperative pain: an efficacy, toxicity and pharmacokinetic trial. ASA abstracts. Anesthesiology 65: A210

Prescott L F, Nimmo W S, Heading R C 1977 Drug absorption interactions In: Grahame-Smith (ed) Drug interactions. Macmillan, London, p 45

Rawlins M D 1981 In: Prescott L F, Nimmo W S (eds) Drug absorption (Proceedings of the Edinburgh International Conference). Adis Press, Auckland, pp 331–334

Reasbeck P G, Rice M L, Reasbeck J V 1982 Double-blind controlled trial of indomethacin as an adjunct to narcotic analgesia after major abdominal surgery. Lancet 2: 115–118

Rowbotham D J, Nimmo W S 1987 Effect of cisapride on morphine-induced delay in gastric emptying. British Journal of Anaesthesia 59: 536–539

Rowland M, Tozer T N 1980 (eds) Clinical pharmacokinetics. Concepts and applications. Lea and Febiger, Philadelphia

Schwartz M L, Meyer M B, Covino B G et al 1974 Antiarrythmic effectiveness of intramuscular lidocaine: influence of different injection sites. Journal of Clinical Pharmacology 14: 77–83

Shah M V, Jones D I, Rosen M 1986 'Patient demand' postoperative analgesia with buprenorphine. British Journal of Anaesthesia 58: 508–511

Simpson K H, Stakes A F 1987 Effect of anxiety on gastric emptying in preoperative patients. British Journal of Anaesthesia 59: 540–544

Vater M, Smith G, Aherne G W, Aitkenhead A R 1984 Pharmacokinetics and analgesic effect of slow-release oral morphine sulphate in volunteers. British Journal of Anaesthesia 56: 521–527

Westerling D, Lindahl S, Andersson K E, Andersson A 1982 Absorption and bioavailability of rectally administered morphine in women. European Journal of Clinical Pharmacology 23: 59–64

Computer-assisted anaesthesia

INTRODUCTION

Lunn & Mushin (1982) found that, overall, the process of anaesthesia is remarkably safe. They did, however, identify areas where current practice could be improved, among them physiological monitoring and the keeping of anaesthetic records. They also noted that potentially fatal mistakes are made by all grades of anaesthetist, and that there has been very little alteration in the pattern of errors over the last 30 years.

Although improvements in training, staffing, and communication will make a contribution to a further reduction in morbidity and mortality associated with anaesthesia, it is arguable that appropriate information technology is capable of improving human performance in the field of anaesthesia, and that such technology is currently available.

The last decade has seen a large amount of research directed towards increasing the safety of anaesthesia by the involvement of computers. The emphasis is very much on assisting, rather than replacing, the anaesthetist.

MONITORING

The conduct of anaesthesia is largely a vigilance task, an area of human performance that is sadly deficient. It was understandable that the initial impact of the computer in the operating theatre was principally in the area of monitoring. Although microprocessors were already a part of sophisticated monitoring systems used in cardiac and neuro-anaesthesia, one of the earliest mass-produced computerised monitors relieved the anaesthetist of the task of taking the blood pressure.

When Ramsey (1979) described the automated oscillometer (the Dinamap, now manufactured by Critikon Inc.), anaesthetists were quick to appreciate the assistance that such a device could offer, particularly during induction of anaesthesia or periods of haemorrhage or hypotension when they were fully occupied in managing the situation. Oscillometry (not to be confused with oscillotonometry, which employs two cuffs) involves inflation of a single cuff to a predetermined pressure, followed by a cycle of decremental deflation, measurement of cuff pressure oscillations, storage of that information, further deflation, further measurement, comparison with the previously stored data, and so on. This repetitive process is ideally suited to microprocessor control, and the Dinamap was found to provide accurate and reproducible data, particularly in relation to mean arterial pressure (Yelderman & Ream 1977). Despite the initial misgivings of some anaesthetists, the non-invasive blood pressure monitor has gained almost universal acceptance.

The ability of the computer to perform large numbers of calculations quickly can be used to adapt what was previously a diagnostic procedure carried out at length, such as electroencephalography, for on-line (that is, continuous) monitoring purposes. Much of the work of electroencephalographic interpretation is based upon identification of the particular frequency components of the EEG waveform present at any time. A number of microprocessor-based EEG monitors have addressed the task not only of analysing the EEG but presenting the information in a comprehensible and useful format. One example, the Cerebral Function Analysing Monitor (CFAM) (Health Care Developments Ltd) processes the EEG via series of asymmetric bandpass filters to derive and display the percentage of EEG activity present respectively in the alpha, beta, theta and delta bands, together with display of the weighted amplitude distribution of the whole EEG signal. Display of a 'suppression band' enables assessment of the proportion of the time that the weighted EEG is below a preset amplitude. A second microprocessor controls the stimulators and amplifiers used in visual, auditory and somatosensory evoked potential monitoring, adjusting the amplifier gain automatically and rejecting artefacts and overload. For a full account of the CFAM, the reader is referred to Maynard & Jenkinson (1984).

The microprocessor is also an integral part of the modern pulse oximeter. The instrument examines the transmission of light from a two-wavelength source through a suitable pulsatile vascular bed (Yelderman & New 1983). The transmitted waveform is processed to isolate the pulsatile component, i.e. that due to arterial blood. Comparison of the transmission at the two different wavelengths of the light source allows calculation of the relative concentrations of oxyhaemoglobin and reduced haemoglobin. This is displayed in digital form as the arterial oxygen saturation, and is usually accompanied by a display of the detected pulse waveform to assist with correct positioning of the sensor. The current status of pulse oximetry has been reviewed by Taylor & Whitwam (1986).

Even if a microprocessor is not strictly necessary to the basic functioning of a monitor, it does enable a number of facilities to be provided, such as digital display, simplified calibration and line-up procedures, printout of data, and interfacing with an external computer. It is this last possibility that permits an attempt at a unified and coherent presentation of all the information that the anaesthetist must assimilate.

Displays and alarms

The modern anaesthetic machine might be described as an ergonomic disaster area. Decades of unco-ordinated development has resulted in a working environment for the anaesthetist in which equipment is stacked on and around the anaesthetic machine, presenting a mixture of meters, digital, analogue, waveform, bar-graph and other displays. Furthermore, little attempt has been made to co-ordinate audible alarms, many of which generate pure tones which can be difficult even to locate.

According to one survey (Cooper et al 1978), nearly 90% of anaesthetic mishaps are the result of human error. The same research attributed one third of these errors to the interaction between the anaesthetist and the anaesthetic machine, and suggested that many such episodes could have been avoided with better equipment design. Reliable as the modern anaesthetic machine is, its operation still leaves unacceptable room for error.

The aircraft designer has long been aware of the possibility of reducing pilot error by good design, and much attention has been given to the presentation of visual information and alarms in aircraft cockpits, such that instruments are logically grouped and their displays are harmonised. Circular dials are designed so that the pointers are vertical in normal operation, making it possible for the pilot to scan several dozen such instruments in a matter of seconds. Nonetheless, errors still occur and designers of aircraft such as the European Airbus have replaced many instruments with multifunction cathode ray tubes, capable of displaying numerical information, as well as checklists and moving map displays. Such a display cannot show all available information simultaneously, and much of the task of monitoring the aircraft's systems has been delegated to the computer, the pilot being presented only with information that he has requested or needs to know (Green 1983). More recently, flight deck audible alarms have been rationalised in an attempt to match the character and the volume of the alarm to the nature of the situation that has arisen, thus reducing the time taken to identify the area of the problem.

Several medical equipment manufacturers have applied similar principles to operating theatre monitoring equipment. The North American Drager Company (Schreiber 1986) has adopted the approach of displaying monitored numeric information in two different forms, both as a multiple bar-graph display and in digital form. The bar graph provides information that can be scanned quickly and reliably, provided the number of bars normally displayed is limited to about five, and they are of appropriate colours, preferably white or yellow. Digitally presented information, on the other hand, is precise and unambiguous, but does take time to read and interpret. Drager have made a conscious attempt not to flood the anaesthetist with information and some 'secondary values' are only available on request unless alarm values are exceeded.

The same manufacturer has also taken a unified look at audible and visual alarms and suggested a three-tier system. An 'advisory' condition is signalled by a continuous yellow light accompanied by a single tone or no tone at all. A 'caution' condition is indicated by a continuous red light and an intermittent repeating tone. The highest level of alarm, a 'warning' condition, produces a flashing red light and a continuous repeating tone. Alarm sounds are designed not to be irritating to staff involved in managing the emergency, and all visual alarms appear on a centralised display, accompanied by identifying information. All audible alarms emanate from a single loudspeaker and can be silenced from a single button, for a period of up to 120 seconds.

In the United Kingdom, The Medical Research Council Applied Psychology Unit has devised a series of seven distinct multitone alarm signals, one of which is intended for general use, and the others for designated areas relating to oxygenation, ventilation, circulation, temperature, drug infusion and artificial perfusion. Each alarm has two versions, a fast or a slow form, depending on the urgency of the condition (Kerr 1986).

On-line operating theatre mass spectrometers such as the Allegheny International SARA (System for Anesthetic and Respiratory Analysis) provide the anaesthetist with information concerning the inspired and end-tidal levels of oxygen, nitrous oxide, carbon dioxide, nitrogen and volatile agent. The SARA system comprises a centrally-located mass spectrometer connected by a network of capillary tubing to every anaesthetising location in an operating suite, up to a maximum of 28. At each location, the system is connected to the airway equipment at the tracheal tube connector or mask elbow. Under computer control, the mass spectrometer samples gas from each location in turn, typically completing a cycle approximately every 90 seconds, and returns data to a terminal on the relevant anaesthetic machine. The data are provided in numerical form at the top of the display screen on the terminal and the user can select a choice of graphic displays, allowing the trend of any of the parameters with time to be observed over periods of from 30 minutes to 16 hours. Reproduction of the carbon dioxide waveform permits confirmation of correct tracheal tube placement. Interfaces on the terminal itself allow direct connection with a variety of associated equipment, including non-invasive blood pressure monitors and pulse oximeters, permitting data from these sources to be displayed on the same screen, and providing a trend facility for that information as well. In addition, discrete results (for example from blood gas or electrolyte analysis) can be entered via a remote terminal in the laboratory for display on the same monitor.

The central processing of all monitored information in this fashion also allows one or more master displays which relay the data from each theatre when its sample has been analysed. Information can also be printed out, and the system opens the door to routine logging of all anaesthetics on magnetic disk, so that anaesthetic incidents or mishaps can be analysed and discussed retrospectively. It can also form the basis for the automation of the task that few anaesthetists enjoy, the keeping of the anaesthetic chart.

RECORD KEEPING

It is a truism that the better the anaesthetic record, the less happened during the anaesthetic. Certainly, when a serious incident occurs, the written details of it are invariably compiled retrospectively, and the resulting record may well be inaccurate and incomplete, particularly with respect to the timing of events.

The most important aspect of computerisation of anaesthetic record keeping is the design of the interface between the anaesthetist and the computer. Entering information into a computer manually can easily take longer than writing it down, and a poorly designed system is very unpopular with the users.

The direct interfacing of the computer to the monitoring equipment allows much of the record to be compiled without the assistance of the anaesthetist, but aspects such as the administration of drugs and intravenous fluids, together with descriptions of procedures will always need to be entered by hand. Few anaesthetists can type, and some form of 'menu-driven' program, where the user is offered a screenful of alternatives and makes a selection, for example by touching the appropriate option on the screen with a light-pen or a finger, is usual.

Many such systems have been described (Zollinger et al 1977, Cushman & Bushman 1983, Prentice & Kenny 1984, Rosen & Rosensweig 1985) but tend to suffer from inflexibility as far as the general user is concerned. Ohmeda now offer in the United States a comprehensive automated record-keeping system which permits regular users to design their own menu options by adding and deleting, for instance, the names of drugs. The individual's personal menus are stored on a plug-in cartridge that is inserted into the computer at the beginning of the operating session.

At the start of a case the screen awaits instructions to initiate the record, requests identifying information about patient and anaesthetist, and offers the options of entering information about laboratory results, drugs, inhaled agents, fluids, the breathing system and other comments. When an option has been selected, for example 'drugs', the screen clears to give way to another menu, in this case the drug list. The relevant drug is selected and the user is asked to enter the dose and appropriate units from a numerical menu. This information, together with the time the entry was made, is added to the current record. With practice, the anaesthetic record can be compiled faster than was possible by hand and with great improvements in completeness and legibility.

Unlike many previous systems, where the information is stored on disk and a printed chart is produced at the end of the anaesthetic, the Ohmeda record keeper actually prints the chart as the anaesthetic progresses, on a dot-matrix printer built into the anaesthetic machine, making additions whenever data are acquired from monitors or entered manually. An important feature is that data cannot be altered or entered retrospectively, but, if necessary, the record keeper can be asked to insert a blank line, with a time alongside, for the addition of later hand-written comments. This makes the resulting record very difficult to tamper with or falsify, and such a document may well be acceptable in a court of law. In North America, medico-legal considerations are one of the principal driving forces in the development of automated record-keeping systems.

DELIVERY SYSTEMS

The modern anaesthetic machine is an example of 'mature technology', reflected in the fact that changes in its design in recent years have largely been cosmetic. Its construction confers mechanical reliability at the expense of the potential for human error in its use. The addition of warning devices such as oxygen analysers and disconnection alarms can only go part of the way to a solution of the problem, and several groups of researchers, notably those in Boston, Utah and Arizona, have turned to microprocessor technology to form the basis of a new approach to the anaesthesia delivery system.

The Boston Anesthesia System (BAS) is the product of a development programme that began in the early 1970s (Cooper & Newbower 1984). The result is a computer-based anaesthetic machine that contains no float flowmeters, needle valves, or conventional vaporisers. In particular, gas flow is controlled not by any kind of variable orifice device, but by binary gas flow controllers.

The binary gas flow controller comprises an array of fixed orifice valves, usually eight in number, each of which can be open or shut (Boaden & Hutton 1986). The cross-sectional area of each valve in turn is such that the flow through it is exactly twice that of the previous one. If, for example, the flow rate through the smallest valve is 50 ml/min, then the maximum possible flow (all valves in use) would be 12 750 ml/min. By using the valves in combination, a total of 255 different total flows can be produced, with a resolution equal to the flow in the smallest valve. Furthermore, if the orifices are designed such that the speed of gas through them exceeds the speed of sound, then the flow rate becomes largely independent of fluctuations in downstream pressure. The significance of the number eight is that it corresponds to the number of bits in a binary word, or byte. The flow rate can thus be specified in the form of one computer word. Once the flow required has been selected, the computer handles the task of selecting the appropriate combination of valves, and, in the case of the Boston system, displays the flow rate in the form of a colour-coded bar graph on the anaesthetic machine console.

In addition to separate bar graphs for oxygen and nitrous oxide flows, analagous to flowmeters, the BAS designers allow selection of an alternative display, showing total gas flow and nitrous oxide concentration. A third bar graph indicates volatile anaesthetic concentration and a label beneath it is automatically illuminated to show the identity of the agent used, which is supplied in a pin-indexed canister which plugs into the vaporising system (see below). Two remaining bar graphs show expired oxygen concentration and airway pressure. The remainder of the display area is reserved for warnings and alarm messages. These are generated by the computer as it checks various aspects of the system's function ten times a second. A total of 16 different specific warnings may be given to the user.

Conventional vaporisers are replaced on the BAS by a modification of a car fuel-injector, which delivers liquid anaesthetic directly into the gas stream in boluses of approximately 5 microlitres, as the gas flows through a passive evaporator coil. The frequency of the pulses from the injector determines the final concentration of volatile anaesthetic delivered. The exact size of the bolus injected with each pulse depends on the physical properties of the agent in use, and a calibration factor allowing for this is stored in the computer. The identity of the agent in use is determined by a magnetic sensing device which reads a code on the canister as it is plugged in.

Palayiwa et al (1986) have adopted a different approach to the digital control of gas flow and vapour concentration. Solenoid valves that pulse open for a set time have their frequency of opening regulated by a microprocessor in accordance with the required gas flow. The pulsatile flow that results is smoothed and the gases are mixed in a swirl chamber with a surge-damping device. The high frequency of the valve operation (up to 8 Hz) raises the question of long-term reliability of such a device. The authors predict a valve life of approximately 5 years.

Computer mediation of all essential functions of the anaesthetic machine, as exemplified by the Boston Anesthesia System, enables all the control settings to be made available to a record-keeping system via an external interface, but, as importantly for the future, it permits complete control of the machine settings by an external computer.

COMPUTERISED ANAESTHETIC MANAGEMENT

The involvement of the computer in the management of an anaesthetic does not necessarily imply that the computer is making therapeutic decisions based on events. For example, if the pharmacokinetic profile of a drug is known with sufficient accuracy, a computer, armed with suitable data about a particular patient, can use a pharmacokinetic model to project plasma concentrations of the drug with different dose regimes, or it can control the rate of infusion of the drug in an attempt to produce a stable plasma concentration. Much work along these lines has been done with infusions of comparatively short-acting analgesics such as fentanyl and alfentanil. Alvis et al (1985) described the application of three-compartment model of fentanyl pharmacokinetics which formed part of an interactive program intended to provide a steady plasma concentration while allowing the anaesthetist to raise the plasma fentanyl concentration during periods of surgical stimulation. With some patient variation, the measured fentanyl levels achieved in a group of patients undergoing coronary artery surgery correlated well with the desired levels, and this was reflected in greater cardiovascular stability compared with a control group given boluses of fentanyl at the discretion of the anaesthetist.

The usefulness or otherwise of such a technique entirely depends on the accuracy and applicability of the pharmacokinetic data on which it is based. Reilly et al (1985) performed computer simulations of predicted plasma fentanyl concentrations resulting from three different dosage regimes, taking their pharmacokinetic data from seven separate studies. They found that different groups of researchers had produced values for the volume of distribution of fentanyl ranging from 4.4 to 59.7 litres, and estimates of the elimination half-life varying between 141 and 853 minutes. Total body clearance of fentanyl had been variously calculated at between 160 and 1530 ml/min. Inserting different workers' data in turn into their program simulating a constant rate of infusion produced estimates of a steady-state plasma fentanyl concentration that differed by as much as an order of magnitude. Set the task of predicting when a supplemental dose of fentanyl would be required following an initial 500 μg bolus, their computer predicted times between 13 and 360 minutes.

Ausems et al (1985) used computer simulation and interactive computer control of alfentanil infusions based on their own pharmacokinetic studies, and succeeded in predicting or producing plasma levels with an error ranging from 22.2% to 32.5%. They suggested that it is unwise to rely entirely on the computer to predict an individual's alfentanil requirements, but that it is of assistance in obtaining relatively stable plasma concentrations.

The behaviour of the volatile anaesthetics within the body is more predictable and better understood, and several groups of workers have devised complex computer models of anaesthetic uptake. In Cardiff, Chilcoat et al (1984) have used one such model as the basis for a computer program aimed at producing a steady brain concentration of halothane. The program makes extensive use of the concepts of feedforward and feedback. The model requires information concerning total body mass, cardiac output, alveolar ventilation and the blood/gas partition coefficient for the individual. The variables, that is cardiac output and alveolar ventilation, are measured as the anaesthetic progresses, and used to modify the program's predictions and adjust the delivered concentration of halothane before the change in brain concentration occurs. Brain concentration cannot easily be measured, but arterial concentration can, and half-hourly arterial halothane measurement allowed data to be fed back into the control program to permit a scaling factor for the individual's response to be applied to subsequent calculations. In dogs, the program was able to deliver a measured-to-computed arterial halothane tension ratio that had a standard deviation of 9.2%.

'Closing the loop'

End-tidal concentration of a volatile agent is, of course, not the same thing as 'depth of anaesthesia', particularly in the early stages of anaesthesia. It is however, conveniently easy to measure non-invasively, and has been made the basis for closed-loop control of anaesthetic administration by a number of different groups. Systems described vary from simple control circuits that inject liquid volatile anaesthetic into a closed circuit until the desired end-tidal concentration is attained (Hawes et al 1982), to more sophisticated adaptive programs, which modify themselves in the light of results. Tatnall et al (1981) made use of the fact that for the first eight to ten breaths of an anaesthetic the mixed venous levels of volatile agent are negligible. This allowed simplification of the equation governing anaesthetic transport, and permitted computer calculation of its rate constants in that individual based on the observed relationship of inspired and alveolar concentrations during that period.

Instead of attempting to project anaesthetic uptake, Hayes et al (1984) have applied a pure feedback technique, called proportional integral derivative (PID) control, to regulate enflurane delivery from a computerised anaesthetic machine. PID control is a method of computer-processing an error signal, in this case, that derived from a comparison of the measured end-tidal enflurane concentration with that desired. Processing is carried out via three separate pathways, each producing an output voltage that is proportional to a different aspect of the error signal, respectively its absolute value, its integral with respect to time (reflecting accumulated error), and its differential derivative with respect to time (rate of change). The outputs from all three pathways are summed and the resulting control signal used to regulate the enflurane delivery system. The system described by the authors was able, with some overshoot, to maintain a steady end-tidal enflurane concentration to within 0.1%.

The stable control of arterial pressure with infusions of short-acting vasodilators such as sodium nitroprusside and nitroglycerine is an area where a suitable computer program can often out-perform a human operator, even one devoting his entire attention to the task. Although most of the systems described are based on PID controllers, the fine adjustment of the algorithm is often the result of trial and error. Stern et al (1985) have described a self-tuning controller able to estimate and take account of the 'dead time' between the change of rate of the infusion and the change of arterial pressure, and thus reduce the likelihood of overshoot. Despite this capability, the authors make the point that stability of such a system under all conditions is very difficult to guarantee, and suggest the use of supervisory programs able to monitor the quality of control actually being achieved.

The evoked electromyogram provides a suitable basis for the computer control of infusions of muscle relaxants, particularly the newer short-acting non-depolarising drugs atracurium and vecuronium, although the technique has been described with pancuronium (Asbury & Linkens 1986) and suxamethonium (Ritchie et al 1985). Asbury and Linkens describe the use of a simple proportional controller based on the rectified and integrated EMG (RIEMG). The RIEMG is a d.c. voltage which is compared with the desired RIEMG to produce the error signal used to drive the infusion pump. The quality of control is inferior to a PID controller but was more than adequate to produce a stable level of blockade in their patients.

Hazards

Failure of a computer or its program is always a disaster for the user. Modern microcomputers are extremely reliable given a stable and interference-free power supply which is, at least in principle, relatively easy to ensure. Failure of software to do what is required of it under all circumstances is a real possibility, and in medical applications particularly, the performance of a program is constantly audited and checked for errors by supervisory programs to ensure fail-safe operation.

Conclusion

The arrival of the computer on the anaesthetic machine will not threaten the existence of the anaesthetist, who will always remain in overall charge of therapeutic decisions. It could, however improve the implementation of those decisions, which must have implications for patient safety.

REFERENCES

Alvis J M, Reves J G, Spain J A, Sheppard L C 1985 Computer-assisted continuous infusion of the intravenous analgesic fentanyl during general anaesthesia — an interactive system. IEEE Transactions on Biomedical Engineering 32: 323–329
Asbury A J, Linkens D A 1986 Clinical automatic control of neuromuscular blockade. Anaesthesia 41: 316–320
Ausems M E, Stanski D R, Hug C C 1985 An evaluation of the accuracy of pharmacokinetic data for the computer assisted infusion of alfentanil. British Journal of Anaesthesia 57: 1217–1225
Boaden R W, Hutton P 1986 The digital control of anaesthetic gas flow. Anaesthesia 41: 413–418
Chilcoat R T, Lunn J N, Mapleson W W 1984 Computer assistance in the control of depth of anaesthesia. British Journal of Anaesthesia 56: 1417–1432
Cooper J B, Newbower R S 1984 The Boston Anesthesia System. Contemporary Anesthesia Practice 8: 207–219

Cooper J B, Newbower R S, Long C D 1978 Preventable anesthesia mishaps — a human factors study. Anesthesiology 49: 399–406

Cushman J, Bushman J A 1983 The semi-automated production of anaesthetic records. British Journal of Anaesthesia 55: 240P–241P

Green R 1983 Aviation psychology. In: Aviation medicine. British Medical Association, London, pp 61–74

Hawes D W, Ross J A S, White D C, Wloch R T 1982 Servo control of closed circuit anaesthesia. British Journal of Anaesthesia 54: 229P–230P

Hayes J K, Westenskow D R, East T D, Jordan W S 1984 Computer-controlled anesthesia delivery system. Medical Instrumentation 18: 224–231

Kerr J H 1986 Alarms and excursions. Anaesthesia 41: 807–808

Lunn J N, Mushin W W 1982 Mortality associated with anaesthesia. Association of Anaesthetists of Great Britain and Ireland, London

Maynard D E, Jenkinson J L 1984 The cerebral function analysing monitor. Anaesthesia 39: 678–690

Palayiwa E, Hahn C E W, Sugg B R, Lindsay-Scott D, Tyrrell P J 1986 A microprocessor-controlled gas mixing device. British Journal of Anaesthesia 58: 1041–1047

Prentice J W, Kenny G N C 1984 Microcomputer-based anaesthetic record system. British Journal of Anaesthesia 56: 1433–1437

Ramsey M 1979 Noninvasive automatic determination of mean arterial pressure. Medical and Biological Engineering and Computing 17: 11–18

Reilly C S, Wood A J J, Wood M 1985 Variability of fentanyl pharmacokinetics in man. Computer predicted plasma concentrations for three intravenous dosage regimens. Anaesthesia 40: 837–843

Ritchie G, Ebert J P, Jannet T C, Kissin I, Sheppard L C 1985 A microcomputer based controller for neuromuscular block during surgery. Annals of Biomedical Engineering 13: 3–15

Rosen A S, Rosensweig W 1985 Computerized anesthesia record. Anesthesiology 62: 100

Schreiber P J 1986 Electronic surveillance during anaesthesia. North American Drager

Stern K S, Chizeck H J, Walker B K, Krishnaprasad P S, Dauchot P J, Katona P G 1985 The self-tuning controller: comparison with human performance in the control of arterial pressure. Annals of Biomedical Engineering 13: 341–357

Tatnall M L, Morris P, West P G 1981 Controlled anaesthesia: an approach using patient characteristics identified during uptake. British Journal of Anaesthesia 53: 1019–1026

Taylor M B, Whitwam J G 1986 The current status of pulse oximetry. Anaesthesia 41: 943–949

Yelderman M, New W 1983 Evaluation of pulse oximetry. Anesthesiology 59: 349–352

Yelderman M, Ream A K 1977 Bio-engineering symposium. San Diego, California.

Zollinger R M, Kreul J F, Schneider A J L 1977 Man-made versus computer-generated anaesthesia records. Journal of Surgical Research 22: 419–424

Controversies in cardiac surgery

INTRODUCTION

This chapter examines some of the controversial topics in surgery for acquired heart disease. Although the mortality for the majority of elective adult operations is low (e.g., for elective coronary artery surgery 1%, single valve replacement 4–5%, valve repair 1–2%), there is still a need to direct attention to the reduction of morbidity. The pattern of cardiac surgery is changing and therefore newer surgical procedures are discussed.

BLEEDING AFTER CARDIOPULMONARY BYPASS

The increasing number of coronary artery operations has directed the attention of many to reducing the donor blood requirement. The cell-separator which allows retransfusion of washed packed red blood cells during and after cardiopulmonary bypass (CPB), appears to be a useful adjunct particularly for difficult repeat ('re-do') procedures (Mayer et al 1985). Occasionally abnormal bleeding may occur after CPB and there is evidence to implicate an acquired defect in the formation of the platelet plug, which in turn may be due to reduced levels of von Willebrand's factor. This can be corrected by transfusion of cryoprecipitate or injection of desmopressin acetate (Harker 1986, Salzman et al 1986).

DAMAGING EFFECTS OF CARDIOPULMONARY BYPASS

Most patients have no ill effects after cardiopulmonary bypass but until recently few detailed studies of organ function had been made. As assessment becomes more critical, even slight impairment of function in different organs can be detected. There is increased capillary permeability, an increase in interstitial fluid, leucocytosis and fever, renal dysfunction, peripheral and probably central vasoconstriction. The red cells are more readily broken down resulting in haemoglobinaemia, haemoglobinurea and anaemia and possibly an increased susceptibility to infection. This used to be referred to globally as the 'post-pump syndrome'. Complications such as severe pulmonary oedema with normal left atrial pressure, bleeding diatheses or transient subtle neurological complications are now more widely recognised as events associated with CPB.

The most likely mechanisms for residual morbidity and mortality following coronary artery surgery are:

1. The exposure of blood to an abnormal environment.
2. Altered arterial blood flow patterns.

Abnormal exposure of blood

This usually occurs when blood is exposed to non-endothelial surfaces, the most important of which is the oxygenator. In a bubble oxygenator, the non-physiological surface is gas which is generally 100% oxygen but this is less of a problem in the membrane oxygenator. A recent development has been that of the microporous hollow fibre membrane oxygenator (Ennema 1983) which preserves red blood cells and platelets. There is a general trend towards the use of membrane oxygenators and it will be interesting to predict the routine use of the microporous hollow fibre oxygenator. The heat exchanger, de-bubbling and filtering devices are also abnormal surfaces but the bypass tubes and cannulae are less important as the bonding layer is small.

These non-physiological surfaces have effects on platelets which clump and embolise, leading to a reduction in the number of circulating platelets and the ability to aggregate. Platelet aggregates have been demonstrated at the end of cardiopulmonary bypass in both membrane oxygenator (Edmunds et al 1978) and in bubble oxygenators (Friedenberg et al 1978, Harker 1986, Hope et al 1981). Platelet damage and depletion might be prevented if it could be rendered non-functional during CPB and if the process were reversible. One method that appears to be helpful in achieving this aim is the coating of the surface of a membrane oxygenator with albumin (Addonizio et al 1979). Other studies have examined the use of an infusion of prostacyclin during CPB, but this process has not been adopted into routine cardiac surgical practice (Addonizio et al 1978, Longmore et al 1981, Di Sesa et al 1984).

Damage to the proteins which are part of the humoral amplification systems has more widespread results involving the following four systems; coagulation, complement, fibrinolysis and kallikrein-bradykinin. Thus, even in the presence of adequate blood levels during CPB, microcoagulation continues resulting in consumption of the coagulation factors to a varying degree (Kalter et al 1979, Kirklin et al 1983).

During CPB complement activation occurs (Hammerschmidt et al 1981, Boscoe et al 1983) and almost certainly interacts with damaged white cells and platelet clumps. Activation occurs via the alternative pathway (Kirklin et al 1986) adding in some patients to the whole body inflammatory reaction (Nordstrom et al 1978).

The adverse effects of complement activation are twofold:

1. The depletion of complement necessary for a normal immune response.
2. The adverse effects of the intravascular production of the anaphylotoxins.

Altered arterial flow patterns

The second major mechanism is that of altered arterial flow patterns. During total cardiopulmonary bypass with the heart not beating, arterial blood flow is non-pulsatile. Intuitively it might be expected that pulsatile flow would be advantageous, but whether there are fewer functional derangements compared with non-pulsatile flow is still controversial (see Mavroudis 1978).

It is interesting to note that Bixler et al (1979) in an experimental model found that non-pulsatile perfusion at a mean pressure of 50 mmHg in the hypertrophied fibrillating heart resulted in subendocardial ischaemia whereas pulsatile flow did not. When the mean perfusion pressure was raised to 80 mmHg neither pulsatile nor non-pulsatile flow resulted in subendocardial ischaemia. There is therefore insufficient evidence to support the view that pulsatile flow during cardiopulmonary bypass for routine short perfusions offers significant advantages. It may be beneficial in severely ill patients with end-stage cardiac disease.

HAEMOFILTRATION

The management of fluid balance of patients in renal failure before, during and after CPB can be problematical. Although the use of peritoneal dialysis is established, its efficiency for fluid removal is poor. It also tends to lead to splinting of the diaphragm which is an undesirable effect in the presence of already reduced ventilatory function. Finally there is also a very real risk of peritonitis.

The alternative technique of haemodialysis which can remove large volumes of extracellular fluid is usually contra-indicated in cardiac surgical patients postoperatively because of the adverse haemodynamic effects.

A recently introduced technique is that of haemofiltration which may be employed during cardiac surgery on patients in renal failure (Magilligan 1985), to stabilise patients adequately for valve surgery or for heart transplantation (Hakim et al 1985, Fauchald et al 1986) or in the management of refractory heart failure. The technique employs hydrostatic pressure and a compact highly permeable membrane which produces an ultrafiltrate of blood containing water, electrolytes and substances whose molecular weight is less that 6000. Arterial to venous communication may be used or venous to venous with a blood pump.

CEREBRAL DAMAGE ASSOCIATED WITH CORONARY BYPASS SURGERY

As the frequency of coronary artery surgery has increased and the mortality of the operation has fallen to less than 2% in most cardiac centres, more attention is now focused on postoperative problems such as neurological complications. Shaw et al (1985) reported neurological dysfunction in the first week after CPB in a prospective study of 312 patients undergoing coronary surgery; 235 patients (79%) showed some form of deterioration although it was not often serious enough to distress the patient or interfere with their everyday activities on the ward. Death occurred in one patient (0.3%) and severe disability as a result of neurological dysfunction in four patients (1.3%). Aberg et al (1982) noted that 91% of patients had an increased level of adenylate kinase in cerebrospinal fluid postoperatively. Raymond et al (1984) reported on psychometric testing in a group of 31 patients receiving coronary bypass grafts and a control group of 16 patients undergoing general surgery (12 of whom had major vascular surgery). The coronary bypass group showed significant deterioration after operation in several psychometric tests but these abnormalities were not present in the control group (Raymond et al 1984). In contrast Smith et al (1986) found minor neuropsychological defects to be common in both CPB and control groups.

Clearly the detection of brain damage during cardiopulmonary bypass is unsatisfactory. Monitoring of CSF adenylate kinase is probably unacceptable for routine use but some have found the modified EEG useful (Pryor 1985, Bolsin 1986). Postoperative coma is especially sinister carrying a high probability of death (Furlan & Breuer 1984). Although the incidence of minor neurological abnormalities is disconcertingly high, the incidence of major disability remains low. The incidence of peri-operative stroke is 4.8% with permanent neurological disability in 1.3% (Shaw et al 1985). The corresponding figures from the Cleveland clinic observed by Breuer et al (1981) were respectively 5.2% and 2%.

The management of patients with a history of previous stroke or with a carotid bruit undergoing CPB remains controversial. In a large prospective study of patients undergoing CPB, Ivey et al (1984) found that there were no focal neurological events in any of the 82 patients with an asymptomatic carotid bruit. They suggested that most patients who have a history of neurological symptoms should undergo arteriography and have either combined or staged procedures, the latter being preferred. This is the first study in which the hypothesis of a favourable outcome of asymptomatic carotid bruit has been prospectively tested in patients undergoing CPB. These results have been confirmed by a retrospective study of Breuer et al (1981).

MYOCARDIAL PROTECTION

1. Cardioplegia

Although it is now common practice to administer cold crystalloid cardio-plegic solution, many modifications have emerged over the last 5 years with regard to content of this solution and its administration. Initially it was believed that infusion of a cardioplegic solution completely inhibited myocardial metabolism, but it now appears that there is still a low level of mitochondrial activity requiring energy at 15–20°C. These requirements can be met by oxygenating the crystalloid solutions. There also have been developments in blood cardioplegia involving the use of pump oxygenated blood modified by adding potassium (Roberts et al 1982, Iverson et al 1984). There is no doubt that myocardial protection is improved with oxygenated solutions (Bodenhamer et al 1983), but whether better results are obtained with crystalloid solutions or blood remains uncertain. The use of blood cardioplegia allows for greater oxygen consumption by the arrested heart (Bing et al 1984).

2. Drugs

A number of studies have demonstrated a beneficial effect of calcium channel blockers such as verapamil or nifedipine (Nayler et al 1980, Macgovern et al 1981, Lange et al 1984). This enhancement is presumably due to blocking of the slow channel transport of calcium into the cell during re-perfusion. Other studies have shown that propranolol in the cardioplegic solution has a beneficial effect (Kanter et al 1981). Some surgeons add hydrocortisone to the cardioplegic solution (Appelbaum et al 1981). The amino acid L-glutamate has been shown experimentally to improve aerobic and anaerobic metabolism when added to a blood cardioplegic solution, and this has been supported in a careful clinical study (Rosenkranz et al 1983).

Shortly after the onset of myocardial ischaemia there is a rapid decrease in myocardial pH and a simultaneous decrease in molecular oxygen accompanied by production of cytotoxic oxygen-free radicals. Superoxide anion scavengers such as superoxide dismutase in combination with mannitol have been shown to be beneficial experimentally (Gardner et al 1983) and may become clinically useful.

3. Infants

Controversy continues about the optimal method for myocardial protection in very young infants. It appears that:

1. The myocardium of young infants is different from that of adults.
2. The frequent use of atriotomies and ventriculotomies raises the possibility that cut coronary arteries and air emboli may be as important in

producing myocardial damage as is the period of global myocardial ischaemia (Bull et al 1984).

NEW SURGICAL PROCEDURES

Arrhythmia surgery

The number of surgical procedures used for the treatment of refractory arrhythmias has developed markedly since 1978. A paradox has arisen whereby most supraventricular tachycardias (SVT) can be readily diagnosed but the surgical procedures for their correction are complex and not easily mastered. On the other hand, ventricular arrhythmias are often difficult to diagnose and their basic mechanisms are poorly understood. Yet almost any surgical intervention designed to treat ventricular tachycardia will either ablate or isolate the arrhythmia and will relieve the patient's symptoms or enhance the effect of anti-arrhythmic drugs.

The indications for arrhythmic surgery are firstly the failure of medical treatment, secondly recurrent SVT in young patients with Wolff-Parkinson-White syndrome (WPW) and thirdly spontaneous atrial fibrillation associated with accessory pathways or AV node bypass tracts. Patients who are intolerant to drugs are a further indication. Others have reported the use of catheter-delivered electric shocks to accessory pathways for the treatment of WPW syndrome (Ward & Camm 1985). This remains experimental at present. Guiraudon et al (1978) reported the technique of encircling endocardial ventriculotomy (EEV). Later, Josephson et al (1979) described the technique of subendocardial resection now termed endocardial resection procedure (ERP). EEV has now been abandoned because of unacceptably high incidence of low cardiac output postoperatively. Most surgeons now use ERP with a surgical cure rate of 60% and a further 25% of patients being controlled more easily with drugs than pre-operatively (Cox 1985).

TRANSPLANTATION

1. Heart

Over the last 5 years there has been a resurgence of interest in heart transplantation and important developments in heart-lung transplantation, the main reason being the recent results from Stanford University, California where in 1968 the 1-year survival for heart transplantation was 22%. In 1982 it was 88% and it has since remained at that level (Oyer et al 1982, Jamieson et al 1984). Much of this recent success has been attributed to the use of cyclosporin. The advantage of cyclosporin is its specific immunosuppressive effect compared to the overall immunosuppressive action of azathioprine. Furthermore, with cyclosporin, graft rejection can be prevented with the administration of minimal doses of steroids (Cavarocchi et al 1985, Yacoub et al 1985). There is evidence that use of cyclosporin is associated with less severe rejection episodes and less serious infections than with azathioprine (Griffith et al 1984).

With the increasing numbers of successful cardiac transplant recipients these patients may very well require general anaesthesia for other unrelated procedures. It is therefore reassuring to find that the transplanted chronically denervated and non-rejecting heart has normal systolic function and a normal contractile reserve (Borow et al 1985).

Heterotopic heart transplantation was introduced in 1975 by Barnard and Allsman. The transplanted heart is used usually to assist the left ventricle. Barnard & Cooper (1981) have recently reported good results in 46 patients. The method has its advantages and may be considered for certain patients with pulmonary hypertension.

2. Heart-lung

Heart-lung transplantation remains an innovative procedure for highly selected patients. Reitz et al (1980) reported long term survival in primates after heart-lung allotransplantation with cyclosporin immunosuppression. This was followed by a series of successful heart-lung transplants in patients at Stanford (Reitz et al 1982). In the UK there has been extensive development of this procedure both at Papworth and Harefield hospitals.

There appear to be two unique postoperative complications. The first involves a triad of impaired gas exchange, lung shadows on chest X-ray and reduced lung compliance occurring between the first and fourth postoperative days and generally referred to as the re-implantation response. It is thought that this is related to transient ischaemia of the allografted organ. The second complication relates to obliterative bronchiolitis which is characterised by small airways obstruction and may occur in up to 35% of patients within 18 months of operation. It is of interest that rejection is less frequent after heart-lung transplantation than after heart transplantation.

CARDIAC ASSIST DEVICES

The incidence of cardiac failure after open heart surgery has diminished markedly in the last 20 years. Patients with postoperative left ventricular failure have been successfully treated with conventional drug therapy and the intra-aortic balloon pump (IABP) (Pennington et al 1983). However a small group of patients fail to respond to these measures and require a more complete form of circulatory support. The criteria for circulatory support have been outlined by Norman et al (1977). They are applicable to patients with IABP support and optimal filling pressures; cardiac index < 2.0 l.min^{-1}.m^{-1}, systemic vascular resistance > 2100 dynes s.$^{-1}$cm^{-5}, left or right atrial pressure above 20 mmHg and urine output < 20 ml. h^{-1} despite inotropic and vasodilator support. Most of these temporary assist devices are pneumatically driven. The quality of materials is good enough to guarantee an implant time free of thrombus for up to 1 month. In general the function of assist devices is limited by the size of the cannula.

The assist device most commonly used is the Pierce-Donachy Thoratec VAD. It uses Bjork-Shiley inlet and outlet valves and has a stroke volume of 65 ml with an ejection fraction of approximately 75%. The cannula system allows cannulation of either ventricle, either atrium and the aorta or pulmonary artery. It provides pulsatile flow and has been used successfully without heparin. Pierce et al (1981) reported 17 patients who could not be weaned from bypass, eight of whom with left ventricular assist had eventual recovery and were discharged from hospital.

For patients who develop cardiogenic shock while awaiting cardiac transplantation or following acute myocardial infarction, extracorporeal membrane oxygenation (ECMO) is useful (Bartlett et al 1977). The disadvantage of ECMO is the need for anticoagulants.

The place of the artificial heart remains experimental (Relman 1986).

REFERENCES

Aberg T, Tyden H, Ronquist G, Ahlumo P, Bergstrom K 1982 Release of adenylate kinase into the cerebrospinal fluid during open heart surgery and its relation to post-operative intellectual function. Lancet 1: 1139–1142

Addonizio V P, Strauss J F, Macarack E J, Colman R W, Edmunds H Jr 1978 Preservation of platelet number and function with prostaglandin E during total cardiopulmonary bypass in rhesus monkeys. Surgery 83: 619–625

Addonizio V P, Macarak E J, Nicolaou K C, Edmunds L H Jr, Colman R W 1979 Effects of prostacyclin and albumin on platelet loss during in vitro simulation of extracorporeal circulation. Blood 53: 1033–1042

Appelbaum A, Gosman M S, Raz S, Ovil Y, Borman J B 1981 Protective effect of hydrocortisone on the myocardium during anoxic arrest. Israel Journal of Medical Sciences 17: 8–11

Barnard C N, Cooper D K C 1981 Clinical transplantation of the heart: a review of 13 years personal experience. Journal of The Royal Society of Medicine 74: 670–674

Bartlett R H, Gazziniga A B, Fong S W, Jefferies M R, Rookh H V, Haiduc N 1977 Extracorporeal membrane oxygenator support for cardiopulmonary failure: experience in 28 cases. Journal of Thoracic and Cardiovascular Surgery 73: 375–386

Bing O H, La Rai P J, Franklin A, Stroughton F J, Weintraub R M 1984 Mechanism of myocardial protection during blood potassium cardioplegia: a comparison of crystalloid red cell and methaemoglobin solutions. Circulation 70 (suppl. I): 184–190

Bixler T J, Magee P G, Flaherty J T, Goldman R A, Gott V L 1979 Beneficial effects of pulsatile perfusion in the hypertrophied ventricle during ventricular fibrillation. Circulation 60: 141–146

Bodenhamer R M, Deboer L W V, Geffin G A et al 1983 Enhanced myocardial protection during ischaemic arrest: oxygenation of a crystalloid cardioplegic solution. Journal of Thoracic and Cardiovascular Surgery 85: 769–780

Bolsin S N 1986 Detection of neurological damage during cardiopulmonary bypass. Anaesthesia 41: 61–66

Borow K M, Neuman N A, Arensman F W, Yacoub M H 1985 Left ventricular contractility and contractile reserve in humans after cardiac transplantation. Circulation 71: 866–872

Boscoe M J, Yewdall V M, Thompson M A, Cameron J S 1983 Complement activation during cardiopulmonary bypass: quantitative study of effects of methylprednisolone and pulsatile flow. British Medical Journal 287: 1747–1750

Breuer A C, Furlan A J, Hansen M R et al 1981 Neurologic complications of open heart surgery: computer-assisted analysis of 531 patients. Cleveland Clinic Quarterly 48: 205–206

Bull C, Cooper J, Stark J 1984 Cardioplegic protection of the child's heart. Journal of Thoracic and Cardiovascular Surgery 88: 287–293

Cavarocchi N, Hakim M, Cory-Pearce R, English T A H, Wallwork J 1985 A prospective randomised trial of cyclosporine and low-dose prednisolone versus cyclosporine and azathioprine. Journal of Heart Transplantation IV: 591

Cox J L 1985 The status of surgery for cardiac arrhythmias. Circulation 71: 413–417

Di Sesa V J, Huval W, Lelcuk S et al 1984 Disadvantages of prostacyclin infusion during cardiopulmonary bypass: a double blind study of 50 patients having coronary revascularisation. Annals of Thoracic Surgery 38: 514–519

Edmunds L H, Saxena N C, Hillyer P, Wilson T J 1978 Relationship between platelet count and cardiotomy suction return. Annals of Thoracic Surgery 25: 306–310

Ennema J J, Mook P H, Elstradt J M 1983 A new hollow-fibre membrane oxygenator with an integral heat exchanger. Thoracic and Cardiovascular Surgery 31: 350–354

Fauchald P, Forfang K, Amlie J 1986 An evaluation of ultrafiltration as treatment of therapy-resistant cardiac oedema. Acta Medica Scandinavica 219: 47–52

Friedenberg W R, Myers W O, Plotka E D et al 1978 Platelet dysfunction associated with cardiopulmonary bypass. Annals of Thoracic Surgery 25: 298–305

Furlan A J, Breuer A C 1984 Central nervous system complications of open heart surgery. Stroke 15: 912–915

Gardner T J, Stewart J R, Casale A S, Downey J M, Chambers D E 1983 Reduction of myocardial ischaemia injury with oxygen-derived free radical scavengers. Surgery 94: 423–427

Griffith B P, Hardesty P L, Bahnson B T 1984 Powerful but limited immunosuppression for cardiac transplantation with cyclosporine and low-dose steroid. Journal of Thoracic and Cardiovascular Surgery 87: 35–42

Guiraudon G, Fontaine G, Frank R, Escande G, Etievent P, Cabrol C 1978 Encircling endocardial ventriculotomy: a new surgical treatment for life threatening ventricular tachycardias resistant to medical treatment following myocardial infarction. Annals of Thoracic Surgery 26: 438–444

Hakim M, Wheeldon D, Bethune D W, Milstein B B, English T A, Wallwork J 1985 Haemodialysis and haemofiltration on cardiopulmonary bypass. Thorax 40: 101–106

Hammerschmidt D E, Stroncek D F, Bowers T K et al Complement activation and neutropenia occurring during cardiopulmonary bypass. Journal of Thoracic and Cardiovascular Surgery 81: 370–377

Harker L A 1986 Bleeding after cardiopulmonary bypass. New England Journal of Medicine 314: 1446–1448

Harker L A, Malpass T W, Branson H E, Hessel E A, Slichter S J Mechanisms of abnormal bleeding in patients undergoing cardiopulmonary bypass: acquired transient platelet dysfunction associated with selective d-granule release. Blood 56: 824–834

Hope A F, Heyns A D, Lotter M G et al 1981 Kinetics and sites of sequestration of indium lll-labelled human platelets during cardiopulmonary bypass. Journal of Thoracic and Cardiovascular Surgery 81: 880–886

Iverson L I, Young J N, Ennix C L et al 1984 Myocardial protection: a comparison of cold blood and cold crystalloid cardioplegia. Journal of Thoracic and Cardiovascular Surgery 87: 509–516

Ivey T D, Strandness E, Williams D B, Langlois Y, Misbach G A, Kruse A P 1984 Management of patients with carotid bruit undergoing cardiopulmonary bypass. Journal of Thoracic and Cardiovascular Surgery 87: 183–189

Jamieson S W, Oyer P, Baldwin J, Stinson E B, Shumway N 1984 Heart transplantation for end-stage ischaemic heart disease: the Stanford experience. Journal of Heart Transplantation III: 224–229

Josephson M E, Harken A H, Horowitz L N 1979 Endocardial excision: a new surgical technique for the treatment of ventricular tachycardia. Circulation 60: 1430–1439

Kalter R D, Saul C M, Wetstein L, Soriano C, Reiss R F 1979 Cardiopulmonary bypass: associated hemostatic abnormalities. Journal of Thoracic and Cardiovascular Surgery 77: 427–435

Kanter K R, Flaherty J T, Bulkley B H, Gott V L, Gardner T J 1981 Beneficial effects of adding propranolol to multidose potassium cardioplegia circulation 64 (suppl. II): 84–90

Kirklin J K, Westaby S, Blackstone E H, Kirlin J W, Chenoweth D E, Pacifico A D 1983
Complement and the damaging effects of cardiopulmonary bypass. Journal of Thoracic
and Cardiovascular Surgery 86: 845–857

Kirklin J K, Chenoweth D E, Naftel D C et al 1986 Effects of protamine administration
after cardiopulmonary bypass on complement, blood elements and the haemodynamic
state. Annals of Thoracic Surgery 41: 193–199

Lange R, Ingwall J, Hale S L, Alker K J, Braunwald E, Kloner A 1984 Preservation of
high-energy phosphates by verapamil in reperfused myocardium circulation 70: 734–741

Longmore D B, Bennett J G, Hoyle P M et al 1981 Prostacyclin administration during
cardiopulmonary bypass in man. Lancet 1: 800–804

Macgovern G J, Dixon C M, Burkholder J A 1981 Improved myocardial protection with
nifedipine and potassium-based cardioplegia. Journal of Thoracic and Cardiovascular
Surgery 82: 239–244

Magilligan D J 1985 Indications for ultrafiltration in the cardiac surgical patient. Journal of
Thoracic and Cardiovascular Surgery 89: 183–189

Mavroudis C 1978 To pulse or not to pulse. Annals of Thoracic Surgery 25: 259–271

Mayer E D, Welsch M, Tanzeem A et al 1985 Reduction of post-operative donor blood
requirement by use of the cell separator. Scandinavian Journal of Thoracic &
Cardiovascular Surgery 19: 165–171

Nayler W G, Ferrari R, Williams A 1980 Protective effect of pre-treatment with verapamil,
nifedipine and propranolol on mitochondrial function in the ischaemic and reperfused
myocardium. American Journal of Cardiology 46: 242–248

Nordstrom L, Fletcher R, Pavek K 1978 Shock of anaphylactoid type induced protamine: a
continuous cardiorespiratory record. Acta Anaesthesiologica Scandinavica 22: 195–201

Norman J C, Cooley D A, Igo S R et al 1977 Prognostic indices for survival during post-
cardiotomy intra-aortic balloon pumping. Journal of Thoracic and Cardiovascular Surgery
74: 709–720

Oyer P E, Stinson E B, Jamieson S W, Bieber C P, Shumway N 1982 One year experience
with cyclosporine-A in clinical heart transplantation. Journal of Heart Transplantation
1: 285–288

Pennington D G, Swartz M T, Godd J E, Merjavy J P, Kaiser G C 1983 Intra-aortic
balloon pumping in cardiac surgical patients — a 9 year experience. Annals of Thoracic
Surgery 36: 125–131

Pierce W S, Parr G V S, Myers J L, Pae W E Jr, Bull A P, Waldhausen J A 1981
Ventricular-assist pumping in patients with cardiogenic shock after cardiac operations.
New England Journal of Medicine 305: 1606–1610

Prior P F 1985 EEG monitoring and evoked potentials in brain ischaemia. British Journal
of Anaesthesia 57: 63–81

Raymond M, Conklin C, Schaeffer J, Newstadt G, Matloff J M, Gray R J 1984 Coping
with transient intellectual dysfunction after coronary bypass surgery. Heart lung
13: 531–539

Reitz B A, Burton N A, Jamieson S W et al 1980 Heart and lung transplantation:
autotransplantation and allotransplantation in primates with extended survival. Journal of
Thoracic and Cardiovascular Surgery 80: 360–372

Reitz B A, Wallwork J L, Hunt S A et al 1982 Heart lung transplantation: successful
therapy for patients with pulmonary vascular disease. New England Journal of Medicine
306: 557–564

Relman A S 1986 Artificial hearts — permanent and temporary. New England Journal of
Medicine 314: 644–645

Roberts A J, Moran J M, Sanders J H et al 1982 Clinical evaluation of the relative
effectiveness of multidose crystalloid and cold blood potassium cardioplegia in coronary
artery bypass graft surgery: a non-randomised matched-pair analysis. Annals of Thoracic
Surgery 33: 421–433

Rosenkranz E R, Buckberg G D, Laks H, Mulder D G 1983 Warm induction of
cardioplegia with glutamate-enriched blood in coronary patients with cardiogenic shock
who are dependent on inotropic drugs and intra-aortic balloon support. Journal of
Thoracic and Cardiovascular Surgery 86: 507–518

Salzman E W, Weinstein M J, Weintraub R M et al 1986 Treatment with desmopressin
acetate to reduce blood loss after cardiac surgery: a double-blind randomised study. New
England Journal of Medicine 314: 1402–1406

Shaw P J, Bates D, Cartlidge N E F, Heaviside D, Julian D G, Shaw D A 1985 Early neurological complications of coronary artery bypass surgery. British Medical Journal 291: 1384–1387

Smith P L, Treasure T, Newman S P et al 1986 Cerebral consequences of cardiopulmonary bypass. Lancet 1: 823–825

Ward D E, Camm A J 1985 Treatment of tachycardias associated with the Wolff-Parkinson-White syndrome by transvenous electrical ablation of accessory pathways. British Heart Journal 53: 64–68

Yacoub M, Alvizatos P, Khaghani A, Mitchell A 1985 The use of cyclosporine, azathioprine and antithymocyte globulin with or without low-dose steroids for immunosuppression of cardiac transplant patients. Transplantation Proceedings XVII: 221–223

The pathophysiology and treatment of adult respiratory distress syndrome (ARDS)

INTRODUCTION

In 1967 a syndrome of lung dysfunction was described which was characterised by severe hypoxaemia, patchy bilateral pulmonary infiltrates on chest X-ray, and low pulmonary compliance (Asbaugh et al 1967). Two years later a further report by the same authors provided the label 'adult respiratory distress syndrome' (Asbaugh et al 1969). Since then this term has become widely used to convey the clinical manifestations of the implied disorder, namely pulmonary oedema resulting from increased permeability of the alveolar-capillary barrier. The evidence for such a process was later to be based upon ultrastructural studies of the alveolar-capillary barrier (Bachofen & Weibel 1977), the occurrence of alveolar oedema formation with a normal plasma oncotic pressure and normal left ventricular function (Swan et al 1970, Weil et al 1978), and an increased protein concentration in oedema fluid (Fein et al 1979).

PHYSIOLOGY OF THE ALVEOLAR-CAPILLARY BARRIER

This barrier includes a layer of surfactant, the alveolar epithelium, the capillary endothelium and their basement membranes which enclose the interstitial space. The fine details of the structure of the barrier together with recent studies of its solute permeability have recently been described (Barrowcliffe & Jones 1987). A diagrammatic representation of the structure, together with the factors which influence the net fluid flux across the barrier, is shown in Fig. 13.1a. A common representation of Starling's concept of these factors oversimplifies them in three ways. The apparent osmotic pressure gradient ($\Delta\pi$) must be modified to take into account the efficacy of the barrier as a semipermeable membrane. This is described by the reflection coefficient (σ) so that $\sigma \times \Delta\pi$ describes the effective gradient of osmotic pressure. If the barrier is an ideal semipermeable membrane then the reflection coefficient of the barrier for a given solute is unity (i.e., 100% of solute molecules impinging on the barrier are reflected from it). When the membrane becomes progressively more leaky to the solute, σ falls towards zero. Thus the situation in ARDS is a leaky barrier where the

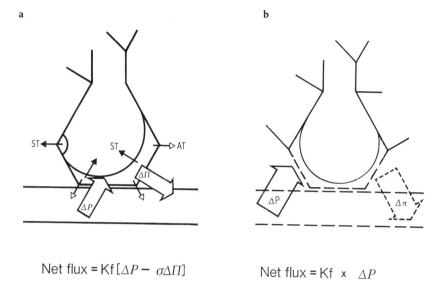

Net flux = $Kf[\Delta P - \sigma \Delta \Pi]$ Net flux = $Kf \times \Delta P$

Fig. 13.1(a) The balance of active and passive forces across the alveolar wall. Δ and $\Delta \pi$ represent the gradient of hydrostatic and osmotic pressure between the alveolar and capillary lumina. ST and AT represent surface tension and active transport. Notice that ST may act in two directions. Small collections of liquid in the 'corners' of alveoli may act as pumps which remove liquid from the alveolar lumen. The Starling equation for liquid flux across the alveolar wall summarises some of the forces, where Kf is the hydraulic conductivity and σ the reflection coefficient of the wall, but does not include ST and AT. **(b)** The alveolar wall is so leaky that the reflection coefficient has fallen to zero and the effective osmotic pressure ($\sigma \times \Delta \pi$) is nil. In this situation the hydrostatic pressure gradient is no longer opposed by an osmotic gradient and the alveoli will tend to flood.

reflection coefficient for protein in many alveoli may be near zero and as a consequence there is no effective colloid osmotic pressure gradient in these alveoli. This is shown in Fig. 13.1b where the hydrostatic pressure gradient across the capillary wall is no longer opposed by an osmotic pressure gradient, and this emphasises the basic principle in management which is to minimise the hydrostatic pressure in the pulmonary capillaries. Although this figure only shows the forces across the endothelium the integrity of the epithelium may be even more important from the point of view of maintaining a fluid-free alveolar space.

The other factors not included in the Starling equation are active transport of solute, both crystalloid and colloid, and the effects of surface forces. Surfactant reduces the surface tension which exerts a force tending to pull liquid into the alveolar space. However a recent concept of surfactant action suggests that because the surfactant acts as a water-repellent layer (Hills 1987) it may promote alveolar dryness by the formation of convex droplets which act as 'corner pumps'. Surfactant deficiency promotes alveolar collapse by increasing the forces tending to close the alveoli; it causes alveolar flooding by abolishing the action of corner pumps and also causes a considerable increase in solute permeability of the alveolar barrier (Robertson et al 1985, Evander et al 1987). Active transport is an important factor in maintaining the large concentration gradient of solute across the barrier which, if the reflection coefficient is near unity, results in a highly protective gradient of osmotic pressure which keeps the alveoli free of fluid.

Thus from the physiological point of view, ARDS results from a breakdown in the integrity of the barrier, particularly of the epithelium, a reduction in the reflection coefficient of both the epithelial and endothelial components, and an increased flux of protein into the alveolar space which denatures surfactant (Ikegami et al 1984) and promotes further flooding and alveolar collapse.

AETIOLOGY

There is a formidable list of disorders which may lead to ARDS. These may be most conveniently subdivided into: physical, chemical, microbiological and activation of host defence (Table 13.1).

The most common causes include aspiration of gastric contents (roughly one third of reliably witnessed aspirations may develop the syndrome); serious infections including pneumonias; lung contusion, and the combination of trauma, blood loss, hypotension and massive transfusion (Fowler et al 1983, Pepe 1986). An impression is emerging of the fundamental problem of sepsis in ARDS (Niederman & Fein 1980, Bell et al 1983, Seidenfield et al 1986). The term 'sepsis syndrome' has been coined to describe what used to be known as septicaemic shock (Weinberg et al 1984, Pepe 1986). The source of infection is frequently intra-abdominal, and positive blood cultures do not have to be obtained to make the diagnosis. ARDS is reported to arise in 25–60% of such selected cases (Kaplan et al 1979, Fein et al 1983, Weinberg et al 1984, Pepe 1986).

A recent prospective study in Los Angeles indicated that 2% of all patients acutely ill develop ARDS, although the inclusion of AIDS patients with pneumocystis pneumonia may invalidate extrapolation of this figure to the UK at present (Baumann et al 1986). In various high risk groups identified within North American hospitals 7% developed the syndrome (Fowler et al 1983). An estimate has been made that the annual incidence of ARDS in that country is 150 000 (Respiratory Disease Task Force 1972), which represents 0.06% of the population. It seems unlikely that the incidence is as great as this in the United Kingdom. For example, if this figure is applied to Leeds (populaton 450 000), then 270 cases would be expected per annum, which is more than three times the number of cases seen in the intensive care units in that city. Whilst some of this discrepancy may be explained by the varying incidence of such predispositions as AIDS or cardiopulmonary bypass, a major problem with such surveys is that there are no rigid diagnostic criteria which must be fulfilled.

Table 13.1 Factors associated with the development of ARDS

Physical	Chemical	Microbiological	Activation of host defence
Inhalation:	Inhalation:	Virus pneumonia	Complement
Hydrogen ions (gastric contents)	Smoke (acrolein, aldehydes, etc.)	Bacterial pneumonia	Neutrophils
Water (fresh, sea)	Oxygen, ozone, nitrogen oxides	Endo- and exotoxaemia	Macrophages
Dusts	Dusts (organic, inorganic)	Fungi	Eicosanoids
Irradiation	Corrosive chemicals	Malaria	Vasoactive amines
Blast injury	Systemic drugs and chemicals:		Polypeptides (kinins)
High inflation pressure	Aspirin		Coagulation factors
Air embolism	Chemotherapy (bleomycin, busulphan, etc.)		Lysosomal enzymes
	Heroin		Free radicals
	Nitrofurantoin		Transfusion reaction
	Paraquat		Cardiopulmonary bypass
	Metabolic disorders:		Anaphylaxis
	Uraemia		
	Diabetes		
	Pancreatitis		
	Fat embolism		

MECHANISMS OF LUNG INJURY

The variety of pathogenetic mechanisms of ARDS, recently the subject of editorial comment (Lancet 1986) is almost as long as the list of clinical disorders which predispose to the syndrome. Eosinophils (Hallgren et al 1987) and platelets (Heffner et al 1987) have been implicated in the pathophysiology. Activation of complement, particularly the C5a component, has been shown in ARDS (Robbins et al 1987). The most exhaustively studied mechanism implicates the neutrophil as a crucial causative factor, although another recent editorial (Rinaldo & Rogers 1986) has emphasised the deficiencies in this approach. Further advances in treatment are likely to depend upon elucidation of specific mechanisms of lung injury. Thus a final common path for many mediators is the production of oxygen-derived free radical species which inactivate proteins, cause lipid peroxidation, destroy nucleic acids and kill cells (Fantone & Ward 1982, Travis 1987). Patients with ARDS may have either enhanced or depleted free radical scavenging systems, and in these circumstances the safe level of oxygen is unknown. The administration of free radical scavengers (for example the vitamins C and E and enzymes superoxide dismutase and catalase) has been suggested and Travis (1987) has advocated the use of garlic! It has been shown that the administration of an aerosol of heparin and dimethyl sulphoxide (a free radical scavenger) following smoke inhalation, lethal to a group of control animals, resulted in the survival of all treated animals (Brown et al 1985). Surfactant depletion is an important mechanism causing pulmonary oedema in ARDS. The delivery of surfactant via the airways as a therapy of infantile respiratory distress syndrome is now giving promising results (Avery et al 1986, Ten Centre Study Group 1987), and it has been suggested that its use be extended to ARDS (Robertson 1984).

Diagnostic criteria

Some of the diagnostic tests used in patients with severe lung injury are shown in Table 13.2. All authorities agree that to make a diagnosis of ARDS there must be marked hypoxaemia, the severity of which can be expressed as physiological shunt, arterial:alveolar oxygen tension ratio, or most simply a statement of the PaO_2 at a defined inspired O_2 fraction.

The chest X-ray manifestations are almost always bilateral, patchy and peripheral, characteristically sparing cardio- and costophrenic angles (Milne et al 1985). Some workers advocate the use of pulmonary angiography as a prognostic guide.

Patients with ARDS usually have values of total static pulmonary compliance below 50 ml/cm H_2O (Fowler et al 1983), typically 20–30 ml/cm H_2O, but because the contribution of chest wall compliance may be difficult to assess, and the lung disorder may be patchy, this measurement is often considered of little value.

Table 13.2   Tests of function following lung injury

1. Gas exchange (P(A-a)O_2 difference, V/Q distributions)

2. Radiography (chest X-ray, angiography)

3. Mechanics (compliance)

4. Alveolar liquid analysis (pulmonary oedema protein, alveolar lavage)

5. Pulmonary artery pressures (wedge pressure)

6. Lung permeability (^{99m}Tc-labelled DTPA, labelled protein)

7. Lung metabolism

8. Lung water (thermodilution, CT scan)

9. Lung inflammation (labelled neutrophils, gallium, biopsy)

When pulmonary oedema fluid can be collected (which is infrequent), an oedema fluid protein to plasma protein ratio above 0.7 is consistent with ARDS, below 0.4 with haemodynamic oedema, whilst between these values the two causes may coexist (Fein et al 1979, Sprung et al 1981). Discrimination may be further improved by measuring globulin ratios. Other mediators of lung injury may be identified in lung lavage fluid in patients who are believed to be developing ARDS (Fein et al 1986).

A pulmonary artery catheter (PAC) enables the measurement of wedge pressure, and most studies exclude ARDS if this exceeds 12–15 mmHg, although some account should be taken of plasma oncotic pressure (Guyton & Lindsay 1959, Weil et al 1978). Also, seriously ill patients, including those with ARDS, frequently suffer from myocardial depression (Unger et al 1975, Zapol & Snider 1977), which will increase the wedge pressure and accelerate the formation of pulmonary oedema, especially with concurrent fluid overload (Stein et al 1974). Furthermore, it is possible for patients to spuriously fulfill conventional criteria for diagnosis of ARDS when their alveolar-capillary barrier function is unimpaired. This can occur when myocardial depression is transient, due for example to myocardial ischaemia (Timmis et al 1981), so that by the time a PAC is inserted the wedge pressure has fallen to normal, whereas pulmonary oedema may take many hours to resolve.

A marked increase in pulmonary venous resistance and hence pulmonary capillary pressure can cause a haemodynamic form of pulmonary oedema with a normal wedge pressure. Pulmonary venoconstriction may be mediated by some compounds that have been implicated in the pathogenesis of ARDS, such as histamine and arachidonic acid metabolites (Malik et al 1985). An accompanying increase in alveolar-capillary barrier permeability, and/or pulmonary hypertension, will greatly increase the rate of pulmonary oedema formation. These effects are difficult to quantify because the conventional measurement of left heart filling pressure using the Swan-Ganz balloon occlusion method, by stopping blood flow, obscures the effect of an increased pulmonary venomotor tone. However, a technique has recently been described that allows estimation of pulmonary capillary pressure using a pulmonary artery catheter (Holloway et al 1983), and application in patients is promising (Cope et al 1986). Robin (1985), in a critical analysis of the clinical usefulness of the PAC, concluded that there is little evidence of any proven value, and Rinaldo (1986) believes that the hazards of PACs justify use only in complex cases. Nevertheless if an increase in venomotor tone is an important part of the pathophysiology of the disorder attempts may need to be made to reduce tone and to monitor the efficacy of such therapy.

Methods to measure solute permeability of the alveolar-capillary barrier provide the latest diagnostic advances which await detailed clinical evaluation. The labelled hydrophilic solute ^{99m}Tc-labelled DTPA is a widely available tracer which in this application is administered as an aerosol and provides a measure of alveolar epithelial permeability. In contrast the accumulation of radiolabelled protein in the lung may give some measure of capillary endothelial permeability. Both methods reveal abnormalities in ARDS patients indicative of permeability defects in the alveolar-capillary barrier (Gorin et al 1980, Jones 1984, Mason et al 1985, Basran et al 1985, Braude et al 1986).

The techniques have been extensively reviewed (Barrowcliffe & Jones 1987) and the basis of the method is shown in Fig.13.2. The ^{99m}Tc-labelled DTPA method relies on the fact that the alveolar epithelium presents a more formidable barrier to the permeation of water soluble molecules than does the pulmonary capillary endothelium. The normal half-time clearance rate from lung to blood ($T_{1/2}$) is about 60 minutes but in a variety of conditions the $T_{1/2LB}$ becomes considerably reduced indicating a greatly increased permeability of the epithelium. Examples of such diseases are ARDS, hyaline membrane disease and the application of positive end-expiratory pressure (PEEP). The shape of the clearance curve, either mono-

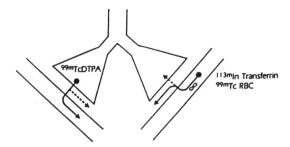

Fig. 13.2 Two minimally invasive methods for measuring indices of solute permeability of the alveolar-capillary barrier. The clearance from lung of technetium-labelled DTPA given by aerosol measures principally epithelial permeability. The accumulation within the lung of indium-labelled transferrin (or albumin), standardised for pulmonary blood volume, provides an index of protein leak of the endothelium and eventually the epithelium. In both methods either a gamma camera or a scintillation probe is used to measure changing lung radioactivity. Reproduced with permission of *Thorax*.

or multi-exponential may be used to discriminate between some of these conditions. For example ARDS, hyaline membrane disease and interstitial lung disease all tend to have multi-exponential clearance curves. The technique has also been used to demonstrate that breathing as little as 50% oxygen for 45 hours will cause an increase in alveolar permeability to both ^{99m}Tc-labelled DTPA and protein (Griffith et al 1986). An accelerated solute clearance (^{99m}Tc-labelled DTPA) has been shown in patients with *Pneumocystis carinii* pneumonia and this may be a useful screening technique in AIDS patients (Mason et al 1987).

The accumulation of protein in the lung may be a test of endothelial permeability and has been rigorously studied by Dauber et al (1985) in animal models. They showed that following mild lung injury, protein accumulation occurred in the lung prior to an increase in lung water and that with increasing severity of lung injury there was a comparable increase in protein and water accumulation. A typical result of such a study is shown in Fig. 13.3.

The sequential changes and relative sensitivity of various tests of progressive lung injury have recently been studied. It was found that ^{99m}Tc-labelled DTPA was the first test to show a change; this was followed some hours later by accumulation of lung water then by a change in lung metabolism. During recovery from lung injury there was a parallel recovery in ^{99m}Tc-labelled DTPA permeability and lung water but with a persistent abnormality of lung metabolism (Minty et al 1987). Tennenberg et al (1987) also showed that the ^{99m}Tc-labelled DTPA technique was a useful method for predicting the development of ARDS, there being a 6–12 hour delay

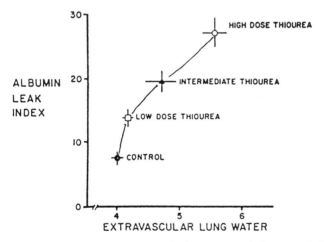

Fig. 13.3 The relationship between extravascular lung water and the accumulation of albumin in the lung. With minimal lung injury induced by low dose Thiourea there is an increase in albumin leak prior to a change in lung water. With more severe lung injury there is a linear relationship between albumin leak and increased lung water. Reproduced with permission of *Journal of Applied Physiology* from Dauber et al (1985).

following the development of an abnormal permeability test and the development of ARDS. This approach seems the most promising in terms of evaluating the fundamental disorder in ARDS, that is to quantify the degree of a breakdown in the integrity of the alveolar-capillary barrier.

Measurements of lung water have long been the goal of clinical physiologists investigating ARDS. An excellent review of the relative merits of a range of techniques is presented by Staub (1986). These include radiography, soluble gas and indicator dilution methods, computed tomography and NMR. It is our opinion that, with the exception of the chest radiograph, lung water measurements are not useful in clinical practice.

Studies of lung inflammation in ARDS using labelled neutrophils have, as one might expect, shown neutrophil accumulation in the lung (Fein et al 1987). However this does not necessarily imply a causal relationship between neutrophil accumulation and lung injury (Flick 1986) and lung biopsy is clearly important in the search for specific microorganisms such as cytomegalovirus and pneumocystis.

TREATMENT

Successful treatment is based upon an increased awareness of the value of careful fluid balance, and a readiness to treat circulatory failure with inotropes rather than volume loading. Because of the loss of the protective gradient of osmotic pressure *it is crucial to avoid volume overloading* which increases pulmonary microvascular pressure. Other therapies to reduce lung water and improve gas exchange include *diuretics*, especially if there has been prior volume overload, and *vasodilators* to reduce pulmonary microvascular pressure, although the latter drugs may increase ventilation/perfusion mismatch and thus hypoxaemia. The role of prostaglandin E1 is now being extensively studied as a therapeutic agent in ARDS. Monitoring of the pulmonary artery and wedge pressures, at least in the early stages of the disease, is of considerable value but is not without risk and expense, and we feel is unnecessary in the majority of our patients.

The pulse oximeter is very useful in managing oxygen delivery in the ARDS patient with severe gas exchange abnormalities. In particular it is a useful aid in reducing the risks of barotrauma by finding an optimum oxygen saturation with the lowest possible airway pressure. Measuring mixed venous oxygen to 'optimise' PEEP may have no rational basis in ARDS, because a recent study (Kariman & Burns 1985) has demonstrated that peripheral oxygen extraction is abnormal in the established syndrome, varying greatly with the supply rather than with the presumed demand.

The dangers of barotrauma caused by the application of large tidal volumes and excessively high levels of positive end-expiratory pressure to normal and to structurally disorganised lungs are being increasingly recognised (Slavin et al 1982, Kolobov et al 1987).

Measurement of the static lung compliance curve commonly reveals an inflection point early in the course of ARDS, which indicates both whether PEEP is necessary, and the optimum value (Holzapfel et al 1983). Ventilating ARDS patients has been shown to produce better gas exchange in the prone position than in the supine and this has been confirmed in animal models of lung injury (Albert et al 1987). More complex manoeuvres such as high frequency ventilation (Butler et al 1980, Hamilton et al 1983) or extracorporeal CO_2 removal (Gattinoni et al 1980, 1984), which permit the lungs to be 'rested', may have attracted more attention than their real worth. Kawano et al (1987) showed that the conventional mechanical ventilation of surfactant-depleted lungs caused a progressive lung injury in contrast to the effect of high frequency ventilation where no such effect occurred. However in subsequent experiments they prevented this type of lung injury by prior neutrophil depletion which emphasises a role for neutrophils in the evolution of lung injury.

There is little good evidence for the use of steroids. Properly designed trials demonstrate that steroids given to patients who have aspirated increase the incidence of gram-negative pneumonia and worsen outcome (Wolfe et al 1977). A high risk group of surgical patients developed more infective complications and pulmonary dysfunction if given high doses of methyl prednisolone (Weigelt et al 1985), and preliminary analysis of results of a multicentre trial in the USA has led the major promoter and manufacturer of this drug to rescind sepsis as an indication for its administration. Although steroids were used in fire victims in the Falklands campaign, based on animal studies subsequently reported by Beeley et al (1986), other studies do not show any benefit in smoke inhalation alone (Robinson et al 1982) or in combination with burns (Moylan & Alexander 1978). The only circumstance in which there is reasonable evidence for their benefit is for the prophylaxis and treatment of fat embolism following major fractures (Shier et al 1977, Alho et al 1978, Schonfield et al 1983).

Outcome

A recent report (Montgomery et al 1985) suggests that respiratory failure is the cause of death in only 16% of ARDS: early deaths (before 3 days) were due to the underlying cause, whilst later deaths (after 3 days) were due to sepsis and multi-organ failure. However other authors (Fowler et al 1985) indicate that respiratory failure is responsible for 75% of deaths.

Despite the improvements in the management of patients in intensive care in the last 15–20 years it would appear from numerous studies (Asbaugh et al 1969, Asbaugh & Petty 1972; Petty & Newman 1978; Montgomery et al 1985) that there has been no significant reduction in the mortality of about 60%. However, it has been suggested that most patients with ARDS in risk groups such as trauma are treated successfully and survive, and that there has been a bias towards entering sicker patients into ARDS trials (Rinaldo 1986).

CONCLUSION

Over a decade ago, Murray (1975) questioned the value of grouping together an extremely heterogeneous group of patients under the label 'adult respiratory distress syndrome'. It is naive to anticipate a unifying pathogenesis, so that this approach may have hindered the realisation of effective specific treatment. An analysis of disease based upon aetiology generally clarifies rational treatment, and a return to classifying increased permeability pulmonary oedema by cause might aid this process. Finally, it would also be preferable to quantify the severity of lung injury by estimation of alveolar-capillary barrier permeability, rather than describing non-specific measurements such as lung water or gas exchange, which are so susceptible to the effects of myocardial depression, renal impairment and fluid overload. This would then provide a more precise end-point by which genuine improvements in lung function could be gauged.

REFERENCES

Albert R K, Ceasa D, Sanderson M, Robertson A T, Hlastala M P 1987 Prone position improves arterial oxygenation and reduces shunt in oleic acid induced acute lung injury. American Review of Respiratory Disease 135: 628–633

Alho A, Saikku K, Eerola P, Koskinen M, Hamalainen M 1978 Corticosteroids in patients with a high risk of fat embolism syndrome. Surgery, Gynecology and Obstetrics 147: 358–362

Asbaugh D G, Bigelow D B, Petty T L, Levine B E 1967 Acute respiratory distress in adults. Lancet ii: 319–323.

Asbaugh D G, Petty T L 1972 Sepsis complicating the adult respiratory distress syndrome. Surgery, Gynecology and Obstetrics 136: 865–869

Asbaugh D G, Petty T L, Bigelow D A, Harris T M 1969 Continuous positive pressure breathing (CPBB) in adult respiratory distress syndrome. Journal of Thoracic and Cardiovascular Surgery 57: 31–41

Avery M E, Taeusch H W, Floros J 1986 Surfactant replacement. New England Journal of Medicine 315: 825–826

Bachofen M, Weibel E R 1977 Alterations of the gas exchange apparatus in adult respiratory insufficiency associated with septicaemia. American Review of Respiratory Disease 116: 589–615

Barrowcliffe M P, Jones J G 1987 Solute permeability of the alveolar-capillary barrier. Thorax 42: 1–10

Basran G S, Byrne A J, Hardy J G 1985 A non-invasive technique for monitoring lung vascular permeability in man. Nuclear Medicine Communications 6: 3–10

Baumann W R, Jung R C, Koss M, Boylen T, Navarro L, Sharma O P 1986 Incidence and mortality of adult respiratory distress syndrome: a prospective analysis from a large metropolitan hospital. Critical Care Medicine 14: 1–4

Beeley J M, Crow J, Jones J G, Minty B, Lynch R D, Pryce D P 1986 Mortality and lung histopathology after inhalation lung injury: the effect of corticosteroids. American Review of Respiratory Disease 133: 191–196

Bell R C, Coalson J J, Smith J D, Johanson W G 1983 Multiple organ system failure and infection in adult respiratory distress syndrome. Annals of Internal Medicine 99: 293–298

Braude S, Nolop K B, Hughes J M B, Barnes P, Royston D 1986 Comparison of lung vascular and epithelial permeability indices in the adult respiratory distress syndrome. American Review of Respiratory Disease 133: 1002–1005

Brown M, Desai M, Herndon D N et al 1985 The use of dimethyl sulfoxide and heparin in the treatment of smoke inhalation injury. Anesthesiology 63: A112

Butler W J, Bohn D J, Bryan A C, Froese A B 1980 Ventilation by high frequency oscillation in humans. Anesthesia and Analgesia 59: 577–584

Cope D K, Allison R C, Parmentier J L, Miller J N, Taylor A E 1986 Measurement of effective pulmonary capillary pressure using the pressure profile after pulmonary artery occlusion. Critical Care Medicine 14: 16–22

Dauber I M, Pluss W T, Van Grondelle A, Trow R S, Weill J V 1985 Specificity and sensitivity of non invasive measurement of pulmonary vascular protein leak. Journal of Applied Physiology 59: 564–574

Evander E, Wollmer P, Jonson B, Lachmann B 1987 Pulmonary clearance of inhaled ^{99m}Tc-DTPA: effects of surfactant depletion by lung lavage. Journal of Applied Physiology 62: 1611–1614

Fantone J C, Ward P A 1982 Role of oxygen-derived free radicals and metabolites in leucocyte-dependent inflammatory reactions. American Journal of Pathology 107: 397–418

Fein A, Grossman R F, Jones J G et al 1979 The value of edema fluid protein measurement in patients with pulmonary edema. American Journal of Medicine 67: 32–38

Fein A, Lippman M, Holtzman H, Eliraz A, Goldberg S K 1983 The risk factors, incidence, and prognosis of ARDS following septicaemia. Chest 83: 40–42

Fein A, Wiener-Kronish J P, Niederman M, Matthay M A 1986 Pathophysiology of the adult respiratory distress syndrome. Critical Care Clinics 2: 429–453

Flick M R 1986 Mechanisms of acute lung injury. Critical Care Clinics 2: 455–470

Fowler A, Hamman R F, Good J T et al 1983 Adult respiratory distress syndrome: a risk with common predispositions. Annals of Internal Medicine 98: 593–597

Fowler A, Hamman R F, Zerbe G O, Benson K N, Hyers T M 1985 Adult respiratory distress syndrome: prognosis after onset. American Review of Respiratory Disease 132: 472–478

Gattinoni L, Agostini A, Pesenti A et al 1980 Treatment of acute respiratory failure with low frequency positive pressure ventilation and extra-corporeal removal of CO_2. Lancet ii: 292–294

Gattinoni L, Pesenti A, Caspani L et al 1984 The role of total static lung compliance in the management of severe ARDS unresponsive to conventional treatment. Intensive Care Medicine 10: 121–126

Gorin A B, Kohler J, Denardo G 1980 Non-invasive measurement of pulmonary transvascular protein flux in normal man. Journal of Clinical Investigation 66: 869–877

Griffith D E, Holden W E, Morris J F, Min L K, Krishnamurthy G T 1986 Effects of common therapeutic concentrations of oxygen on lung clearance of ^{99m}TcDTPA and bronchoalveolar lavage albumin concentration. American Review of Respiratory Disease 134: 233–237

Guyton A C, Lindsey A W 1959 Effect of elevated left atrial pressure and decreased plasma protein concentration on the development of pulmonary edema. Circulation Research 7: 649–657

Hallgren R, Samuelsson T, Venge P, Modig J 1987 Eosinophilic activation in the lung is related to lung damage in ARDS. American Review of Respiratory Disease 135: 639–642

Hamilton P P, Onayemi A, Smyth J A et al 1983 Comparison of conventional and high frequency ventilation: oxygenation and lung pathology. Journal of Applied Physiology 55: 131–138

Heffner J E, Sahn S A, Repine J E 1987 The role of platelets in the adult respiratory distress syndrome. American Review of Respiratory Disease 135: 482–497

Hills B A 1987 Bursting the alveolar bubble. Anaesthesia 42: 467–469

Holloway H, Perry M, Downey J, Parker J, Taylor A 1983 Estimation of effective pulmonary capillary pressure in intact lungs. Journal of Applied Physiology 54: 846–851

Holzapfel L, Robert D, Perrin F, Blanc P L, Palmier B, Guerin C 1983 Static pressure-volume curves and effect of positive end-expiratory pressure on gas exchange in adult respiratory distress syndrome. Critical Care Medicine 11: 591–597

Ikegami M, Jobe A, Jacobs H, Lam R 1984 A protein from airways of premature lambs that inhibits surfactant function. Journal of Applied Physiology 57: 1134–1142

Jones J G, Royston D, Minty B D 1983 Changes in alveolar-capillary barrier function in animals and humans. American Review of Respiratory Disease 127: S51–59

Jones J G 1984 Mechanisms and measurement of injury to the alveolar-capillary barrier. In:

Jones J G (ed) Effects of anesthesia and surgery on pulmonary mechanisms and gas exchange. International Anesthesiology Clinics 22: 131–148. Little, Brown & Co, Boston

Kaplan R L, Sahn S A, Petty T L 1979 Incidence and outcome of the respiratory distress syndrome in gram negative sepsis. Archives of Internal Medicine 139: 867–868

Kariman K, Burns S R 1985 Regulation of tissue oxygen extraction is disturbed in adult respiratory distress syndrome. American Review of Respiratory Disease 132: 109–114

Kawano T, Mori S, Cybulsky M et al 1987 Effect of granulocyte depletion in a ventilated surfactant depleted lung. Journal of Applied Physiology 62: 27–33

Kolobov T, Muretti M P, Fumagalli R et al 1987 Severe impairment in lung function induced by high peak airway pressure during mechanical ventilation: an experimental study. American Review of Respiratory Disease 135: 312–315

Lancet Editorial 1986 Adult respiratory distress syndrome. Lancet i: 301–303

Malik A B, Selig W M, Burhop K E 1985 Cellular and humoral mediators of pulmonary edema. Lung 163: 193–219

Mason G R, Effros R M, Uszler J M, Mena I 1985 Small solute clearance from the lungs of patients with cardiogenic and noncardiogenic pulmonary edema. Chest 88: 327–334

Mason G R, Duane G B, Mena I, Effros R M 1987 Accelerated solute clearance in P. carinii pneumonia. American Review of Respiratory Disease 135: 864–868

Milne E C, Pistolesi M, Miniati M, Guintini C 1985 The radiologic distinction of cardiogenic and noncardiogenic edema. American Journal of Roentgenology 144: 879–894

Minty B D, Scudder C M, Grantham C J, Jones J G, Bakhle Y S 1987 Sequential changes in lung metabolism, permeability, and edema after ANTU. Journal of Applied Physiology 62: 491–496

Montgomery A B, Stager M A, Carrico C J, Hudson L D 1985 Cause of mortality in patients with the adult respiratory distress syndrome. American Review of Respiratory Disease 132: 472–478

Moylan J A, Alexander L G 1978 Diagnosis and treatment of inhalation injury. World Journal of Surgery 2: 185–191

Murray J F 1975 The adult respiratory disease syndrome (may it rest in peace). American Journal of Respiratory Disease 111: 716–718

Niederman M S, Fein A M 1986 The interaction of infection and the adult respiratory distress syndrome. Critical Care Clinics 2: 471–495

Pepe P E 1986 The clinical entity of adult respiratory distress syndrome: definition, prediction and prognosis. Critical Care Clinics 2: 377–404

Petty T L, Newman J H 1978 Adult respiratory distress syndrome. Western Journal of Medicine 128: 399–407

Respiratory Diseases Task Force 1972 Report on problems, research approaches, needs. The Lung Program, National Heart & Lung Institute DHEW, Publication No. (NIH) 73–432, Washington DC, pp 165–180

Rinaldo J E 1986 The prognosis of the adult respiratory distress syndrome. Chest 90: 470–471

Rinaldo J E, Rogers R M 1986 Adult respiratory distress syndrome. New England Journal Medicine 315: 578–580

Robbins R A, Russ W D, Rasmussen J K, Clayton M M 1987 Activation of the complement system in the adult respiratory distress syndrome. American Review of Respiratory Disease 135: 651–659

Robertson B 1984 Surfactant replacement in neonatal and adult respiratory distress syndrome. European Journal of Anaesthesiology 1: 335–343

Robertson B, Berry D, Curstedt T et al 1985 Leakage of protein in the immature rabbit lung: effect of surfactant replacement. Respiratory Physiology 61: 265–276

Robin E D 1985 The cult of the Swan-Ganz catheter. Overuse and abuse of pulmonary flow catheters. Annals of Internal Medicine 103: 445–449

Robinson N B, Hudson L D, Reim M et al 1982 Steroid therapy following isolated smoke inhalation injury. Journal of Trauma 22: 876–879

Schonfield S A, Ploysongsang Y, Dilisio R et al 1983 Fat embolism prophylaxis with corticosteroids. Annals of Internal Medicine 99: 438–443

Seidenfield J J, Pohl D F, Bell R C, Harris G D, Johanson W G 1986 Incidence, site, and outcome of infections in patients with the adult respiratory distress syndrome. American Review of Respiratory Disease 134: 12–16

Shier M R, Wilson R F, James R E, Riddle J, Mammen E F, Pedersen H E 1977 Fat embolism prophylaxis: a study of four treatment modalities. Journal of Trauma 17: 621–628

Slavin G, Nunn J F, Crow J 1982 Bronchiolectasis — a complication of artificial ventilation. British Medical Journal 285: 931–934

Sprung C L, Rackow E G, Fein A M, Jacob A I, Isikoff S K 1981 The spectrum of pulmonary edema; differentiation of cardiogenic, intermediate and non-cardiogenic forms of pulmonary edema. American Review of Respiratory Disease 124: 718–722

Staub N C 1986 Clinical use of lung water measurements: report of a workshop. Chest 90: 588–594

Stein L, Beraud J-J, Cavinilles J, da Luz P, Weil M H, Shubin H 1974 Pulmonary edema during fluid infusion in the absence of heart failure. Journal of the American Medical Association 229: 65–68

Swan H J C, Ganz W, Forrester J, Marcus H, Diamond G, Chonette D 1970 Catheterisation of the heart in man with use of a flow-directed balloon-tipped catheter. New England Journal of Medicine 283: 447–451

Ten Centre Study Group 1987 Ten centre trial of artificial surfactant (artificial lung expanding compound) in very premature babies. British Medical Journal 294: 991–996

Tennenberg S D, Jacobs M P, Solomkin J S, Ehlers N A, Hurst J M 1987 Increased pulmonary alveolar-capillary permeability in patients at risk for the adult respiratory distress syndrome. Critical Care Medicine 15: 409 (Abstr)

Timmis A D, Fowler M B, Burwood R J, Gishen P, Vincent R, Chamberlain D A 1981 Pulmonary oedema without critical increase in left atrial pressure in acute myocardial infarction. British Medical Journal 283: 636–638

Travis J 1987 Oxidants and antioxidants in the lung. American Review of Respiratory Disease 135: 773–774

Unger K M, Shibel E M, Moser K M 1975 Detection of left ventricular failure in patients with adult respiratory distress syndrome. Chest 67: 8–13

Weigelt J A, Norcross J F, Borman K R, Snyder W H 1985 Early steroid therapy for respiratory failure. Archives of Surgery 120: 536–540

Weil M H, Henning R J, Morissette M, Michaels S 1978 Relationship between colloid osmotic pressure and pulmonary artery wedge pressure in patients with acute cardiorespiratory failure. American Journal of Medicine 64: 643–650

Weinberg P F, Matthay M A, Webster R O, Roskos K V, Goldstein I M, Murray J F 1984 Biologically active products of complement and acute lung injury in patients with the sepsis syndrome. American Review of Respiratory Disease 130: 791–796

Wolfe J E, Bone R C, Ruth W E 1977 Effects of corticosteroids in the treatment of patients with gastric aspiration. American Journal of Medicine 63: 719–722

Zapol W M, Snider M T 1977 Pulmonary hypertension in severe acute respiratory failure. New England Journal of Medicine 296: 476–480

Advances in ENT anaesthesia

The scope of ENT surgery has expanded considerably within the last few years. The introduction of the operating microscope and more recently the laser, have greatly facilitated surgery of both the larynx and the ear. The success of these surgical advances has become possible with better understanding of the relevant pathology and simultaneous advances in anaesthesia and pharmacology.

CONTROLLED HYPOTENSION

A reduction in blood pressure is essential for reconstructive surgery of the middle ear and control of bleeding has not only made this surgery feasible but increased greatly the chances of success. While smooth and properly administered anaesthesia is important, specific pharmacological agents are commonly used to achieve a fall in blood pressure.

Ganglion blocking agents

Trimetaphan is the commonly used agent from this group of drugs. Its hypotensive effect is mainly due to ganglion blocking action although impaired myocardial contractility with a fall in cardiac output also contributes (Adams & Hewitt 1982). It has a rapid onset and short duration of action undergoing hydrolysis by plasma cholinesterase and is administered by continuous infusion as a 0.1% solution. Trimetaphan however suffers from disadvantages such as tachycardia and resistance in some patients.

Sodium nitroprusside

This agent acts directly on the smooth musculature of the vessels, producing dilatation predominantly in the resistance vessels. It has no direct effect on myocardium and cardiac output is usually well maintained. Tachycardia may occur particularly in the young. Its popularity stems from its rapid transient action, easy controllability and rapid reversal of hypotension on stopping the drug administration. It is used as a 0.01% solution in 5% dextrose. The solutions are unstable if exposed to light and should be wrapped in aluminium or similar foil. The overall total dose should be limited to a maximum of 1.5 mg.kg^{-1} and the maximum rate of administration should not exceed 10 μg.kg^{-1}.min^{-1} in order to avoid toxicity.

Resistance and rebound hypertension may occasionally occur due to increased activity of the renin-angiotensin and sympatho-adrenal systems (Fahmy et al 1979, Khambatta et al 1979). The toxic effects of the drug are due to histotoxic hypoxia and metabolic acidosis due to release of cyanide (Vessey & Cole 1975). The signs of toxicity include tachycardia, progressive cardiovascular collapse, persistent hypotension even after stopping the drug administration and progressive metabolic acidosis. The treatment is administration of sodium bicarbonate and 50% sodium thiosulphate i.v. (25 ml) slowly and assessing the metabolic changes by frequent blood gas analysis and estimation of blood lactate. In resistant cases cobalt edetate 300 mg has been recommended (Cole 1979).

Trimetaphan-nitroprusside mixture

In order to avoid the undesirable and potentially toxic effects of both trimetaphan and nitroprusside it has been suggested that a combination of the two drugs (Dinmore 1977, MacRae et al 1981) in a ratio of 10:1 (125 mg trimetaphan and 12.5 mg sodium nitroprusside in 500 ml of 5% dextrose) should be used. The combination is synergistic rather than simply additive. The effects based on haemodynamic studies resemble those of nitroprusside but hypotension is achieved at a much reduced dosage thus avoiding toxicity particularly in resistant cases (Wildsmith et al 1983). However, tachycardia can still occur.

Nitroglycerine

The predominant action of nitroglycerine is dilatation of peripheral veins. Hypotension occurs as a result of a decrease both in the cardiac index as well as the systemic vascular resistance (Guggiari et al 1985). The heart rate remains stable or shows a small increase. Post-hypotensive rebound increase in blood pressure is uncommon due to a smaller increase in plasma renin activity in comparison to sodium nitroprusside (Guggiari et al 1985).

The drug is administered in a continuous infusion as a 0.01% solution and is stored in glass bottles or rigid polyethylene infusion packs as loss of activity occurs in contact with polyvinyl chloride. The usual dose is between 0.5 and 5.0 μg.kg^{-1}.min^{-1} the dose being titrated to the required levels of hypotension. The hypotensive effect is achieved relatively slowly, in 4–5 minutes, and may occasionally be unpredictable and difficult to obtain. Sodium nitroprusside in a dose of 2 μg.kg^{-1}.min^{-1} has been used to supplement its hypotensive effect (Guggiari et al 1985).

Adenosine and adenosine triphosphate (ATP)

The vasodilatory action of purines, adenosine and adenine nucleotides has been known since late 1920s (Drury & Szent-Gyorgyi 1929) and the use of ATP as a hypotensive agent has been recently examined both in experimental animals and in man (Hoffman et al 1982, Fukunaga et al 1982a,b). The hypotensive effect of intravenous ATP is due to its degradation to adenosine (Sollevi et al 1984a); hence interest is now focused on the use of adenosine as a hypotensive agent. Hypotension is produced by a profound decrease in peripheral vascular resistance accompanied by an increase in cardiac output (Sollevi et al 1984b), with minimal change in the heart rate. There is an overall reduction of myocardial work (Owall et al 1986). The fall in blood pressure is rapidly attained and is rapidly reversible upon discontinuation due to a very short plasma half-life of 10–20 seconds (Fredholm & Sollevi 1981). A considerable advantage of adenosine over ATP is the lack of phosphate and uric acid accumulation seen with the latter drug. The approximate dose is about 0.4 mg.kg^{-1}.min^{-1} but this can be reduced by simultaneous administration of dipyridamole, an adenosine uptake inhibitor (Sollevi et al 1984b).

Adrenergic receptor blocking drugs

These act by decreasing the heart rate, reducing the velocity and force of contraction and slowing conduction and are mainly used as adjuvants particularly in situations where induced hypotension is associated with considerable increases in heart rate. Small doses of propranolol (1–2 mg) or practolol (5–10 mg) i.v. are often used in combination with other drugs. Labetalol which has both alpha and beta blocking action (predominantly the latter) and acts by reducing both the peripheral vascular resistance and the cardiac output (Richards 1976) is sometimes used on its own in a dose of 0.2–0.5 mg.kg^{-1} to produce moderate degrees of hypotension.

Other agents

Potent volatile anaesthetic agents such as halothane and enflurane are widely used for lowering the arterial pressure either on their own or to supplement the effects of other hypotensive drugs. Their hypotensive effect is mainly due to a reduction in cardiac output (Adams & Hewitt 1982).

General anaesthesia for microsurgery of the ear

While many methods can be employed for producing hypotension, it is important not to overlook the accepted principles of safe anaesthesia. A limit, to which the blood pressure will be lowered, should be set at the beginning, particularly in patients with hypertension, coronary artery disease, pulmonary disease and in the elderly. Occasionally, reliance may have to be placed on local infiltration with vasoconstrictors.

Anticholinergic premedicants are avoided and anaesthesia is induced with an intravenous agent. The choice of the muscle relaxant depends upon whether ventilation is spontaneous or controlled. The advantages of spontaneous ventilation are maintenance of adequate cerebral and coronary blood flows, a well maintained cerebral arteriovenous pressure gradient due to maintenance of the negative intrathoracic pressure, the use of regular breathing as a sign of adequate cerebral perfusion and avoiding an increase in dead-space:tidal-volume ratio. However, oxygenation may occasionally be inadequate from combined effects of respiratory depression and ventilation-perfusion mismatch in the lungs and hypercarbia may produce increased wound bleeding and cardiac dysrhythmias. On balance it is better to use controlled ventilation but taking precautions to avoid hypocarbia. Sodium nitroprusside is the most widely used agent for inducing hypotension. The aim is to reduce the systolic arterial pressure to 60–70 mmHg. Occasionally if the consumption of nitroprusside appears to be high supplementation of hypotensive effect may be obtained by inhalational agents or the addition of adrenergic receptor blocking drugs.

Monitoring during hypotensive anaesthesia should include continuous monitoring of the arterial pressure, preferably using an intra-arterial cannula particularly where potent agents such as nitroprusside are used. ECG for heart rate and rhythm and ST segment and T-wave changes, end-tidal carbon dioxide concentrations or arterial carbon dioxide tension, central venous pressure and if necessary urine output in selected cases should be monitored throughout. A cerebral function monitor may be used to detect dangerous decreases in cerebral blood flow and cerebral activity. Pulse oximeters are now becoming available and would provide a continuous non-invasive measurement of oxygen saturation and it is likely that these will become standard monitoring in patients whose blood pressure is deliberately lowered.

The complications of inducing hypotension are mainly related to the level to which the arterial pressure is lowered and are reduced by careful attention to detail. Arterial pressure should be allowed to rise immediately if signs of myocardial ischaemia appear. Urine output may be temporarily depressed but improves once the arterial pressure rises. The incidence of cerebral complications is similarly low in carefully controlled hypotension (Pasch & Huk 1986).

NITROUS OXIDE AND MIDDLE EAR PRESSURE

Nitrous oxide diffuses into air-filled cavities including the middle ear in proportion to its partial pressure at a much greater rate than nitrogen can diffuse out. Inhalation of 67% nitrous oxide in oxygen increases the middle ear pressure in adults at a rate of 0.15 kPa.min^{-1} (15 mm H_2O) reaching peak values in about 15 min sometimes in excess of 6.0 kPa (600 mm H_2O) (Mann et al 9185, O'Neill 1985). The rate of pressure rise may be even greater in children (Casey & Drake-Lee 1982). Although the pressure falls rapidly once nitrous oxide is discontinued, negative pressure in the middle ear cavity may persist for a day or more (Blackstock & Gettes 1986).

Except in the occasional situation where the rise in pressure may force an otherwise irreversible atelectatic tympanic membrane into its normal contour and position (Graham & Knight 1981), the rise in pressure in the middle ear may be sufficient to rupture the tympanic membrane (Man et al 1980). The harmful effects of nitrous oxide administration however, arise in the postoperative period due to development of negative pressure in the middle ear cavity giving rise to pain, impaired hearing, and nausea and vomiting (Normandin et al 1982, Mann et al 1985, Blackstock & Gettes 1986). More serious however is the risk of tympanic membrane graft displacement or even the displacement of reconstructed ossicles. Since it takes about 40–60 minutes after stopping nitrous oxide to reverse the pressure changes (Jahrsdoerfer 1981, Mann et al 1985), it is advisable not to use nitrous oxide, particularly in the presence of pre-operative Eustachian tube blockage.

AIRWAY OBSTRUCTION IN CHILDREN

Airway obstruction in children is a potentially serious problem which may need urgent attention. The diagnosis is based mostly on clinical signs such as chest and suprasternal retraction and stridor during inspiration in conditions like epiglottitis, laryngotracheobronchitis, laryngomalacia and choanal atresia or prolonged forced expiration and wheeze with foreign bodies in the trachea or bronchi. In either case the respiratory rate is increased and the child is very anxious and restless. It is likely that some degree of hypoxia and hypercarbia are present in a child presenting with these signs.

Acute epiglottitis

Acute epiglottitis is a rare but dangerous condition occurring in children 5 to 6 years old with occasional reports in adults (Bishop 1981, Baines et al 1984, Muller & Fliegel 1985). Presenting symptoms in the early stages include fever and refusal to take food or drink as in other febrile states. However quite soon the child is seen sitting up and leaning forward with drooling of saliva due to pain on swallowing, and a thick muffled voice. Swelling of the epiglottitis and ary-epiglottic folds may be seen in the lateral X- rays of the neck but should not be carried out as an urgent measure for establishing the diagnosis unless the child is supervised at all times. The most common organism cultured is *Haemophilus influenzae B* (Baines et al 1984).

Severe respiratory obstruction can develop very quickly in acute epiglottitis. Such a child should be taken to the operating theatre straightaway in the sitting position. No attempt should be made at cannulation of a vein at this stage. Anaesthesia is induced gently by inhalation of halothane in 100% oxygen in the sitting position. Ventilation is assisted as soon as feasible and venous access secured and atropine administered if required. Intubation should be carried out initially under direct vision with a generally smaller than usual oral tube changed subsequently to a nasotracheal tube. In severe cases with the epiglottis looking like a red cherry, the only pointer to the glottic opening may be the expulsion of small bubbles of air from the trachea through the oedematous glottic tissues; this sign may be enhanced by gently compressing the chest wall. In such situations the airway may be initially secured by the passage of a small rigid bronchoscope. The nasotracheal tube may have to be left in situ for 1 to 3 days and until a leak can be detected around it. Tracheostomy, although commonly used at one time, is rarely required (Baines et al 1984). All children are given ampicillin or chloramphenicol intravenously and allowed warm humidified oxygen-enriched air to breathe. Conservative management without intubation may be employed in less severe cases but only if constant attention and expert assistance are available at all times.

Laryngotracheobronchitis

Acute laryngotracheobronchitis is a viral infection usually affecting children under 3 years of age and can be confused with acute epiglottitis. The onset in laryngotracheobronchitis is, however, more gradual starting with an upper respiratory infection followed by stridor, increased respiratory rate, tachycardia and restlessness. Respiratory problems may be further increased by secondary bacterial infection. There is usually no sore throat, dysphagia or drooling and the child does not appear very toxic. The treatment for less severe cases may be the administration of humidified oxygen in a mist tent. Inhalation of 20% racemic adrenaline provides a means of shrinking the mucosa but may need to be repeated. If the severity of airway obstruction increases treatment should be instituted on the same lines as for acute epiglottitis.

Laryngomalacia

This transient form of stridor is due to abnormal flaccidity of the laryngeal tissues. The flaccid epiglottis or ary-epiglottic folds are drawn into the glottis during inspiration. The condition improves with growth of the infant and usually disappears by 2 years of age.

Congenital subglottic stenosis

Congenital subglottic stenosis may become manifest at 2 to 3 months of age with a characteristic 'brassy' stridor and a respiratory infection which is difficult to clear. The diagnosis is confirmed by bronchoscopy. A child who survives the first 2 or 3 months will perhaps reach adult life. Tracheal dilatation is not helpful and tracheostomy is necessary if the airway is inadequate.

Congenital cysts and tumours of larynx

Congenital cysts are rare but can result in respiratory obstruction at birth or soon afterwards and these may obscure the normal anatomy. It is usually possible to pass a tracheal tube which must be kept in place till the cyst is evacuated. Emergency tracheostomy is required only very rarely.

Cystic hygromas may sometimes present as respiratory obstruction due to pressure on the larynx and trachea. Inhalational induction is usually employed and muscle relaxants should be avoided if there is any difficulty in ventilation. Rarely awake intubation may be necessary.

Foreign bodies

Inhalation of foreign bodies must be considered as a cause of airway obstruction in children up to 3 or 4 years old particularly when choking, coughing or wheezing are of a very sudden onset. The signs and symptoms vary from simple hoarseness to severe asphyxia and sudden death. A single foreign body lodged beyond the carina rarely causes acute respiratory distress and may present after considerable delay with chronic cough, localised pneumonia or wheezing. However, a foreign body lodged in the larynx or trachea or multiple foreign bodies involving both bronchi will cause severe respiratory obstruction. The most common foreign body is peanuts and these should be removed promptly as these may not only fragment but also produce intense inflammation with swelling and oedema.

The diagnosis is confirmed by antero-posterior and lateral chest X-rays or fluoroscopic examination revealing distended areas of the lungs or atelectasis distal to the obstruction.

Atropine should be given to decrease salivary and bronchial secretions and to obtund vagal reflexes during endoscopy. Foreign bodies are usually removed by rigid bronchoscopy but a flexible fibreoptic bronchoscope has also been used for this purpose (Laurence & Burton 1986). Induction with halothane in a high oxygen concentration with spontaneous ventilation is a safe method of anaesthesia. Anaesthesia is continued via the side arm of the bronchoscope. Breath holding and bronchial or chest wall spasm are overcome by deepening anaesthesia and instilling lignocaine down the bronchoscope or administration of suxamethonium, particularly when the endoscopist is attempting to grip and manipulate a large foreign body through the vocal cords.

An alternative technique of anaesthesia for bronchoscopic removal of foreign bodies, which can give at least as good operating conditions is to

use the jet injector. This requires of course that the patient be fully paralysed throughout the procedure.

Following bronchoscopy for removal of foreign bodies the child should
be nursed in a highly humid atmosphere for at least 24 hours and if
respiratory distress or stridor persist, oxygen and steroids should be given.

Foreign bodies lodged firmly in the lower part of the trachea are of
particular danger because even a tracheostomy may be of no help in
regaining a patent airway. Such cases have been managed on cardiopulmonary bypass by cannulation of the femoral vessels under local anaesthesia
before induction of general anaesthesia (Maharaj et al 1983).

MICROSURGERY OF THE LARYNX

Although local anaesthesia combined with sedation is occasionally used for
microlaryngoscopy, general anaesthesia provides good patient comfort. The
main problem in microsurgery of the larynx is the sharing of the airway by
the surgeon and the anaesthetist and close co-operation between the two is
essential. The problematic cases are those with proliferative laryngeal
tumours accompanied by oedema, leading to significant narrowing of the
airway. A local anaesthetic technique employing spraying the mouth,
pharynx and larynx with lignocaine may be advisable in these cases to carry
out a preliminary laryngoscopy and assessment of laryngeal space available
for intubation. The majority of the patients, however, do not pose these
problems. General anaesthesia is induced using an intravenous or an inhalational agent, the agents used thereafter depending upon the method of
airway maintenance.

Anaesthesia using tracheal intubation

Although intubation facilitates easy maintenance of general anaesthesia with
a safe airway it may interfere with the surgeon's access to the lesion. A
smaller diameter tube (5.0–6.0 mm) has often to be used, necessitating
controlled ventilation. A higher concentration of oxygen (up to 50%) is
employed. Muscle relaxation can be maintained with a continuous infusion
of suxamethonium or the use of a small dose of one of the newer relatively
short acting agents, atracurium or vecuronium.

Anaesthesia using tracheal catheter

To avoid the interference from a tube it has been suggested that oxygen
and the anaesthetic agents should be insufflated down a 14 FG or a similar
catheter sited above the carina (Hadaway et al 1982, Young & Robinson
1983). Once anaesthesia has been induced and deepened using conventional
techniques, the larynx and trachea are sprayed with 4% lignocaine and the
intratracheal catheter inserted. General anaestheisa is maintained with an

inhalational agent in a high oxygen concentration or with intravenous agents (Liscombe 1982) with the patient breathing spontaneously. The superior laryngeal nerves may also be blocked. The disadvantages of this method are that it allows movement of the vocal cords and there is an unprotected lower airway.

Anaesthesia using jet ventilation

In this technique there is neither a tracheal tube nor a catheter down the larynx, thus allowing unobstructed access for the surgeon. The basic equipment for jet ventilation is shown in Figure 14.1 (Morrison et al 1985). Either oxygen or an oxygen-nitrous oxide mixture using a blender is used as the driving gas entraining variable amounts of air depending upon the duration of gas flow and the position of the tip of the injector. The cords should be fully relaxed with the line of the jet in the same axis as the trachea and with no mechanical obstruction to outflow of the air. For relatively larger tumours, a tracheal tube can be used initially for removal of the bulk of the tumour, followed by jet ventilation to remove the remainder. Jet ventilation systems may not ensure adequate ventilation in patients with low lung compliance, marked obstructive airway disease and severe obesity, where it is preferable to use a tracheal tube. Some form of intravenous supplementation such as small doses of opiates or infusions of methohexi-

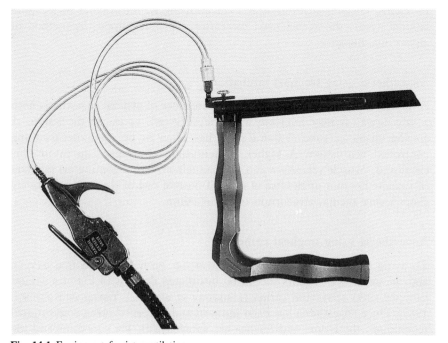

Fig. 14.1 Equipment for jet ventilation

tone or propofol are necessary to maintain anaesthesia. Muscle relaxation is again usually provided with suxamethonium.

Anaesthesia using high frequency ventilation

Use of high frequency ventilation has been recently suggested for ventilation during laryngoscopy (Smith 1982). Respiratory rates of 60–100 per minute and a ventilator driving pressure of 40–140 kPa are commonly used. The gas is delivered via a stiff catheter 3.5–4.0 mm in diameter passed through the nose or mouth and placed well below the vocal cords (Babinski et al 1980). The main advantages of this technique are the maintenance of a low airway pressure and good cardiovascular stability as well as a lower risk of surgical emphysema and barotrauma (Fischler et al 1985). Anaesthesia is maintained in the same way as for jet ventilation. The method is not widely available and conventional jet ventilation is the most frequently used method of airway maintenance during routine laryngoscopies lasting 20–30 minutes.

Airway maintenance and anaesthesia for laser surgery

Lasers are used in otolaryngology mostly for excision of various laryngeal and tracheobronchial lesions and less frequently in tympanoplasty, myringotomy, stapedectomy, choanal atresia, subglottic stenosis and soft tissue lesions in the neck. Lasers are accurate and precise in focal tissue removal and provide a bloodless field with minimal tissue reaction, postoperative pain and oedema.

Lasers (light amplification by stimulated emission of radiation) are associated with the production of a beam of intense, highly coherent monochromatic radiation focused on a very small spot with a high power density, which can vaporise the tissues or any other material. The lasers used in laryngeal and tracheobronchial surgery are either the carbon dioxide (CO_2) or the neodymium-yttrium-aluminium-garnett (NdYAG) type. The wavelength of the CO_2 laser is 10.6 μm and is strongly absorbed within the first 200 μm of any tissue traversed and can therefore damage all soft tissue cells. The beam is invisible and is not transmitted by fibreoptics and hence travels only in a straight line. Although these lasers have outputs of up to 50 W, commonly used power levels vary between 10 and 25 W in intermittent mode for 100–200 ms at a distance of about 400 mm. NdYAG laser can travel through flexible fibres 1 mm in diameter and has a wavelength of 1.06 μm and is also invisible. The output of 90 W is higher than that from a CO_2 laser. A pilot beam produces a red spot aimed at the lesion. The distance between the fibre tip and the target is 5–10 mm using a power of about 30 W for 0.7–1.0 s for coagulation and 40–70 W for 0.3 s once every 2 s for excision.

The considerations in the use of lasers are the safety of the operating room personnel, the patients and the equipment used. The high intensity invisible beam is reflected by mirror-like metal surfaces changing its direction and deflecting it onto an unintended target with the eye being the most vulnerable. All theatre staff should wear protective glasses and the patient's eyes should be closed and covered with moist pads. Matt black metal surfaces should be used to reduce the chances of beam reflection.

The problems of anaesthesia for laser surgery of the airway are mainly related to fire hazards (Healy et al 1984). The laser beam is capable of igniting all rubber and plastic material even in the absence of 100% oxygen and even when the tracheal tube is not in the direct path of the laser beam (Hirschman & Smith 1980). Several means are employed to overcome this problem. Ordinary tracheal tubes may be wrapped in muslin kept moist at all times; however, the muslin wraps are bulky, can come off easily and dry out. Flexible metal tubes (Norton & DeVos 1978) or vinyl plastic tubes coated with dental acrylic (Kumar & Frost 1981) have been used but such tubes are thick-walled and traumatic or rigid and bulky. The non-flammable 'laser shield' tube (made by Xomed USA) is a silicone-lined laser proof plastic tube but this can also ignite particularly in the region of the cuff. Bivona Inc. of the USA are introducing a silicone-lined plastic Fome-cuf (foam cuff) endotracheal tube (Fig. 14.2) in which the cuff is made of foam and thus unaffected if the laser accidentally hits the cuff region. The most commonly used tube, however, is a conventional red rubber tube slightly smaller than normal and wrapped in aluminium or copper foil in a spiral manner as far down as the cuff (Fig. 14.3). Although these have disadvantages such as causing trauma or accidental occlusion of the tube by the foil, careful wrapping can prevent most of these problems. Use of a mixture of oxygen and helium further decreases the chances of ignition

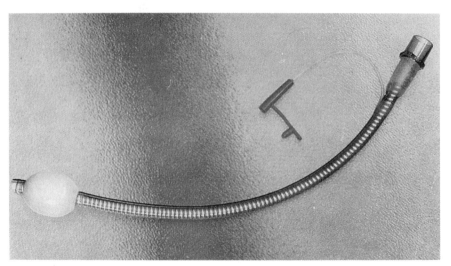

Fig. 14.2 Fome-cuf tracheal tube for laser surgery (picture courtesy of Bivona Inc, USA)

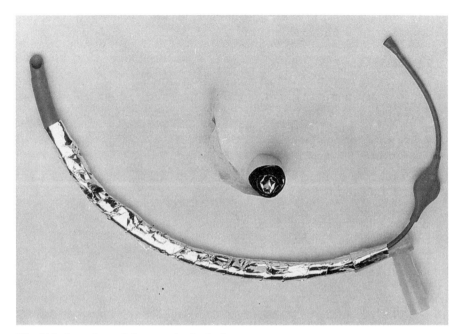

Fig. 14.3 An ordinary foil-wrapped tube for laser surgery

(Pashayan & Gravenstein 1985). In practice complete protection of the tubes is impossible and these should be lightly taped and be accessible throughout so that immediate extubation is possible in case of ignition (Vourc'h et al 1979). The cuff may be inflated with saline solution to limit the damage in case it is accidentally hit by the laser beam. If ignition occurs during the procedure, immediate bronchoscopy should be carried out to assess the damage and necessary treatment such as steroid and antibiotic administration, humidification of inhaled gases and tracheostomy with or without assisted ventilation instituted. Unrecognised complications may include perforations of the main trachea or one of the bronchi (Ganfield & Chapin 1982, Emery 1986).

The alternatives to the use of tracheal tubes are the use of an insufflation technique or jet ventilation. With insufflation techniques and spontaneous ventilation, there is however no control of the airway and the vocal cords are not immobile. Jet (venturi) ventilation has the advantages of providing good surgical access with an unobstructed view and adequate ventilation. The jet can be kept within the laryngoscope or a foil-wrapped catheter can be placed below the vocal cords as used by Rontal et al (1985).

Anaesthesia during laser surgery depends upon the technique of airway maintenance. If a tracheal tube is used anaesthesia can be maintained with nitrous oxide or nitrogen or helium in oxygen with the addition of a potent volatile agent following an intravenous or inhalational induction. Muscle relaxation is maintained either with suxamethonium by intermittent administration or by continuous infusion or with one of the newer agents, atracurium or vecuronium. The anaesthetic management using jet ventilation is as for microlaryngoscopy described earlier.

Anaesthesia for NdYAG laser surgery is usually maintained in the same way, jet ventilation being most commonly used (Vourc'h et al 1980, Sia et al 1985). Since the NdYAG laser beam can travel in optical fibres, the localisation is much easier with less chance of ignition of tracheal tubes. Unmarked polyvinyl-chloride tubes are preferable where intubation is carried out since these are slightly more resistant than foil-wrapped red rubber tubes to damage by the NdYAG laser (Geffin et al 1986).

Monitoring during microlaryngoscopy or laser surgery apart from the ECG and blood pressure monitoring should where possible include oximetry and capnography. Transient sinus tachycardia, ventricular ectopic beats and ischaemic changes are often observed during endoscopy. Prophylactic intravenous practolol in a dose of 0.15 mg. kg^{-1} may help to reduce the occurrence of sinus tachycardia and junctional rhythms (Sarnivaara et al 1986): moderate doses of fentanyl or alfentanil may prevent the increases in arterial pressure and rate pressure product (Wark et al 1986).

BRONCHOSCOPY

Bronchoscopy is an invaluable diagnostic and therapeutic procedure useful in many life-threatening situations. The introduction of the flexible fibreoptic bronchoscope (Ikeda 1970) has markedly changed the practice of diagnostic bronchoscopy. The management of patients for rigid bronchoscopy is a standard procedure described elsewhere recently (Morrison et al 1985) and the discussion here is limited to fibreoptic bronchoscopy.

The fibreoptic bronchoscope (Fig. 14.4A) is made up of fibreoptic bundles transmitting the light from a light source to the tip of the bronchoscope and the image from the distal telescopic end to the eyepiece. In addition there is a lumen for suction and all are made up as a flexible rod-like structure. Its smaller size and flexibility allow its introduction into the tracheobronchial tree well beyond the range of the rigid bronchoscopes, particularly in those with distorted anatomy. The disadvantages are the need of experience, inability to ventilate through it and the possibility of taking only relatively small biopsies. The first fibreoptic bronchoscopes were suitable only for adults, but instruments with external diameters as small as 2.0 mm are now available.

Fibreoptic bronchoscopy is commonly carried out under local anaesthesia. The instrument is usually passed through the nose after surface anaesthesia of the nose, nasopharynx and oropharynx with 1–2 ml of 4% lignocaine from a hand nebuliser. The instrument is advanced far enough to visualise the vocal cords and is advanced through them after spraying more lignocaine to anaesthetise the larynx, trachea and bronchi. The

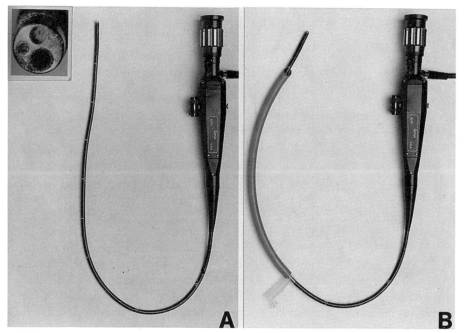

Fig. 14.4 A Fibreoptic bronchoscope with the inset showing the tip and **B** the endoscope with a tracheal tube over it

procedure is usually well tolerated and doses of lignocaine up to 370 mg have been shown to be safe (Sutherland et al 1985).

If general anaesthesia has to be administered, the bronchoscope is passed through a tracheal tube (Fig. 14.4**B**) about 2.0 mm wider than the scope using the space between the tube and the endoscope for ventilation and anaesthesia. An alternative is to pass the fibreoptic bronchoscope through a rigid bronchoscope which can be left in and used for ventilation in case of difficulty. Anaesthesia and ventilation are maintained using an intravenous technique and jet ventilation.

A natural extension of the use of fibreoptic bronchoscopes and more recently the fibreoptic laryngoscope has been in cases of difficult tracheal intubation. A fibreoptic rhinoscope 25 cm long and 3.7 mm in diameter normally used for intubating children has also been used in difficult intubations in the adult (Eriksen 1986). The fibreoptic endoscopy needs considerable skill and practice and should be used as a planned procedure. It is not feasible for use in urgent situations with increasing respiratory obstruction where cricothyrotomy, rigid bronchoscopy or tracheostomy may be more appropriate. Following a definite step by step protocol based on properly carried out training routines is important for ensuring success (Ovassapian et al 1983, Davies & Holloway 1986). The procedure is preferably performed in the awake patient with topical anaesthesia. The tracheal tube cut to the right length is threaded over the well lubricated endoscope which is passed as close as possible in the midline and once in the pharynx the tip is flexed upwards to bring the vocal cords into view. The tip of the endoscope is passed into the trachea through the glottis following straightening of the tip and the tracheal tube is threaded over it and the endoscope removed following fixation of the tube.

THE LARYNGEAL MASK AIRWAY

The laryngeal mask airway (Fig. 14.5A) is a unique and a different way of securing the airway and may be useful in some situations where intubation is difficult. An airtight seal is obtained by an elliptical cuff inflated in the hypopharynx around the perimeter of the larynx (Fig. 14.5B). The first prototypes were described in 1983 (Brain 1983) and results on its efficacy published by Brain (1983) and Brain et al (1985).

In the original prototypes the rubber cuff of a Goldman paediatric dental mask was stretched onto the diagonally cut endotracheal end of a Portex 10 mm clear plastic tube and fixed in position using acrylic glue. The pilot tube for inflating the elliptical cuff was attached to the inflation port of the cuff on the mask. The device is inserted like a Guedel airway. If there is

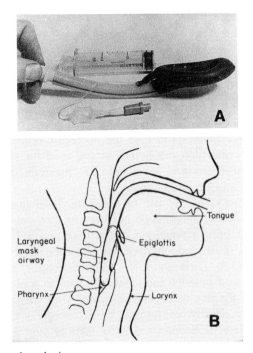

Fig. 14.5 A Laryngeal mask airway;
B diagrammatic representation of the laryngeal mask airway covering the laryngeal inlet (reproduced from Brain et al (1985) with permission of the publishers)

downward displacement of the epiglottis, the laryngeal mask airway can be inserted over a specially constructed introducer which guarantees correct positioning of the epiglottis (Brain et al 1985).

The laryngeal mask airway is useful where there is difficulty in maintaining the airway with a face mask or as a less invasive alternative to tracheal intubation and can be used during both spontaneous and controlled ventilation. The advantages are no trauma to the cords or trachea and no interference with mucociliary clearance. It can be introduced without a muscle relaxant under moderate depth of anaesthesia and can be left in place until the protective reflexes have returned. Portex Ltd are further developing the device.

POST-INTUBATION LARYNGEAL PARALYSIS

Varying degrees of pain in the throat and neck are not uncommon following tracheal intubation but are usually transient. Of greater importance however is hoarseness (Editorial 1986). While hoarseness is usually not due to vocal cord paralysis (Walts et al 1980) and may be due to nodules, granulomas or injury to laryngeal or surrounding mucosa, or due to surgical procedures, Cavo (1985) from an extensive search of the literature, found about 30 case reports of true vocal cord paralysis as a result of peripheral nerve damage following intubation.

Dissection of cadaveric specimens by Ellis & Pallister (1975) and Cavo (1985) localised the most vulnerable area to about 6–10 mm below the level of the posterior end of the free edge of the true vocal cords where the anterior branch of the recurrent laryngeal nerve may be compressed by an inflated cuff while passing medial to the rigid thyroid lamina.

The compression of the nerve may be due to an irregular or overinflated cuff placed just below the vocal cords (Renault et al 1985), or the diffusion of nitrous oxide from the anaesthetic gas mixture into a cuff filled with air with a significant rise (Fig. 14.6) in intracuff pressure (Raeder et al 1985, Cavo 1985). Coughing, straining and head movements may also raise the intracuff pressure. Other contributing factors may be the material from which the tube itself is made with red rubber tubes being more harmful (Lindholm & Carrol 1975) and the apparent mismatch between the cross-sectional shapes of the tube and the subglottic area (Mackenzie et al 1982), most tracheal tubes being circular and the human trachea elliptical at the glottic level.

The commonest presentation of vocal cord paralysis is hoarseness without respiratory distress even with bilateral involvement since the cords remain paralysed in their intermediate position due to exclusive paralysis of the adductors. Some simple precautions such as adequate general or local anaesthesia and proper muscle relaxation prior to intubation should be on the minds of all who practise intubation. Thin large diameter compliant cuffs which generally 'just seal' are preferable since these exert relatively

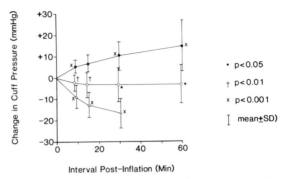

Fig. 14.6 Intracuff pressure changes following inflation with air ●——●, nitrous oxide and oxygen mixture ○——○, and nitrous oxide △——△. The patients have been breathing nitrous oxide and oxygen (reproduced from Cavo (1985) with permission of the publishers)

low intracuff pressures on surrounding structures (Bernhard et al 1985). An intracuff pressure of 25–30 cm H_2O (2.5–3.0 kPa, approximately 18–22 mmHg) will ensure adequate sealing of the airway without compromising the tracheal mucosal perfusion (Mehta & Mickiewicz 1985). The cuffs should not be overinflated beyond the point of just preventing air leak It may be advisable to inflate the cuff with the same mixture of anaesthetic gases as that used for anaesthetizing the patient, as Cavo (1985) has shown that this maintains the intracuff pressure at a constant level (Fig. 14.6). Depending on circumstances, cuffs may be periodically deflated and re-inflated to minimise any possible pressure effects or else a pressure-sensitive relief valve may be connected to the cuff. Alternatively the cuff may be inflated with saline but this may occasionally spill into the tracheobronchial tree if the cuff ruptures accidentally. Any irregularly inflating cuff should not be used and the cuff should be completely deflated prior to extubation.

The problems of inflation of the cuff are compounded by improper placement of the tube in the trachea. A distance of 1.5 cm between the true vocal cords and the upper limit of the cuff ensures that no undue pressure is exerted in the most vulnerable area (Cavo 1985). The tracheal tubes could be made with a mark about 1.5–2.0 cm above the cuff so that this point would be left at the level of the true vocal cords at the time of intubation. Alternatively the tracheal tube could be marked at this level just prior to intubation.

INTRACRANIAL SURGERY

Surgery for the decompression of facial nerve and for the removal of acoustic neuromas has been carried out by ENT surgeons for many years. In some centres however ENT surgeons are increasingly undertaking surgery of the pituitary fossa. The principles of anaesthesia are the same as for any type of intracranial surgery and have recently been described elsewhere (Ingram 1985).

REFERENCES

Adams A P, Hewitt P B 1982 Clinical pharmacology of hypotensive agents. International Anesthesiology Clinics 20: 95–109

Babinski M, Smith R B, Klain M 1980 High frequency jet ventilation for laryngoscopy. Anesthesiology 52: 178–180

Baines D B, Wark H, Overton J H 1984 Acute epiglottitis in children. Anaesthesia and Intensive Care 13: 25–28

Bernhard W N, Yost L, Joynes D, Cothalis S, Turndorf H 1985 Intracuff pressures in endotracheal and tracheostomy tubes; related cuff physical characteristics. Chest 87: 720–725

Bishop M J 1981 Epiglottitis in the adult. Anesthesiology 55: 701–702

Blackstock D, Gettes M A 1986 Negative pressure in the middle ear in children after nitrous oxide anaesthesia. Canadian Anaesthetists' Society Journal 33: 32–35

Brain A I J 1983 The laryngeal mask — a new concept in airway management. British Journal of Anaesthesia 55: 801–805

Brain A I J, McGhee T D, McAteer E J, Thomas A, Abu-Saad M A W, Bushman J A 1985 The laryngeal mask airway: development and preliminary trials of a new type of airway. Anaesthesia 40: 356–361

Casey W F, Drake-Lee A B 1982 Nitrous oxide and middle ear pressure: a study of induction methods in children. Anaesthesia 37: 896–900

Cavo J W 1985 True vocal cord paralysis following intubation. Laryngoscope 95: 1352–1359

Cole P 1979 Sodium nitroprusside. In: Langton-Hewer C, Atkinson R S (eds) Recent advances in anaesthesia and analgesia 13, Churchill Livingstone, Edinburgh, pp 139–149

Davies N J H, Holloway T E 1986 Training in fibreoptic intubation. Anaesthesia 41: 1265

Dinmore P 1977 Combined use of trimetaphan and sodium nitroprusside. British Journal of Anaesthesia 49: 1070

Drury A N, Szent-Gyorgyi A 1929 The physiological activity of adenine compounds with especial reference to their action upon the mammalian heart. Journal of Physiology (London) 68: 213–237

Editorial 1986 Laryngeal paralysis after endotracheal intubation. Lancet 1: 536–537

Ellis P D M, Pallister W K 1975 Recurrent laryngeal nerve palsy and endotracheal intubation. Journal of Laryngology and Otology 89: 823–826

Emery R A 1986 Laser perforation of a main stem bronchus. Anesthesiology 64: 120–122

Eriksen S 1986 The fibreoptic rhinoscope in adult intubation. Anesthesiology 64: 128–129

Fahmy N R, Sunder N, Moss J, Slater E, Lappas D G 1979 Tachyphylaxis to nitroprusside. Role of renin-angiotensin system and catecholamines in its development. Anesthesiology 51: S72

Fischler M, Seigneur F, Bourreli B, Melchior J C, Lavaud C Vourc'h G 1985 Jet ventilation using low or high frequencies during bronchoscopy. British Journal of Anaesthesia 57: 382–388

Fredholm B B, Sollevi A 1981 The release of adenosine and inosine from canine subcutaneous adipose tissue by nerve stimulation and noradrenaline. Journal of Physiology (London) 313: 351–367

Fukunaga A F, Flacke W E, Bloor B C 1982a Hypotensive effects of adenosine and adenosine triphosphate compared with sodium nitroprusside. Anesthesia and Analgesia 61: 273–278

Fukunaga A F, Ikeda K, Matsuda I 1982b ATP-induced hypotensive anesthesia during surgery. Anesthesiology 57: A65

Ganfield R A, Chapin J W 1982 Pneumothorax with upper airway laser surgery. Anesthesiology 56: 398–399

Geffin B, Shapshay S M, Bellack G S, Hobin K, Setzer S E 1986 Flammability of endotracheal tubes during Nd-YAG laser application in the airway. Anesthesiology 65: 511–515

Graham M D, Knight P R 1981 Atelectatic tympanic membrane reversal by nitrous oxide supplemented anesthesia and polyethylene ventilation tube insertion. Laryngoscope 91: 1469–1471

Guggiari M, Dagreon F, Lienhart A et al 1985 Use of nitroglycerine to produce controlled decreases in mean arterial pressure to less than 50 mmHg. British Journal of Anaesthesia 57: 142–147

Hadaway E G, Page J, Shortbridge R T 1982 Anaesthesia for microsurgery of the larynx. Annals of the Royal College of Surgeons of England 64: 279–280

Healy G B, Strong M S, Shapshay S, Vaughan C, Jako G 1984 Complications of CO_2 laser surgery of the aerodigestive tract: Experience of 4416 cases. Otolaryngology Head Neck Surgery 92: 13–18

Hirshman C, Smith J 1980 Indirect ignition of the endotracheal tube during carbon dioxide laser surgery. Archives of Otolaryngology 106: 639–641

Hoffman W E, Satinover I, Miletich D J, Albrecht R F, Gans B J 1982 Cardiovascular changes during sodium nitroprusside or adenosine triphosphate infusion in the rat. Anesthesia and Analgesia 61: 99–103

Ikeda S 1970 Flexible bronchofiberoscope. Annals of Otology, Rhinology and Laryngology 79: 916–923

Ingram G S 1985 Neurosurgical anaesthesia. Kaufman L (ed) Anaesthesia review 3 Churchill Livingstone, Edinburgh, pp 99–109

Jahrsdoerfer R A 1981 Anesthesia in otologic surgery. Otolaryngologic Clinics of North America 14: 699–704

Khambatta H J, Stone J G, Khan E 1979 Hypertension during anesthesia on discontinuation of sodium nitroprusside induced hypotension. Anesthesiology 51: 127–130

Kumar A, Frost E 1981 Prevention of fire hazard during laser microsurgery. Anesthesiology 54: 350

Laurence A S, Burton A 1986 Removal of inhaled peanut using a fibreoptic bronchoscope. Anaesthesia 41: 1269–1270

Lindholm C E, Carrol R G 1975 Evaluation of tube deformation pressure in vitro. Critical Care Medicine 2: 196–199

Liscombe R M 1982 Anaesthesia for microsurgery of the larynx. Annals of the Royal College of Surgeons of England 64: 430

Mackenzie C F, Hallisey J, Clark D, Steinberg S, Helrich M 1982 Adult tracheal and laryngeal dimensions as an indicator for correct tracheal tube size. Anesthesiology 57: A500

MacRae W R, Wildsmith J A W, Dale B A B 1981 Induced hypotension with a mixture of sodium nitroprusside and trimetaphan camsylate. Anaesthesia 36: 312–315

Maharaj R J, Whitton I, Blyth D 1983 Emergency extracorporeal oxygenation for an intratracheal foreign body. Anaesthesia 38: 471–474

Man A, Segal S, Ezra S 1980 Ear injury caused by elevated intratympanic pressure during general anaesthesia. Acta Anaesthesiologica Scandinavica 24: 224–226

Mann M S, Woodsford P V, Jones R M 1985 Anaesthetic carrier gases: their effect on middle-ear pressure perioperatively. Anaesthesia 40: 8–11

Mehta S, Mickiewicz M 1985 Pressure in large volume, low pressure cuffs: its significance, measurement and regulation. Intensive Care Medicine 11: 267–272

Morrison J D, Mirakhur R K, Craig H J L 1985 Anaesthesia for eye, ear, nose and throat surgery, 2nd edn. Churchill Livingstone, Edinburgh, pp 51–80

Muller B J, Fliegel J E 1985 Acute epiglottitis in a 79-year-old man. Canadian Anaesthetists' Society Journal 32: 415–417

Normandin N, Perreault L, Plamondon L et al 1982 Change in the tympano-ossicular system under general anaesthesia with nitrous oxide and oxygen. Canadian Anaesthetists' Society Journal 29: 498–499

Norton M L, DeVos P 1978 New endotracheal tube for laser surgery of the larynx. Annals of Otology, Rhinology, Laryngology 87: 554–557

O'Neill G 1985 Prediction of postoperative middle ear pressure changes after general anaesthesia with nitrous oxide. Acta Otolaryngologica 100: 51–57

Ovassapian A, Dykes M H M, Golmon M E 1983 A training programme for fibreoptic nasotracheal intubation. Use of model and live patients. Anaesthesia 38: 795–798

Owall A, Sollevi A, Rudehill A, Sylven C 1986 Effect of adenosine-induced controlled hypotension on canine myocardial performance, blood flow and metabolism. Acta Anaesthesiologica Scandinavica 30: 167–172

Pasch T, Huk W 1986 Cerebral complications following induced hypotension. European Journal of Anaesthesiology 3: 299–312

Pashayan A G, Gravenstein J S 1985 Helium retards endotracheal tube fires from carbon dioxide lasers. Anesthesiology 62: 274–277

Raeder J C, Borchgrevink P C, Sellevold O M 1985 Tracheal tube cuff pressures: the effects of different gas mixtures. Anaesthesia 40: 444–447

Renault J, Wesoluch M, Souron R 1985 Laryngeal paralysis after intratracheal intubation. Annales Francaises d'Anesthesie et de Reanimation (Paris) 4: 75–76

Richards D A 1976 Pharmacological effects of labetalol in man. British Journal of Clinical Pharmacology 3: 721S–723S

Rontal E, Rontal M, Wenokur M E, Southfield M I 1985 Jet insufflation anesthesia for endolaryngeal laser surgery: A review of 318 consecutive cases. Laryngoscope 96: 990–992

Sarnivaara L, Kentala E, Kautto U-M, Yrjola H 1986 Electrocardiographic changes during microlaryngoscopy in practalol-pretreated patients under balanced anaesthesia. Acta Anaesthesiologica Scandinavica 30: 128–131

Sia R L, Edens E T, Overbeek J J M, Rashkovsky O M 1985 Three years' anaesthetic experience with the Groningen Nd YAG laser coagulation technique. Anaesthesia 40: 904–906

Smith R B 1982 Ventilation at high respiratory frequencies. Anaesthesia 37: 1011–1018

Sollevi A, Lagerkranser M, Andreen M, Irestedt L 1984a Relationship between arterial and venous adenosine levels and vasodilatation during ATP — and adenosine infusion in dogs. Acta Physiologica Scandinavica 120: 171–176

Sollevi A, Lagerkranser M, Irestedt L, Gordon E, Lindquist C 1984b Controlled hypotension with adenosine in cerebral aneurysm surgery. Anesthesiology 61: 400–405

Sutherland A D, Santamaria J D, Nana A 1985 Patient comfort and plasma lignocaine concentrations during fibreoptic bronchoscopy. Anaesthesia and Intensive Care 13: 370–374

Vessey C J, Cole P V 1975 Nitroprusside and cyanide. British Journal of Anaesthesia 47: 1115

Vourc'h G, Tannieres M L, Freche G 1979 Anaesthesia for microsurgery of the larynx using a carbon dioxide laser. Anaesthesia 34: 53–57

Vourc'h G, Tannieres M L, Toty T, Personne C 1980 Anaesthetic management of tracheal surgery using the neodymium-yttrium-aluminium-garnet laser. British Journal of Anaesthesia 52: 993–997

Walts L F, Calcaterra T, Cohen A 1980 Vocal cord function following short term endotracheal intubation. Clinical Otolaryngology 5: 103–105

Wark K J, Lyons J, Feneck R O 1986 The haemodynamic effects of bronchoscopy. Effect of pretreatment with fentanyl and alfentanil. Anaesthesia 41: 162–167

Wildsmith J A W, Sinclair C J, Thorn J, MacRae W R, Fagan D, Scott D B 1983 Haemodynamic effects of induced hypotension with a nitroprusside-trimetaphan mixture. British Journal of Anaesthesia 55: 381–389

Young P N, Robinson J M 1983 Anaesthesia for microsurgery of the larynx. Annals of the Royal College of Surgeons of England 65: 135

Ophthalmic anaesthesia

INTRODUCTION

Although operations on the eye had been performed without anaesthesia for many centuries, it is less than 100 years since topical local anaesthetic agents were introduced. In 1884 Karl Koller performed operations on the eye using cocaine following the advice of Sigmund Freud. Later that year Herman Knapp described the method of retrobulbar anaesthesia, a technique which is still in use for ophthalmic surgery. Its use is especially valuable in patients with major cardiovascular disease. However the procedure may be associated with complications including retrobulbar haemorrhage, retinal vascular occlusion and scleral puncture (Feibel 1985). In the past 20 years improved optics in microscopes, anaesthetic techniques, and greater control of intra-ocular pressure (IOP) during surgery have led to the development of superior microsurgical techniques in ophthalmic surgery.

Ophthalmic operations can be divided into those which are intra-ocular, extra-ocular or both intra- and extra-ocular. They may be subdivided as follows:

1. Anterior segment
   a. Cataract extractions
   b. Glaucoma surgery
   c. Corneal surgery
2. Posterior segment
   a. Retinal detachments
   b. Vitrectomies
3. Strabismus surgery
4. Lacrimal surgery
5. Oculoplastic surgery
6. Orbital surgery
7. Ophthalmic oncology
   a. Retinoblastoma
   b. Uveal melanoma
8. Ocular trauma
   a. Penetrating eye injuries

This chapter will only review current concepts and recent literature on control of the intra-ocular pressure (IOP) and anaesthesia for anterior and posterior segment surgery and penetrating eye injuries.

INTRA-OCULAR PRESSURE

The IOP is the tension exerted by the ocular contents on the corneo-scleral envelope and its control is a major factor influencing the outcome of intra-ocular operations, which may be open, closed or mixed. In closed operations such as vitrectomies, intra-operative control of IOP is maintained by techniques involving intravitreal infusion, whereas during open (cataract extractions) or mixed operations (major ocular trauma) it is greatly influenced by general anaesthesia.

Cunningham & Barry (1986) have listed the requirements for open mixed operations as follows.

1. A stationary eye with extra-ocular muscle akinesis
2. Airway control with adequate alveolar ventilation
3. Cardiovascular stability with avoidance of stimuli likely to raise central venous pressure
4. Controlled IOP before, during and after surgery

Prior to surgical incision, a low–normal IOP is desirable; sudden decompression of a hypertensive eye may be catastrophic, with iris or lens prolapse, and vitreous loss from expulsive choroidal haemorrhage.

Factors affecting IOP

There are four major factors affecting the IOP.

1. Aqueous humour fluid dynamics
2. Choroidal blood volume
3. Vitreous volume and extra-ocular muscle tone
4. Scleral rigidity

Aqueous humour fluid dynamics

Alterations in the above play a minor role in the acute changes that occur in IOP during surgery. However, in the treatment of acute glaucoma, where there is a sudden loss of vision, intense meiosis, acetazolamide and oral glycerol tend to lower IOP dramatically (Smith 1983). Acetazolamide has a significant effect on the production of aqueous humour, but the exact mode of action of β- adrenergic blocking agents in reducing IOP is not known (McDonald et al 1977, Benson & Epstein 1981).

Choroidal blood volume

The choroidal blood volume is the single most important factor influencing changes in IOP during general anaesthesia. Many attempts have been made to measure choroidal thickness in vivo. Coleman & Lizzi (1979) using ultrasonography were able to distinguish between the retinal, choroidal and scleral thicknesses. We have found no evidence corroborating these results by other workers. Restori (1987) failed to measure choroidal thickness using the methods described by Coleman & Lizzi. However, Canning & Restori (1987) successfully demonstrated the variations in the velocity of blood flow in the ophthalmic arteries during anaesthesia.

Blood pressure (BP). The choroidal blood flow remains relatively constant throughout a wide range of perfusion pressures. However, sudden increases in systolic blood pressure do cause transient increases in IOP.

Central venous pressure (CVP). An increase in CVP is associated with an instantaneous and substantial rise in IOP. This may occur during light anaesthesia when there is straining or bucking on the endotracheal tube.

Hvidberg et al (1981) found that altering the posture from Trendelenburg to a 'head-up' position was linked with changes in CVP and IOP, producing a significant fall in both parameters.

pH, $PaCO_2$, PaO_2. Respiratory and metabolic acidosis, and alkalosis, have opposing effects on IOP. Samuel & Beaugie (1974) noticed, in patients without ophthalmic symptoms, that increasing the $PaCO_2$ resulted in a linear increase in IOP while the CVP remained constant. Smith et al (1974) confirmed these findings by maintaining a constant CVP at different values of $PaCO_2$. Hyperbaric oxygen tensions have been shown by Saltzman et al (1965) to cause a reduction in IOP due to profound vasoconstriction.

Vitreous volume and extra-ocular muscle tone

A combination of haemodynamic and hormonal control of the vascular and extra-ocular muscle tones is involved in the complex central control of IOP. In addition, Von Sallmann & Lowenstein (1955) demonstrated that stimulation of various centres in the cat diencephalon produced alterations in IOP.

Effect of anaesthetic agents on IOP

Most of the premedicant drugs have little effect on the IOP. Diazepam appears to lower the IOP and therefore benzodiazepines are favoured as premedicant drugs in ophthalmic anaesthesia (Al-Abrak 1978). Intramuscular morphine also decreases IOP (Holloway 1980). Intramuscular anticholinergic agents do not appear to alter IOP (Murphy 1985).

All the induction agents, except ketamine, lower IOP. Mirakhur et al (1987) found that propofol caused a greater reduction in IOP compared with thiopentone. Oji & Holdcroft (1979) found that a significant reduction of IOP was produced using etomidate as the induction agent, while Thompson et al (1982), noticed a greater decrease in IOP after an i.v. infusion of etomidate when compared with halothane.

Presbitero et al (1980) reported a dose-related lowering of IOP during neurolept anaesthesia using droperidol and fentanyl. The fall in IOP after midazolam was similar to that produced by thiopentone and diazepam (Fragen & Hauch 1981).

All inhalation agents save nitrous oxide produce a significant reduction in IOP (Holloway 1980). There are many reports of the effects of trichloroethylene on IOP, but the results are conflicting. Al-Abrak & Samuel (1974) discovered an increase in IOP using trichloroethylene under controlled conditions, but Adams et al (1979) found a slight decrease in IOP during normocapnic ventilation. The medico-legal aspects of repeated use of halothane tend to restrict its usefulness in ophthalmic anaesthesia. However, it still remains one of the most commonly used inhalational anaesthetics and like the two newer drugs, enflurane and isoflurane, causes significant reductions in IOP. During spontaneous respiration, halothane reduced the IOP by 18–33% (Magora & Collins 1961, Mehta 1962, Tammisto et al 1965). During enflurane anaesthesia there was a reduction in IOP by 21–40%. Runciman et al (1978), Radtke & Waldman (1975) and Ansinsch et al (1975) have demonstrated that isoflurane reduces the IOP in a manner similar to that of halothane.

In ventilated patients increasing the concentration of enflurane from 1% to 1.5% was not accompanied with a further lowering of IOP, but resulted in a marked decrease in systolic blood pressure (Zindel et al 1987).

Suxamethonium results in a short lived increase in IOP (Lincoff et al 1955, Adams & Barnett 1966, Cook 1981). Despite this, suxamethonium appears to be an acceptable relaxant for intubation for routine intra-ocular surgery. Pandey et al (1972) found that the IOP had already returned to normal at the onset of surgery. Its use for penetrating ocular trauma is controversial.

Various techniques have been suggested to modify the rise in IOP produced by suxamethonium, but none of these have proved to be completely satisfactory. These have included 'self-taming' with suxamethonium, pre-curarisation and the use of drugs such as hexafluorenium, acetazolamide, lignocaine, diazepam and droperidol. However endotracheal intubation especially under light anaesthesia results in a greater rise in IOP than that produced by suxamethonium.

Non-depolarising muscle relaxants do not increase IOP and in fact may cause a significant reduction (Al-Abrak & Samuel 1974). Tattersall et al (1985) noted a slight decrease in IOP following the use of fazadinium and atracurium when used for intubation. This confirmed the findings of Couch et al (1979) and Maharaj et al (1984). Sia & Rashkovsky (1981) reported similar findings with veccuronium.

Abbot & Samuel (1987) using 200 μg. kg^{-1} of vecuronium obtained satisfactory intubating conditions in all patients, the IOP not rising above the pre-induction level in 70% of the patients. The rise was also influenced by the administration of a small dose of alfentanil.

In spite of ideal anaesthetic conditions, there may be occasions when the posterior segment bulges into the anterior segment which may lead to vitreous loss during cataract surgery. The scleral elasticity in the younger group of patients may also be a contributory factor. It is also possible that there may be an increase in choroidal volume due to choroidal vasodilatation caused by the inhalational agent.

For posterior segment surgery, it is important to have a well controlled IOP with good choroidal vasoconstriction especially in the initial stages. A dilated choroid may result in severe choroidal haemorrhage during vitrectomy (Charles 1981). It may also occur during repeated surgical procedures especially in 'hot' infected eyes.

When bubbles of air, sulphur hexafluoride (SF6) and C3F8 are introduced into the vitreous cavity for internal tamponade of the retina, nitrous oxide should be withdrawn as it is 117 times more soluble than SF6. Stimson & Donlon (1982), using a mathematical model, predicted a three-fold increase in the size of the gas bubble when 70% nitrous oxide was used. Thus IOP and the tamponade effect of the bubble would be increased during surgery and markedly reduced postoperatively (Smith et al 1974). It is common practice amongst ophthalmic anaesthetists to use either total intravenous anaesthesia or inhalational anaesthesia with oxygen-enriched air to ventilate the patient.

OCULAR TRAUMA

Ocular trauma is a singularly challenging aspect of ophthalmic anaesthesia. Its problems are:

1. Associated trauma to other regions, mainly head and neck
2. Full stomach
3. Open eye injury

Improved microsurgical techniques for pars plana vitrectomy results in a considerably improved prognosis for useful vision in eyes previously thought beyond redemption. Cooling (1987) presenting the postoperative visual acuities (VA) in 100 consecutive major ocular trauma vitrectomies at Moorfields Eye Hospital, found only 21 patients (having no useful navigational vision) with VA of below 3/60. 49 patients had VA between 3/60 and 6/12 and 20 patients had VA of 6/12 or above. In this series there were 87 penetrating eye injuries while 13 had injuries as a result of blunt trauma. A complicating factor in 24 eyes was the presence of intra-ocular foreign bodies. In another series 62% of patients with pars plana vitrectomies following ocular trauma achieved visual improvement (Ryan & Allen 1979). De Juaan et al (1984) found no significant differences in two compatible groups of patients with ocular trauma treated with or without vitrectomy. However, among the vitrectomy group, beneficial trends occurred in particular types of injuries in patients with severe trauma and very low initial VA.

These reports indicate the high potential for visual improvement even in very severe eye injuries. This requires maintenance of ideal conditions during eye trauma surgery. Endotracheal intubation however presents problems, in that suxamethonium while providing satisfactory conditions for rapid intubation, especially in the presence of a full stomach, may result in a rise in IOP leading to the extrusion of ocular contents.

Many of the patients with eye injuries primarily admitted to specialist eye hospitals have no associated trauma, and, unless the damage is very serious, the operation can be postponed until the stomach has emptied. In situations where life-threatening generalised trauma complicates severe eye injury, anaesthesia is more urgently required. Cunningham & Barry (1986) concluded that there was no technique that consistently prevented the increase in IOP following suxamethonium.

Libonati et al (1985) reported a series of 250 patients with penetrating eye injuries treated over 10 years at the Wills Eye Hospital in Philadelphia, and suggested that 'despite the theoretical objections to suxamethonium, it was still a valuable part of the rapid sequence induction because of its quick action'. Adults in the series were pretreated with d-tubocurarine but children were induced with halothane and a suxamethonium drip was used to facilitate endotracheal intubation. These findings were supported by Bruce et al (1982) and Bourke (1985). However Weiner & Olk (1986) were opposed to the use of suxamethonium for penetrating eye injury as it might influence the results of surgery in patients to whom there was a potentially good visual outcome. This view was also endorsed by Rich et al (1986).

A major criticism of Libonati et al's paper was that the final postoperative VA has not been reported. Results of studies comparing the use of suxamethonium and non-depolarising muscle relaxants suggest that it would be imprudent to use suxamethonium for penetrating eye injuries. Murphy (1985) reviewed the other intravenous induction agents and found that apart from ketamine there was a significant reduction in IOP. Ketamine appears to be contra-indicated for intra-ocular surgery, although it has a place for paediatric ophthalmological examinations.

Calla et al (1987) found that etomidate produced a greater reduction in IOP than did thiopentone. Propofol, when compared with thiopentone, led to a decrease in IOP following endotracheal intubation especially when an additional small dose of propofol was given prior to intubation (Mirakhur et al 1987); it also led to systemic hypotension especially in geriatric patients.

In patients with penetrating eye injuries, Abbot & Samuel (1987) advised the use of high dose vecuronium (0.2 mg. kg^{-1}) following induction with thiopentone. Using the eyelid reflex as a reference point, outpatients were intubated within 60 seconds without coughing or bucking on the endotracheal tube. 70% of the post-intubation IOPs remained below pre-intubation levels. A subsequent study found that the administration of a small dose of alfentanil (0.015 mg. kg^{-1}) further attenuated the pressure response to intubation. Morton & Hamilton (1986) found that 20 μg. kg^{-1} appears to be the optimal dose to abolish the pressor and heart rate responses to intubation.

Oji & Holdcroft (1979) described the significant reduction in IOP following induction of anaesthesia with etomidate. In fact an intravenous infusion of etomidate lowered the IOP to a greater extent than halothane (Thompson et al 1982). Drenger et al (1985) in a study of 40 children ranging between 1 and 10 years, concluded that 2 mg. kg^{-1} of intravenous lignocaine approximately 2 minutes before endotracheal intubation significantly attenuated the increase in IOP.

Thus anaesthesia for penetrating eye injuries seems best performed with a rapid sequence of induction and intubation technique involving a non-depolarising muscle relaxant. Intravenous alfentanil or lignocaine may attenuate the pressor response following endotracheal intubation. A high dose of vecuronium is preferred to a 'priming technique' which may lead to an unacceptable level of side effects (Sosis 1985).

MONITORING

The conditions in which anaesthesia is administered for ophthalmic surgical procedures demands a high degree of patient monitoring. Continuous monitoring of blood pressure and ECG are routine. In addition, PCO_2 and oxygen saturation are monitored with capnography and pulse oximetry while neuromuscular activity is assessed by the use of a nerve stimulator. Cerebral function monitoring may become standard practice in the future.

MORBIDITY AND MORTALITY

As many of the patients undergoing ophthalmic surgery are elderly, it is not surprising that there have been many reports of central nervous system malfunction following general anaesthesia. Elderly patients may show increased sensitivity to anaesthetic agents (Atkinson & Henthorne 1985). Blundell (1967) reported temporary mental disturbance affecting the intellectual faculties in the elderly. Transient global amnesia, characterised by sudden transitory loss of memory of recent events has also been reported. On the other hand, Karhunen & Jönn (1982) compared memory function postoperatively in patients undergoing cataract extractions. There was a greater loss of memory in those who had the operation under local anaesthesia. Surveys from the USA suggest that morbidity and mortality are similar irrespective of use of either local or general anaesthesia (Duncalf et al 1970, Quigley 1974).

REFERENCES

Abbott M, Samuel J R 1987 High dose vecuronium and penetrating eye injuries. Anaesthesia (in press)

Adams A K, Barnett K C 1966 Anaesthesia and intraocular pressure. Anaesthesia 21: 202–210

Adams A P, Freedman A, Dart J K G 1979 Normal capnic anaesthesia with trichloroethylene. Anaesthesia 34: 526–533

Al-Abrak M H 1978 Diazepam and intraocular pressure. British Journal of Anaesthesia 50: 866

Al-Abrak M H, Samuel J R 1974 Effect of general anaesthesia on the intraocular pressure in man: comparison of tubocurarine and pancuronium in nitrous oxide and oxygen. British Journal of Ophthalmology, 58: 806–810

Ansinsch B, Graves G A, Munson E S, Levy N S 1975 Intraocular pressure in children during isoflurane and halothane anaesthesia. Anesthesiology 42: 167–172

Atkinson A J, Henthorn T K 1985 Thiopentone anaesthesia in the elderly. Anesthesiology 62: 706–707

Benson F G, Epstein D L 1981 Separate and combined effects by timolol maleate and acetazolamide in open angle glaucoma. American Journal of Ophthalmology 92: 788–791

Blundell E 1967 Psychological study of the effects of surgery on 86 elderly patients. British Journal of the Society of Clinical Psychologists 6: 297–303

Bourke D L 1985 Open eye injuries. Anesthesiology 63: 727

Bruce R A, McGoldrick D E, Oppenheimer P 1982 Anaesthesia for ophthalmology. Aescalapius, Birmingham, pp 74–75

Calla S, Gupta N F, Garg I P 1987 Comparison of the effects of etomidate and thiopentone on intraocular pressure. British Journal of Anaesthesia 59: 437–439

Canning C J, Restori M 1987 Personal communication

Charles S 1981 Vitreous microsurgery. Williams & Wilkins, Baltimore

Coleman D J, Lizzi F 1979 In vivo choroidal thickness measurements. American Journal of Ophthalmology 88: 369

Cook J H 1981 The effect of suxamethonium on intraocular pressure. Anaesthesia 36: 359–365

Cooling R J 1987 Personal communication

Couch J A, Eltringham R J, Magauran D M 1979 The effect of thiopentone and fazadinium on intraocular pressure. Anaesthesia 34: 586–591

Cunningham A J, Barry P 1986 Intraocular pressure — physiology and implications for anaesthetic management. Canadian Anaesthetists' Society Journal 33: 195–208

de Juaan E, Sternberg P, Michels R G 1984 Evaluation of vitrectomy in penetrating ocular trauma. Archives of Ophthalmology 102: 1160–1163

Drenger B, Pe'er J, Benezra D, Katzenelson R, Davidson J T 1985 Effect of lidocaine on the increase of intraocular pressure induced by tracheal intubation. Anesthesia and Analgesia 64: 1211–1213

Duncalf E, Gartner S, Carol B 1970 Mortality in association with ophthalmic surgery. American Journal of Ophthalmology 69: 610

Feibel R M 1985 Current concepts in retrobulbar anaesthesia. Survey of Ophthalmology 30: 102–110

Fragen R J, Hauch T 1981 The effect of midazolam maleate and diazepam on intraocular pressure in adults. Arzneimittelforch 31: 2273–2275

Holloway K B 1980 Control of the eye during general anaesthesia for intraocular surgery. British Journal of Anaesthesia 52: 671–679

Hvidberg A, Kessing S V V, Fernandes A 1981 Effect of changes in PCO_2 and body positions on intraocular pressure during general anaesthesia. Acta Ophthalmologica 59: 465–475

Karhunen U, Jönn G 1982 Comparison of memory function following local and general anaesthesia for extraction of senile cataract. Acta Anaesthesiologica Scandinavica 26: 291–296

Libonati M M, Leahy J J, Ellison N 1985 The use of suxamethonium in open eye surgery. Anesthesiology 62: 637–640

Lincoff H A, Ellis C H, Devoe A G et al 1955 The effect of succinylcholine on intraocular pressure. American Journal of Ophthalmology 40: 501–510

McDonald M J, Gore S A, Cullen P M, Phillips C I 1977 Comparison of ocular hypotensive effects of acetazolamide and atenolol. British Journal of Ophthalmology 61: 345–348

Magora F, Collins V J 1961 The influence of general anaesthetic agents on intraocular pressure in man. Archives of Ophthalmology 66: 806–811

Maharaj R J, Humphrey D, Kaplan N et al 1984 Effects of atracurium on intraocular pressure. British Journal of Anaesthesia 56: 459–463

Mechta M 1962 General anaesthesia on intraocular surgery. British Journal of Clinical Practice 16: 339–344

Mirakhur R K, Shepherd W F I, Darrah W C 1987 Propofol or thiopentone: effects on intraocular pressure associated with induction of anaesthesia and tracheal intubation (facilitated by suxamethonium). British Journal of Anaesthesia 59: 431–436

Morton N F, Hamilton W F D 1986 Alfentanyl in an anaesthetic technique for penetrating eye injuries. Anaesthesia 41: 1148–1151

Murphy D S, 1985 Anaesthesia and intraocular pressure. Anesthesia and Analgesia 64: 520–530

Oji E O, Holdcroft A 1979 The ocular effects of etomidate. Anaesthesia 34: 245–249

Pandey K, Badola R P, Kumar S 1972 Time course of intraocular hypertension produced by suxamethonium. British Journal of Anaesthesia 44: 191–196

Presbitero J V, Ruiz R S, Rigor B M, Drouillmet J M, Reilley E L 1980 Intraocular pressure during enflurane and neurolept anaesthesia in adult patients undergoing ophthalmic surgery. Anesthesia and Analgesia 59: 50–54

Quigley H A 1974 Mortality associated with ophthalmic surgery. American Journal of Ophthalmology 77: 517

Radtke N, Waldman J 1975 The influence of enflurane anaesthesia on intraocular pressure in youths. Anesthesia and Analgesia 54: 212–215

Restori M 1987 Personal communication

Rich A L, Witherspoon G D, Morris R E, Feist R M 1986 Use of nondepolarizing agents in penetrating ocular injuries. Anesthesiology 65: 108–109

Rundman J C, Bowen-Wright R M, Welsh N A, Downing J W 1978 Intraocular pressure changes during halothane and enflurane anaesthesia. British Journal of Anaesthesia 50: 371–374

Ryan S J, Allen A W 1979 Pars plana vitrectomy in ocular trauma. American Journal of Ophthalmology 88: 483–491

Saltzman H A, Anderson B, Hart L, Duffy E, Becker H O 1965 The retinal vascular functional response to hyperbaric oxygenation. Hyperbaric oxygenation (proceedings of the second international congress), Livingstone, London, p 202

Samuel J R, Beaugie A 1974 Effect of carbon dioxide on the intraocular pressure in man during general anaesthesia. British Journal of Ophthalmology 58: 62–67

Sia R L, Rashkovsky O M 1981 Org Nc45 and intraocular pressure during anaesthesia. Acta Anaesthetiologica Scandinavica 25: 219–221

Smith G B 1983 Ophthalmic anaesthesia. Edward Arnold, London

Smith R B, Carl B, Linn J G, Nemoto E 1974 Effect of nitrous oxide on air in vitreous. American Journal of Ophthalmology 78: 314–317

Sosis M 1985 A caution on vecuronium priming. Anesthesiology 63: 460

Tammisto T, Halalainen L, Tarkkanen L 1965 Halothane and methoxyflurane in ophthalmic anaesthesia. Acta Anaesthesiologica Scandinavica 9: 173–177

Tattersall M P, Manus N J, Jackson D M 1985 The effect of atracurium and fazadinium on intraocular pressure. A comparative study during induction of general anaesthesia. Anaesthesia 40: 805–807

Thompson M F, Brock-Utne J G, Bean P, Welsh N, Downing J W 1982 Anaesthesia and intraocular pressure: a comparison of total intravenous anaesthesia during etomidate with conventional anaesthesia. Anaesthesia 37: 758–761

Timpson T W, Donlon J V 1982 The interaction of air and sulphur hexafluoride with nitrous oxide; a computer simulation. Anesthesiology 56: 385–388

Von Sallmann L, Lowenstein O 1955 Responses of intraocuar pressure, blood pressure and cutaneous vessels to electrical stimulation in the diencephalon. American Journal of Ophthalmology 39: 11–29

Weiner M J, Olk R J 1986 Anaesthesia for open eye surgery. Anesthesiology 65: 109–110

Zindel G, Meistelmah C, Gaundy J H 1987 Effects of increasing enflurane concentrations in intraocular pressure. British Journal of Anaesthesia 59: 440–443.

Dental anaesthesia

INTRODUCTION

This chapter is primarily concerned with outpatient general anaesthesia for exodontia. Although the traditional dental gas has been administered since the early days of anaesthesia, the technique has become less popular in recent years. The reasons for this decline and the future of dental anaesthesia will be discussed. The place of new agents will be assessed as well as recent research in dental anaesthesia. Reference will be made to sedation involving intravenous and inhalational techniques while the practicality of monitoring in the dental outpatient environment will be evaluated.

INCIDENCE

The only statistically accurate figures for a yearly number of anaesthetics for dentistry in England and Wales are for 1976 (Dinsdale & Dixon 1978). Their survey produced a figure of 1200 000 general anaesthetics outside hospitals. In addition there were 400 000 sedation/analgesic or 'intermediate' administrations mainly for conservation. The Dental Estimates Board (DEB) (1986) figure of 956 170 anaesthetics paid for in 1976 is accounted for by the addition of community dental service patients and patients treated privately, but it includes some sedation procedures.

In 1971 the DEB figure for anaesthetic was 1217 950, in 1975 it was 1056 200 and this fell to 373 730 in 1985. In Sheffield the community dental service figures dropped from 2036 in 1975 to 804 in 1985 (Heesterman 1986). Parbrook (1986) found that in Scotland the number of general anaesthetics given in general dental practice and the community dental service nearly halved between 1975 and 1984. He suggested reasons for this reduction, the salient being the decrease in dental caries, which has occurred in industrialized countries over the last 15 years (Jenkins 1985). Though fluoride toothpaste is probably the major reason for the reduction of dental caries, there are a number of other factors which have played a part in the steady decline of general anaesthesia for dental outpatient surgery. The decline is most marked in the South East: there has been a parallel decline in the North albeit from a higher level (Dinsdale 1983).

Cause of decline

When the Health Service began in 1948, all treatment was free and this, with the derationing of sweets in the early 1950s, produced a vast increase in dental treatment. A conservative estimate put the number of general anaesthetics for exodontia at three million per year at that time, but the figure may have been higher. There are many reasons for the reduction since the '50s, some of which resulted in a gradual decline but others have been more recent.

Preventive measures

Improved dental hygiene has reduced the extent and severity of caries, and this has resulted from better dental education in schools and probably also from the subliminal effects of frequent television commercials for different brands of toothpaste (one of the first advertisements on ITV in 1955 was for Gibbs SR). Where fluoride levels in drinking water are 1 p.p.m. or more, either naturally or by addition, dental decay (caries rate) is much lower than in unfluoridated areas. Fluoridation of water in certain parts of the country such as Anglesey, Birmingham and Watford has produced an impressive decline in the caries rate. Although many parts of the country do not have fluoridated water, it has been appreciated by intelligent members of the public that fluoride tablets or drops will help to preserve their children's teeth and in fact it is now very difficult to buy unfluoridated toothpaste. Topical fluoride is less effective than oral administration. Children appear to retain the toothpaste in their mouths more readily than adults, increasing their exposure to fluoride and they also tend unwittingly to swallow it. The advent of fluoride toothpaste in 1974 has helped the decline in caries and exodontia nationwide, but patients in socio-economic group V from deprived inner-city areas may not be able to afford the toothpaste or the toothbrush.

The introduction of lignocaine in 1948 which was superior in action to those agents hitherto available led to improved patients' acceptance of conservation treatment. In the early 1960s the air rotor drill capable of a speed of 500 000 r.p.m. or more replaced the earlier cord-driven drill, reducing considerably the time to extirpate caries and prepare cavities for filling. Both these improvements have contributed to the comfort and well-being of dental patients, shortened the time spent in the dental surgery and encouraged patients to return for conservative treatment. Not only did this reduce the number of candidates for general anaesthesia directly, but made multiple extractions less common and encouraged the use of local anaesthesia for the extraction of one or two teeth.

In the very nervous patients including those with dental-needle phobia, restorative or conservative treatment can be carried out with intravenous or inhalational sedation techniques. Otherwise the patients might have been inclined to forego treatment and would eventually require multiple extractions under general anaesthesia. Advances in the techniques of intravenous sedation with local anaesthesia have reduced the necessity for extraction of teeth under general anaesthesia.

Improvements in general and public health, and diet following the poverty and poor nutrition of the depressed 1930s have produced a generation with structurally sound teeth. In particular, acute inflammation and infection may now be successfully treated with antibiotics, subsequently allowing the use of local anaesthesia. It thus becomes readily apparent why there has been a decline in the numbers of the 'dental gases' and its popularity has waned with the dentists and patients. However there are other practical and economic reasons.

In the last 30 years the number of patients receiving general anaesthesia in the Charles Clifford Dental Hospital, Sheffield has declined sixfold, whilst the number of students has doubled. The consequences are that it is almost impossible for dental students or even trainee anaesthetists to receive adequate instruction, training and practice in the administration of outpatient dental anaesthesia. Dental surgeons now qualify well able to extract teeth under local anaesthesia but are ill prepared for exodontia under general anaesthesia. In 1985 the General Dental Council (GDC) recommended that students should have practical experience in intravenous and inhalational sedation techniques, in general anaesthesia and resuscitation but 'students should qualify with the full recognition of their limitations in these aspects of pain control which must be recognised as subjects for postgraduate study' (GDC 1985).

A recent postal survey of British dental schools (Padfield 1987) shows a fall in the numbers of patients anaesthetized (mainly for extractions) over the 15 years between 1971 and 1985 (Table 16.1). It will be seen, however, that some departments have noticed a small upturn in cases in the last few years. This probably reflects the decision of the DHSS to stop paying fees for the operator-anaesthetists from 1 April 1983 and the condemnation of the practice by the GDC as constituting 'infamous or disgraceful conduct in a professional respect'. The increased attendance at dental schools may be accounted for by the increasing fees for general dental treatment (in dental surgeries), the retirement of the older group of GPs and GDPs who were expert at dental anaesthesia and the reluctance of younger members of the profession to undertake 'gas' sessions. Retirements have resulted in the loss of knowledge and experience which cannot easily be replaced. SHO posts in anaesthesia for dentists attract applicants in England and Wales, but not in Scotland (Parbrook 1986), and very few of these SHOs administer general anaesthesia in general dental practice, their expertise being devoted to sedation techniques (Hillary 1986, Thompson 1986). In addition, vocational training in general medical practice does not include anaesthesia although some GP trainees have held anaesthetic posts. There may be some younger partners in medical and dental practice who will

Table 16.1 Number of dental anaesthetics administered 1971–1985 (Padfield 1987)

	1971	1972	1973	1974	1975	1976	1977	1978	1979	1980	1981	1982	1983	1984	1985
Birmingham	6272	5386	4830	4198	3649	3367	3000	2880	2563	2411	2303	2170	1828	1900	1859
Bristol	*2340	2257	2178	2180	2012	1787	1792	1783	1732	1823	1652	1545	1537	1656	1493
Leeds	1835	2035	1956	2001	2018	1985	1819	1720	2045	1928	1856	1806	1699	1612	1465
Liverpool	6636	*6290	*5950	*5610	5270	5576	4621	4450	3880	3816	3328	2678	2571	2551	2206
Manchester	4363	4097	3504	4781	4683	4608	3878	3564	3269	2836	2657	2324	2387	2288	2520
Newcastle	3448	3177	2689	2560	2232	1837	1698	1898	1552	1697	1767	1673	1992	2071	1693
Sheffield	3024	3006	2850	2474	2755	2717	2697	2165	1954	1796	1291	1081	1070	968	1251
Total provincial	27 918	26 248	23 957	23 804	22 619	21 877	19 505	18 460	16 995	16 307	14 854	13 277	13 084	13 046	12 487
Dundee	1213	1189	1148	1064	958	898	789	643	606	516	577	559	634	543	684
Edinburgh	3083	2788	2823	2833	2722	2693	2345	2293	2244	2202	2075	2170	2458	2555	2628
Glasgow	3663	3791	4262	4065	3838	3759	3225	2881	2662	2552	2484	2369	2584	2903	3336
Total Scottish	7959	7768	8233	7962	7518	7350	6359	5817	5512	5270	5136	5098	5676	6001	6648
Cardiff	1930	2003	2058	1987	1964	2384	2268	*2080	*1890	*1700	1517	1579	1885	1731	1819
Guy's	*2800	2660	2375	2084	1891	1953	1949	1807	1579	1475	1435	1561	1482	1380	1343
KCH	5373	5506	5062	4761	3843	3848	3254	2951	2542	2471	2255	2253	2306	2091	2068
London	6962	6859	6095	5742	4661	3795	3812	3342	3527	*3350	3164	2799	2630	3023	3325
Royal Dental Hospital	3980	3978	4270	3896	3469	3525	2799	2449	2015	2037	1517	1446	1108	901	463
UCH	6090	5877	5528	5467	5254	5091	4342	3613	2851	2311	2120	1802	1328	1649	1484
Total metropolitan	25 205	24 880	23 330	21 950	19 118	18 212	16 156	14 162	12 514	11 644	10 491	9861	8854	9044	8683
Total anaesthetics in academic units	63 012	60 899	57 578	55 703	51 219	49 823	44 288	40 519	36 911	34 921	31 998	29 815	29 499	29 822	29 637
Dental Estimate Board	1 217 950	1 226 520	1 176 820	1 138 320	1 056 200	956 170 †1.2M	877 040	792 660	703 250	666 440	606 510	548 930	474 350	408 960	373 730

* Indicates approximation.
† Figures for 1976 from Dinsdale & Dixon (1978)

learn the art of 'dental gas' by apprenticeship to one of their seniors who have regular sessions in dental anaesthesia.

As dentists are paid by item of service they may be loathe to purchase their own anaesthetic machine, as this represents a poor return on capital for equipment costing well over £1000. In addition, there are the costs of ancillary equipment including monitors which are now essential for the safe management of general anaesthesia; it may also be desirable to have a defibrillator. Although trainee anaesthetists are taught to undertake preoperative assessment, to have venous access throughout anaesthesia, to monitor the ECG and blood pressure, and to ensure that the patient does not appear to respond to surgical stimuli, it is difficult to achieve these desirable standards in a busy dental surgery or even in some academic units.

However there may be an increased demand for general anaesthesia in the more specialized areas than the traditional 'dental gas', and these include (1) orthodontic surgery in children and (2) day case surgery.

(1) Four quadrant orthodontic extractions in children to prevent overcrowding of teeth may be carried out in one session under general anaesthesia. This is still controversial as the trauma of extracting four adult size molars in 8–12-year-old children can produce such a degree of pain and morbidity that a good relationship achieved between patient and dental practitioner may be undone. Some prefer several sessions of local analgesia with or without sedation, feeling this is a kinder and more humane treatment.

(2) The encouragement of day case surgery and the need to reduce waiting lists, has led to the treatment of impacted wisdom teeth in day case units in district general hospitals and dental hospitals. Fit young patients, who may have to wait for months or years for an inpatient bed, can receive endotracheal general anaesthesia in such a day case unit within a short time of the initial consultation. This is likely to be administered by a specialist anaesthetist who has access to full monitoring facilities. Pre-operative assessment may be carried out in outpatients before the operation and recovery should take place in a dedicated area with nursing staff providing postoperative analgesia as required. Intubation of patients for day case surgery of this nature is increasing, as borne out by the author's postal survey (Padfield 1987).

Parbrook (1986) predicted the demise of general anaesthesia in community and general dental practice within 10 years and in Scotland perhaps as early as 1992. This may be unduly optimistic given the natural conservatism of both professions and the fact that fees are still paid. The demise could be accelerated by ensuring that all dental anaesthetic machines were frequently tested and that maintenance contracts should be compulsory, adding to costs. Studies have shown that there may be gross inaccuracies in the delivery of oxygen and nitrous oxide mixtures in dental anaesthetic practice (Nainby-Luxmoore 1967, Hutchinson 1975).

MORTALITY

Bourne (1957) has steadfastly campaigned against the sitting posture during dental anaesthesia. Although he also advised against any restriction in the amount of inspired oxygen, he has maintained that 80–90% of all dental anaesthetic deaths are caused by fainting in the dental chair (Bourne 1986). Although there is a steady trend towards anaesthetizing patients in the supine posture, it is by no means universal practice in dental hospital or in general dental practice. A number of authorities have disputed Bourne's hypothesis. Coplans & Curson (1973, 1982) and Curson (1985) have analyzed deaths related to anaesthesia and local analgesia with sedation. Both they and Tomlin (1974) have concluded that the deaths that occurred were not primarily related to posture, and that a significant number occurred in the postoperative period and were then associated with cardiovascular collapse.

From the patient's point of view, sitting up with a normal field of vision may be more comfortable than lying flat with visibility restricted to a blank ceiling. Surgical access to the mouth, insertion of the gag and pack and application of the forceps may be easier and more convenient in the upright than in the supine position. For exodontia in the lower right quadrant the surgeon's approach from behind the head of the supine patient, may inconvenience the anaesthetist and cause difficulties in management of the airway. If the patient is lying flat any blood or debris not absorbed by the pack may be carried by gravity to the oropharynx and inhaled; this is less likely in the upright position.

The management of the airway in the supine patient is also aggravated by gravity. Occlusion of the oropharynx by the tongue may be more difficult to prevent and nasopharyngeal airway obstruction may occur in the patient with a large floppy soft palate (Tomlin & Roberts 1981). Thus respiratory obstruction may occur more readily while regurgitation of gastric contents, especially in the obese is an additional hazard. However, apart from the rare event of fainting, it has to be considered that prolonged anaesthesia with potent cardiovascular depressant agents may result in hypotension and possible cerebral hypoxia with the patient in the sitting posture. Although exodontia is associated with stimulation of the cardiovascular system resulting in a rise in blood pressure (Al-Khishali et al 1978), cardiac dysrhythmias also occur and these can result in a fall in cardiac output.

With the decline in the numbers of general anaesthetics administered for outpatient dental extractions there has been an associated reduction in the number of deaths. The statistics are bedevilled with inaccuracies due to the nature of reporting deaths to the Office of Population Census and Surveys and the difficulty of establishing the numbers of anaesthetics actually delivered. However, according to Curson (1985) 23 patients died in the years 1980–1983 compared to 43 in the period of 1970–1973; the figures included hospital inpatients and outpatients, general practice and community dental service. As the numbers of patients actually anaesthetized during these two periods probably more than halved, no progress seems to have been made in reducing the mortality rates. In fact if the figures only for general dental practice are considered, there were 26 deaths in the 1970s and 15 in the 1980s. The total number of anaesthetics and sedation techniques based on figures supplied by the DEB were 4846 980 (1970–1973) and 2296 210 (1980–1983), giving a mortality rate of 1:186 422 and 1:153 080 respectively. The difference is insignificant, although one might have expected there might have been proportionately fewer deaths in more recent years in line with improved training and the general trend of reduction in anaesthetic mortality.

One of the remarkable findings of Coplans & Curson's analysis (1982) was that the use of unsupplemented nitrous oxide and oxygen as a hypoxic mixture, had the lowest mortality rate, significantly lower than a non-hypoxic mixture with volatile supplements. This finding is hardly surprising in that the technique was only amenable for short procedures. The operating conditions were not ideal, but a short procedure even with the hypoxic mixture without the use of more potent inhalational agents such as halothane, could still result in patients leaving the dental surgery after a short interval following the 'dental gas'.

ANAESTHETIC AGENTS

The introduction of halothane in 1956 was an agent of great promise to outpatient dental anaesthesia, as this more potent agent would obviate the need for techniques using a hypoxic mixture of gases. The advent of halothane should at least have promoted the increased safety.

However hepatic damage may occur following repeated exposure to halothane, and records of agents administered in dental surgeries are not readily available. There have also been problems of cardiac dysrhythmias during dental surgery, and a number of studies have compared halothane with enflurane and its stereo-isomer isoflurane. Strunin et al (1979) reported on the use of enflurane and halothane for outpatient dental anaesthesia. There was no difference in induction time, but recovery to eye opening was significantly more rapid from enflurane after an inhalational induction. Ventricular ectopic beats and bradycardia were significantly more common with halothane, but postoperative sequelae were similar. Hoyal et al (1980) found that induction and maintenance with halothane and enflurane were comparable and satisfactory. Although recovery of consciousness was quicker with enflurane, time to full recovery was equal. Rollason et al (1984) studied 120 patients having outpatient dental anaesthesia and found a lower incidence of dysrhythmias with enflurane than previously found with halothane (Rollason & Russell 1980). However, Haden (1985) noted no significant difference in the frequency of dysrhythmias in 49 children having either halothane (25) or enflurane (24) for dental extractions.

The comparison was extended to isoflurane by Casson & Jones (1985) who found that the frequency of arrhythmias during halothane anaesthesia was statistically higher than anaesthesia using either enflurane or isoflurane. They observed that the heart rate was increased more by isoflurane than enflurane, and by enflurane more than by halothane.

Cattermole et al (1986) compared halothane with isoflurane for children during outpatient dental anaesthesia. They also found that isoflurane produced significantly fewer arrhythmias. However, induction with isoflurane was longer and more difficult, echoing Ryder & Wright's study of halothane and enflurane (1981). An American study (Fisher et al 1984) of the three agents in paediatric outpatient anaesthesia concluded that halothane was the smoothest induction agent and isoflurane produced most problems during both induction and recovery, citing coughing and laryngospasm as complications.

McAteer et al (1986) used isoflurane and halothane randomly in 80 outpatient paediatric dental patients. They found that the pungent odour of isoflurane did not cause problems and did not delay induction, but during and after anaesthesia, coughing, salivation and laryngospasm were more frequent than with halothane. Despite the physical properties of isoflurane, recovery was significantly slower than from halothane.

There have been many studies undertaken on the incidence of dysrhythmias in inpatients during the course of dental anaesthesia (Kaufman 1965). Halothane and enflurane have been compared (Wright 1980, Willatts et al 1983) whilst Rodrigo et al (1986) have studied halothane and isoflurane. Their results were in agreement with those of the outpatient studies (see above). A haemodynamic comparison of halothane and isoflurane using echocardiography was carried out in children by Wolf et al (1986) and this showed significant myocardial depression with halothane, whilst myocardial function was well preserved with isoflurane. The studies were carried out before surgery commenced. It appears that dysrhythmias during oral surgery may be reduced by treatment with beta blocking drugs as oral premedication (Hanna et al 1983), intravenously at induction (Whitehead et al 1980) or intra-operatively (Rollason & Russell 1980, Rollason et al 1984).

Intravenous agents

Although propanidid and Althesin showed initial promise for dental anaesthesia, both these drugs were withdrawn in 1983 because of the possible dangers of anaphylactoid reactions. Thus many dental anaesthetists have relied on methohexitone as their intravenous agent of choice. Unfortunately it may cause pain on injection but this may be reduced by using a large vein or by the preliminary injection of a small amount of lignocaine. Etomidate is a rapid and short-acting agent which should be ideal for outpatient dental anaesthesia, but it is more painful on injection, may cause thrombophlebitis and involuntary muscle movements in the unpremedicated outpatient.

Recently propofol has been re-introduced in an aqueous emulsion, which seems to have greatly reduced the possibility of anaphylactoid reactions. McCollum & Dundee (1986) compared propofol with thiopentone, methohexitone and etomidate. For smoothness of induction, propofol was second to thiopentone and superior to the other two agents. The most dangerous properties of propofol are depression of respiration and hypotension. Despite changing the solvent, propofol still remains painful on injection (Walmsley et al 1986), suggesting that it is the drug itself that is irritant. MacKenzie & Grant (1985) found that propofol was a smoother induction agent than both thiopentone and methohexitone, but caused greater cardiovascular and respiratory depression. Recovery was smooth and rapid with fewer side-effects such as nausea and vomiting or headache. A study of the relative potencies of thiopentone and propofol (Grounds et al 1986) estimated that 1 mg of propofol was equivalent to 1.6 mg of thiopentone. Though there may be an increased sensitivity to propofol in the elderly (Dundee et al 1986), this agent seems to be very suitable for outpatient dental anaesthesia. Pain on injection may be minimized by the use of a larger vein or the prior administration of lignocaine; whether thrombophlebitis and venous thrombosis ensues has yet to be elucidated (see Postgraduate Medical Journal (1985) for detailed presentation of propofol).

SEDATION

Intravenous agents

The use of diazepam (Valium, Roche) for intravenous sedation results in pain on injection and the possible sequelae of thrombophlebitis and venous thrombosis. This is due to the solvent (propylene glycol) and these complications can be reduced by presenting the drug as an emulsion, Diazemuls (Rosenbaum 1982). Thus Diazemuls has largely replaced the need for Valium which should now be discarded for intravenous use.

The initial recovery from diazepam is rapid but the long half-life (24 hours) and the 'second peak' effect from enterohepatic recirculation (Baird & Hailey 1972) raise the possibility that resedation might occur and the patient become amnesic for up to 24 hours after treatment.

Midazolam (Hypnovel) is a water-soluble benzodiazepine twice as potent as diazepam. Its solubility is due to a fused imidazole ring not found in other benzodiazepines, allowing midazolam to dissolve in acidic aqueous media for parenteral administration. At normal body pH, however, midazolam becomes highly lipophilic, thus allowing rapid entry into the brain. The fused imidazole ring is speedily oxidized in the liver (much more quickly than the diazepine ring of the other benzodiazepines) producing 1-

and 4-hydroxymidazolam which are excreted in the urine. The distribution half-life of midazolam is half that of diazepam whilst the elimination half-life is ten times shorter (see Reves et al 1985).

Midazolam is not painful on intravenous injection, does not cause thrombophlebitis and has a half-life of 60–90 minutes (Dundee et al 1986). In dentistry Rosenbaum (1985) regarded it as highly suitable as amnesia and recovery time were superior to that of diazepam while venous sequelae were similar to those of Diazemuls. An elegant study by Barker et al (1986) proved the statistical significance of the first two advantages and also of the rapidity and effectiveness of sedation. They confirmed that midazolam was twice as potent as diazepam but warned that there was considerable variation between patients. Because midazolam is supplied as 10 mg in 2 ml solution, patients often receive an overdose. A more dilute solution of 10 mg in 5 ml has allowed easier titration of dosage, although ampoules of 5 mg (equipotent to the 10 mg ampoules of diazepam) would be safer.

The fact that diazepam and midazolam are purely sedatives and have no analgesic powers is often overlooked. Incremental doses in an effort to quieten a suffering patient may lead to full general anaesthesia with consequent loss of protective reflexes. A number of analgesic drugs have been used intravenously in conservative dentistry in this context, including pentazocine (Corall et al 1979) and nalbuphine (Parsons 1986).

A very recent paper (MacKenzie & Grant 1987) describes the use of propofol by infusion at a subanaesthetic dose level as a sedative in association with spinal analgesia for lower limb surgery. It seems likely that propofol will be used in a similar manner as an infusion in dentistry but with caution to avoid the problems encountered in the past with methohexitone.

Oral sedation

Temazepam does not form active metabolites and has a relatively short duration of action. If it is given as a soft gelatin capsule sedation rapidly ensues. It has been compared with intravenous diazepam for outpatient oral surgery, and it was found that the pattern and duration of sedation were similar (O'Boyle et al 1986). Although it is less flexible than intravenous sedation, there appears to be a place for oral sedation in conservative dentistry.

Benzodiazepine antagonism

Two recent double-blind randomized studies have assessed the place of Ro 15-1788 as an antagonist to intravenous diazepam (Kirkegaard et al 1986) and midazolam (Wolff et al 1986). In both studies Ro 15-1788 improved the speed of recovery significantly with little effect on cardiorespiratory function. There was an increased frequency of nausea and vomiting in the latter study. It is probable that Ro 15-1788 will fulfill an antagonist role to benzodiazepines as naloxone with the opioids (Ro 15-1788 is now available as Flumazenil).

Inhalational sedation

'Relative analgesia' has been widely interpreted and it has been suggested that 'inhalational sedation and analgesia' would be a more accurate term (Roberts 1979). The use of nitrous oxide in low concentration (5–30%) to produce sedation in the early part of Guedel's stage I, has been a popular method in North American dental offices for 50 years (Langa 1976). In this country a number of enthusiasts (Lindsay & Roberts 1979, Allen 1985) have tried to popularize the technique, but it depends for success on 'a steady flow of reassuring and encouraging talk to the patient. This establishes and maintains rapport with the patient . . . as . . . semihypnotic suggestion' (Roberts 1979). It is unlikely that many anaesthetists will become directly involved with this method of sedation although it does have its advocates (Manford & Roberts 1980, Edmunds & Rosen 1984).

MONITORING

Since Lunn & Mushin's mortality report (1982) most junior anaesthetists have felt it incumbent to monitor the ECG of every anaesthetized patient. This has presented many problems in a busy outpatient dental clinic. The application of ECG electrodes may arouse anxiety and cause delay. However, with the decline in number of patients and the increase of day case intubated patients, ECG monitoring will become the accepted routine.

Various methods of applying ECG electrodes in a rapid or less frightening manner have been described and used in trial situations but all take time and heighten anxiety. Automatic blood pressure monitors are now reliable if expensive and they are less likely to worry the patient.

Recently Beeby & Thurlow (1986) have evaluated a pulse oximeter during outpatient dental general anaesthesia. They found that it performed satisfactorily in most patients and in some cases provided an early warning of airway obstruction. They felt that it was a considerable advance in the care of the anaesthetized dental patient, and might be useful during both intravenous and inhalational sedation. A similar study using a different oximeter also demonstrated that a reduction in oxygen saturation was detectable before it became clinically apparent (Clapham & Mackie 1986). The pulse oximeter is even easier to apply than the blood pressure cuff and provides a continuous and accurate indication of peripheral perfusion and oxygenation. It seems likely to become an obligatory monitor in this and other spheres of anaesthesia.

POLLUTION

It is almost impossible to prevent pollution of the atmosphere in the dental surgery when general anaesthesia is taking place. A stealthy induction for a child may involve hosing the facial area with anaesthetic gases; leaks around the mask are common and during extractions expired anaesthetic escapes from the mouth. Several different methods have been suggested to reduce pollution but none are entirely successful. In addition, both the patient and the machine will release anaesthetic gas into the atmosphere at the end of surgery. Parbrook & Davis (1979) identified five factors that reduce pollution in the dental surgery. Of these the most efficient is satisfactory room ventilation; an increase in air changes to ten per hour from the normal two will reduce pollution by 80%. Specific ventilation of the area around the patient's head is also helpful as is a reduction in the total flow of anaesthetic agents. Scavenging using a second tube to duct away the expired gas also helped and larger rooms reduced the build-up of anaesthetic gases. They also suggested that at the end of anaesthesia every patient should be given oxygen for at least 1 minute to reduce pollution in the recovery period (and as a safeguard and prophylactic). The use of a scavenging block attached to the nasal mask has also been suggested and the Lack coaxial system in conjunction with an intermittent flow anaesthetic machine at 'on demand' setting has been tested (Padfield & Asbury 1983). Pollution by nitrous oxide during inhalational sedation may be serious (Schuyt et al 1986) as the problem may be overlooked as the technique is often used in poorly ventilated premises.

ANTIBACTERIAL PROPHYLAXIS (ANTIBIOTIC COVER)

Infective endocarditis is still a serious condition and the incidence has not fallen (Drug & Therapeutics Bulletin 1985). Patients at risk include those with congenital heart disease, prosthetic valves and those who have had previous endocarditis or rheumatic heart disease (much rarer today). Bacteraemia is caused by exodontia, but also by scaling and gingival surgery and cannot be prevented, although it may be reduced by chlorhexidine mouthwash (McGowan 1983). The British Society for Antimicrobial Therapy's (BSAC) recommendation (1982) of amoxycillin 1 g intramuscularly 1 hour before surgery, plus 0.5 g orally 6 hours postoperatively is not necessarily practicable in the outpatient environment. 2–3 g orally before surgery is effective, gives high blood levels for 6–8 hours (Drugs & Therapeutics Bulletin 1985) and is kinder. The British National Formulary No. 12 (1986) suggests 3 g oral amoxycillin 4 hours before general anaesthesia and a further 3 g as soon as possible postoperatively. In children, quarter to a half of a 3 g sachet (Amoxil) pre-operatively repeated afterwards is effective, and this is prescribed by the author 1 hour before anaesthesia. In patients who are sensitive to penicillin oral erythromycin 1.5 g 1 hour before surgery and 0.5 g 6 hours later is recommended by BSAC, or intravenous vancomycin 1 g followed by 120 mg gentamicin intravenously (BSAC).

POSTGRADUATE EDUCATION

The Association of Dental Anaesthetists (ADA) held its inaugural meeting at Manchester in April 1977. Since then there have been two meetings a year in a variety of hospitals in different parts of the UK. In 1983 the first volume of its Proceedings was published (Du Pont Pharmaceuticals), and each subsequent year successive volumes have recorded the communications given at the bi-annual meetings. A high proportion of these papers are subsequently published in the recognised dental and anaesthetic journals and reflect a wide spectrum of interests.

The Society for the Advancement of Anaesthesia in Dentistry (SAAD) is much older and plays a more educative role. Founded by the late S. L. Drummond-Jackson in 1957 it has run 90 courses over the intervening years. The most recent courses have consisted of three weekends at short intervals, which aim to give comprehensive instruction in both theoretical and practical aspects of dental sedation and anaesthesia based on the Wylie report (1978). In addition the Society holds update meetings, publishes a lively digest four times a year and awards an annual prize in memory of its founder.

There are a growing number of dental anaesthetists who are members of both SAAD and ADA and the two organizations are complementary rather than antagonistic. Other individuals and bodies such as health authorities arrange postgraduate refresher courses in dental anaesthesia, but Sarll & Goldwater (1985) felt that there was an urgent need to provide suitable courses designed for the dental team: the surgeon, the anaesthetist and the dental surgery assistant.

THE FUTURE

Dental outpatient anaesthesia has been described as 'the last art form in anaesthesia' and every doctor knows the Hippocratic aphorism 'the art is long: life is brief'. If experience is as to intensity and not as to duration, then the intensity of experience in dental outpatient anaesthesia has diminished to such an extent that it is difficult to provide young trainees either medically or dentally qualified with the practical experience they need to become competent anaesthetists. To be a good dental anaesthetist requires a degree of self-confidence founded on practical experience gained in concert with a good dental operator. The young trainee anaesthetist today may be attempting to learn his craft whilst the extractions are carried out by a dental student. In addition, the trainee anaesthetist would expect to have venous access, ECG and blood pressure monitors and might be disconcerted by not having the security of intubation for surgery within the airway.

Perhaps we should look to North America to see what our future might hold. Adelson (1984), a New York dentist, described his operatory for general anaesthesia in which had been performed 27 000 anaesthetics in 32 years since 1951 with 100% safety. He attributed his success and safety to, amongst other factors, 'physical plant approximating a hospital and the use of the newest monitoring devices'. In Toronto, Kay (1983) administered 10 650 general anaesthetics in 18 years in 201 dental offices. He provided a mobile anaesthetic service using a portable Haloxair unit with a trained assistant.

Both of these examples require a considerable initial capital outlay and are expensive to maintain. The return from practice confined entirely to the NHS would be inadequate but with the trend towards more private dentistry it might become financially viable.

REFERENCES

Adelson J J 1984 Restorative dentistry with general anesthesia. A safe, effective office procedure. New York State Dental Journal 50: 433–435

Al-Khishali T, Padfield A, Perks E R, Thornton J A 1978 Cardio-respiratory effects of nitrous oxide: oxygen: halothane anaesthesia administered to dental outpatients in the upright posture. Anaesthesia 32: 184–188

Allen W A 1985 Aspects of relative analgesia. Proceedings of the Association of Dental Anaesthetists 3: 10

Baird E S, Hailey D M 1972 Delayed recovery from a sedative: correlation of the plasma levels of diazepam with clinical effects after oral and IV administration. British Journal of Anaesthesia 44: 803–808

Barker I, Butchart D G M, Gibson J, Lawson J I M, Mackenzie N 1986 IV Sedation for conservative dentistry. A comparison of midazolam and diazepam. British Journal of Anaesthesia 58: 371–377

Beeby C, Thurlow A C 1986 Pulse oximetry during general anaesthesia for dental extractions. British Dental Journal 160: 123–125

Bourne J G 1957 Fainting and cerebral damage: a danger in patients kept upright during dental gas anaesthesia and after surgical operations. Lancet 2: 499–505

Bourne J G 1986 Deaths and posture in the dental chair: a 30 year perspective. Today's Anaesthetist 1: 29–33

British National Formulary 1986 Antibacterial prophylaxis No 12: 188 BMA & PSGB London

British Society for Antimicrobial Therapy Working Party (BSAC) 1982 Lancet 2: 1323

Casson W R, Jones R M 1985 Cardiac rate and rhythm during anaesthesia for dental extraction. A comparison of halothane, enflurane and isoflurane. British Journal of Anaesthesia 57: 476–481

Cattermole R W, Verghese C, Blair I J, Jones C J H, Flynn P J, Sebel P S 1986 Isoflurane and halothane for outpatient dental anaesthesia in children. British Journal of Anaesthesia 58: 385–389

Clapham M C C, Mackie A M 1986 Pulse oximetry. An assessment in anaesthetised dental patients. Anaesthesia 41: 1036–1038

Coplans M P, Curson I 1973 Deaths associated with general dental anaesthesia. British Medical Journal 1: 109–110

Coplans M P, Curson I 1982 Deaths associated with dentistry. British Dental Journal 153: 357–362

Corall I M, Strunin L, Ward M E, Mason S A, Alcalay M 1979 Sedation for outpatient conservative dentistry. A trial of pentazocine supplementation to diazepam and local analgesia techniques. Anaesthesia 34: 855–858

Curson I 1985 Report on deaths associated with dentistry 1980–83. Proceedings of the Association of Dental Anaesthetists 3: 14–15

Dental Estimates Board 1986 Personal communication

Dinsdale R C W 1983 Personal communication: paper at Royal College of Surgeons/ADA meeting

Dinsdale R C W, Dixon R A 1978 Anaesthetic services to dental patients: England and Wales, 1976. British Dental Journal 144: 271–279

Drug and Therapeutics Bulletin 1985 Prophylaxis for endocarditis 23: No 14 July 15

Dundee J W, Robinson F P, McCollum J S C, Patterson C C 1986 Sensitivity to propofol in the elderly. Anaesthesia 41: 482–485

Edmunds D H, Rosen M 1984 Inhalational sedation with 25% nitrous oxide. Report of a field trial. Anaesthesia 39: 138–142

Fisher D M, Robinson S, Brett C, Gregory G A, Perin G 1984 Comparison of enflurane, halothane and isoflurane for outpatient pediatric anesthesia. Anesthesiology 61: A427

General Dental Council 1985 Recommendations concerning the dental curriculum. London

Grounds R M, Moore M, Morgan M 1986 The relative potencies of thiopentone and propofol. European Journal of Anaesthesiology 3: 11–17

Haden R M 1985 Cardiac dysrhythmias during dental surgery: a comparison of halothane and enflurane in children. British Dental Journal 158: 23–24

Hanna M H, Heap D G, Kimberley A P S 1983 Cardiac dysrhythmia associated with general anaesthesia for oral surgery. Anaesthesia 38: 1192–1194

Heesterman R A 1986 Personal communication (District Dental Officer: Sheffield)

Hillary D J 1986 Education for dental anaesthesia. Proceedings of the Association of Dental Anaesthetists 4: 16–17

Hoyal R H A, Prys-Roberts C, Simpson P J 1980 Enflurane in outpatient paediatric dental anaesthesia. A comparison with halothane. British Journal of Anaesthesia 52: 219–222

Hutchinson R I 1975 The accuracy and efficiency of general anaesthetic machines in Dental Practice. British Dental Journal 138: 187–189

Jenkins G N 1985 Recent changes in dental caries. British Medical Journal 291: 1297–1298

Kaufman L 1965 Cardiac arrhythmias in dentistry. Lancet 2: 287

Kay M 1983 General anaesthesia in the private dental office. Canadian Anaesthetists' Society Journal 30: 406–411

Kirkegaard L, Knudsen L, Jensen S, Kruse A 1986 Benzodiazepine antagonist Ro 15-1788. Antagonism of diazepam sedation in outpatients undergoing gastroscopy. Anaesthesia 41: 1184–1188

Langa H 1976 Relative analgesia in dental patients. Saunders, Philadelphia

Lindsay S J E, Roberts G J 1979 Does relative analgesia work? British Dental Journal 147: 206

Lunn J N, Mushin W W 1982 Mortality associated with anaesthesia. The Nuffield Provincial Hospitals Trust, London

McAteer P M, Carter J A, Cooper G M, Prys-Roberts C 1986 Comparison of isoflurane and halothane in outpatient paediatric dental anaesthesia. British Journal of Anaesthesia 58: 390–393

McCollum J S C, Dundee J W 1986 Comparison of induction characteristics of four intravenous agents. Anaesthesia 41: 995–1000

McGowan D A 1985 Bacterial endocarditis and prophylaxis. Proceedings of the Association of Dental Anaesthetists 3: 13–14

MacKenzie N, Grant I S 1985 Comparison of a new emulsion formulation of propofol with methohexitone and thiopentone for induction of anaesthesia in day cases. British Journal of Anaesthesia 57: 725–731

MacKenzie N, Grant I S 1987 Propofol for intravenous sedation. Anaesthesia 42: 3–6

Manford M L M, Roberts G J 1980 Dental treatment in young handicapped patients. An assessment of relative analgesia as an alternative to general anaesthesia. Anaesthesia 35: 1157–1168

Nainby-Luxmoore R C 1967 Some hazards of dental gas machines. Anaesthesia 22: 545–555

O'Boyle C A, Harris D, Barry H 1986 Sedation in outpatient oral surgery. Comparison of temazepam by mouth and diazepam i.v. British Journal of Anaesthesia 58: 378–384

Padfield A 1987 Communication to the Association of Dental Anaesthetists

Padfield A, Asbury A J 1983 Economy and antipollution. The Lack circuit in outpatient dental anaesthesia. Proceedings of the Association of Dental Anaesthetists 1: 10–11

Parbrook G D 1986 Death for anaesthesia in the general and community dental service? British Journal of Anaesthesia 58: 369–370

Parbrook G D, Davis P D 1979 Anaesthetic pollution in the outpatient dental surgery. Anaesthesia 34: 47–52

Parsons J D 1986 The use of nalbuphine (Nubain) and midazolam in sedation for dentistry. SAAD Digest 6: 125–131

Postgraduate Medical Journal 1985 Propofol. A new intravenous anaesthetic. 61 (suppl 3)

Reves J G, Fragen R J, Vinik H R, Greenblatt D J 1985 Midazolam: pharmacology and uses. Anesthesiology 62: 310–324

Roberts G J 1979 Relative analgesia an introduction. Dental Update 6: 271–280

Rodrigo M R C, Moles T M, Lee P K 1986 Comparison of the incidence and nature of cardiac arrhythmias occurring during isoflurane or halothane anaesthesia. Studies during dental surgery. British Journal of Anaesthesia 58: 394–400

Rollason W N, Russell J G 1980 Intravenous metoprolol and cardiac dysrhythmias. Anaesthesia 35: 783–789

Rollason W N, Bennetts F E, Clarke I 1984 Cardiac dysrhythmias during outpatient dental anaesthesia with enflurane. The role of "beta blockade". Acta Anaesthesiologica Scandinavica 28: 497–502

Rosenbaum N L 1982 A new formulation of diazepam for intravenous sedation in dentistry. A clinical evaluation. British Dental Journal 153: 192–193

Rosenbaum N L 1985 The use of midazolam for intravenous sedation in general dental practice. British Dental Journal 158: 139–140

Ryder W, Wright P A 1981 Halothane and enflurane in dental anaesthesia. Anaesthesia 36: 492–497

Sarll D W, Goldwater H L 1985 Training needs of postgraduates in dental general anaesthesia. British Medical Journal 2: 1641–1642

Schuyt H C, Brakel K, Ostendorp S G L M, Schiphorst B J M 1986 Abortions amongst dental personnel exposed to nitrous oxide. Anaesthesia 41: 82–83

Strunin L, Strunin J M, Phipps J A, Corrall I M 1979 A comparison of halothane and enflurane (Ethrane) for outpatient dental anaesthesia. British Dental Journal 147: 299–301

Thompson P W 1986 The Cardiff experience. Proceedings of the Association of Dental Anaesthetists 4: 17

Tomlin P J 1974 Death in outpatient dental anaesthetic practice. Anaesthesia 29: 551–570

Tomlin P J, Roberts J F 1981 The airway in the upright anaesthetised patient. British Dental Journal 150: 312–314

Walmsley A J, McLeod B, Ponte J 1986 The new formulation of ICI 35868 (propofol) as the main agent for minor surgical procedures. European Journal of Anaesthesiology 3: 19–26

Whitehead M H, Whitmarsh V B, Horton J N 1980 Metoprolol in anaesthesia for oral surgery. Anaesthesia 35: 779–782

Willatts D G, Harrison A R, Groom J F, Crowther A 1983 Cardiac arrhythmias during outpatient dental anaesthesia: comparison of halothane and enflurane. British Journal of Anaesthesia 55: 399–403

Wolf W J, Neal M B, Peterson M D 1986 The hemodynamic and cardiovascular effects of isoflurane and halothane anesthesia in children. Anesthesiology 64: 328–333

Wolff J, Carl P, Clausen T G, Mikkelsen B O 1986 Ro 15-1788 for postoperative recovery. A randomised clinical trial in patients undergoing minor surgical procedures under midazolam anaesthesia. Anaesthesia 41: 1001–1006

Wright C J 1980 Dysrhythmias during oral surgery. A comparison between halothane and enflurane anaesthesia. Anaesthesia 35: 775–778

Wylie Report of the Working Party on Training in Dental Anaesthesia 1978 London

Obstetrics

This section is essentially an update to the chapter on anaesthetic factors in obstetrics which appeared in *Anaesthesia Review 3*. It also considers material not discussed in that chapter.

HYPERTENSION IN PREGNANCY

The report on Confidential Enquiry into Maternal Deaths in England and Wales 1979–1981 (1986) revealed that there were 36 deaths in that period from hypertension of pregnancy and this was the commonest cause of death.

There has been confusion regarding the terminology of hypertension in pregnancy and eclampsia but this has been clarified by the classification as set out by The American College of Obstetricians and Gynecologists as follows.

1. Pre-eclampsia and eclampsia
2. Chronic hypertension
3. Chronic hypertension with superimposed pre-eclampsia
4. Late or transient hypertension

   1. Pre-eclampsia occurs in 5–10% of all pregnancies and is associated with hypertension, proteinuria and oedema.
   2. Chronic hypertension may be secondary to renal-artery stenosis, coarctation of the aorta, phaeochromocytoma, primary aldosteronism or renal disease. Pregnancy has little effect on the underlying disorder.
   3. Chronic hypertension with superimposed pre-eclampsia is a medical emergency and is both dangerous for mother and fetus.
   4. In transient hypertension the hypertension develops in late pregnancy but the blood pressure returns to normal within the 10th day following delivery (Lindheimer & Katz 1985).

Treatment of hypertension in pregnancy

Intravenous angiotensin II in normotensive pregnant women is a sensitive indicator of the likelihood of hypertension or pre-eclampsia developing later in pregnancy. In the group of pregnant women who showed an exaggerated response to angiotensin II the administration of low dose aspirin (60 mg per day) starting at 28 weeks' gestation resulted in a reduced incidence of hypertension or pre-eclampsia. The aspirin appears to suppress the production of thromboxane A_2 which is a potent vasoconstrictor and stimulator of platelet aggregation (Wallenburg et al 1986).

Gallery et al (1985) found that oxprenolol was most likely to produce the best results for the fetus and they recommended the use of the beta-blocking agent providing there was no maternal contra-indication. However de Swiet (1985) concluded that the safest drug in the treatment of hypertension in pregnancy was still methyldopa with beta blockers being recommended for short term therapy. Other drugs used for treatment included hydralazine, diazoxide, sodium nitroprusside, labetalol and nifedipine.

Concern has been expressed about the possibility that drugs used for the treatment of maternal hypertension might cross the placental barrier. Patients who were being treated with 100–300 mg of labetalol given three times a day at least a week before delivery with the last dose being given within 12 hours before birth have been studied by MacPherson et al (1986). Although there was transient neonatal hypotension this returned to normal within 24 hours. There were no differences between the infants of treated patients and the control group on the other parameters measured which included heart and respiratory rates, palmar sweating, blood glucose and the metabolic and vasomotor responses to cold stress. Jouppila et al (1986) confirmed the absence of detrimental effects on the fetus by labetalol given intravenously to the mother. Maternal blood pressure decreased but there were no alterations in the blood flow in the intervillous space, the umbilical vein or the fetal descending aorta. Placental vascular resistance decreased. Labetalol was also shown to have no effect on prostacyclin (vasodilator) or on thromboxane A_2 (vasoconstrictor).

For the management of hypertension at term or during labour intravenous hydralazine or diazoxide is advocated. Sedation with diazepam or chlormethiazole is often necessary and there must be adequate pain relief. Epidural blockade can provide adequate control of blood pressure and provide pain relief. The use of magnesium sulphate is recommended in the United States. In a recent retrospective study of pregnancy induced hypertension in 285 women it was shown that epidural blockade compared favourably with local anaesthesia on the incidence of maternal hypotension or fetal well-being as measured by fetal heart rate trace, Apgar score or admission to the neonatal intensive care unit. The duration of the first stage of labour was increased by 50% with epidural bupivacaine (Moore et al 1985). 100 patients were delivered by Caesarean section. 15% had general anaesthesia as opposed to epidural anaesthesia and in the general anaesthesia group there was a significant increase of low Apgar scores, depressed umbilical cord pH and an increased admission to the neonatal intensive care unit. Moore et al (1985) suggested that this was due to poor fetal status prior to anaesthesia and did not necessarily reflect an unfavourable effect of general anaesthesia.

Anaesthetic complications in this series are of interest. Two patients developed prolonged apnoea due to atypical cholinesterase: hypotension and cardiac arrest occurred following Caesarean section with epidural anaesthesia which readily responded to intravenous ephedrine. During general anaesthesia with thiopentone, suxamethonium, nitrous oxide oxygen and low concentrations of halothane there were marked rises of blood pressure which required intravenous sodium nitroprusside and there were other episodes of profound hypotension.

THE UNCONSCIOUS ECLAMPTIC PATIENT

Prolonged unconsciousness may occur as a complication of an eclamptic fit. Richards et al (1986) have described the problems of management in 20 such patients. One of the difficulties in treatment is lack of information on the paraphysiology of the condition. Changes compatible with cerebral oedema were noted on CT scan in 75% of the patients, with cerebral haemorrhage occurring in 9%. The patients were treated in a semi-sitting position and given 20% mannitol (0.5 g/kg) to reduce the increased intracranial pressure with hyperventilation to reduce the arterial PCO_2. If treatment by these means was unsuccessful althesin was given at the rate of 20 μg/kg/min. CSF drainage, 5 ml at a time, was also performed. Postmortem findings in one patient revealed pulmonary oedema, a soft swollen brain, widespread hypoxic ischaemic nerve damage and haemorrhages in the liver and adrenal medulla.

CATECHOLAMINES AND CORTISOL IN PREGNANCY

Catecholamines have been measured in maternal venous and mixed umbilical cord blood (Jones et al 1985). Following epidural analgesia there was a 36% reduction in maternal noradrenaline and a 33% fall in adrenaline. Fetal catecholamine levels were the lowest in patients undergoing Caesarean section under epidural analgesia. During spontaneous vaginal delivery fetal noradrenaline was increased by three- to eightfold but there was little change in adrenaline levels.

During pregnancy the blood pressure, pulse rate and plasma catecholamines may vary in response to changes in posture. In non-pregnant women standing for 10 minutes resulted in a rise in blood pressure, pulse rate and plasma noradrenaline. In pregnant women there was less response to postural change although the diastolic pressure decreased. The pulse rate was variable but the patients as a group showed no change (Whittaker et al 1985). Barron et al (1986) concluded that normal pregnancy altered the cardiovascular and sympathetic response to physiological stimuli. They also noted that during normal pregnancy plasma renin and aldosterone levels were increased.

Serum concentration of total cortisol levels increased linearly during pregnancy, significantly higher levels being found in nulliparous women. Cortisol levels were not influenced by age of the patients (Vleugels et al 1986).

During labour and vaginal delivery Neumark et al (1985) measured plasma adrenaline, noradrenaline and cortisol levels. In patients who had had epidural blockade there was a significant drop in plasma adrenaline and cortisol but there was no significant reduction in noradrenaline. Following delivery the plasma adrenaline and cortisol were still significantly suppressed. In the control group receiving intramuscular pethidine all the hormone levels rose significantly up to delivery and although catecholamines had returned to normal levels 1 hour after delivery cortisol levels took longer to return to normal.

Other hormones

The measurement of other hormones besides cortisol and catecholamines may have implications for anaesthesia. Holst et al (1986) measured the plasma levels of vasoactive intestinal polypeptide which increased significantly during labour and remained elevated for 15 minutes following delivery. Plasma gastro-inhibitory polypeptide decreased significantly between 5 and 30 minutes after delivery. Blood glucose levels increased significantly during labour, delivery and in the early post-partum period. Plasma insulin levels rose significantly within 5 minutes of delivery and stayed at a threefold level for 120 minutes following delivery. These findings may be of interest in relation to inhalation of gastric contents and may also explain the reason for the fall in insulin requirements in diabetic patients following delivery.

Beta-endorphin

Beta-endorphin levels have been studied during labour and delivery by Kofinas et al (1985). During vaginal delivery maternal beta-endorphin levels were significantly higher than in their infants, whereas the reverse applied following Caesarean section. However there was no significant difference between fetal plasma endorphin levels in those patients delivered vaginally or by Caesarean section but the stress of labour and delivery produced a marked increase in maternal beta-endorphin release. The high level of beta-endorphin at vaginal delivery may provide some degree of analgesia.

PAIN RELIEF

The use of intrathecal morphine was discussed in *Anaesthesia Review 3* (see

p. 151), a troublesome side effect being pruritus. Dailey et al (1985) advocated the use of a bolus injection of naloxone (0.4 mg) followed by an infusion of 0.4–0.6 mg/h, which successfully reduced the incidence of pruritis but had little effect on nausea, vomiting, sleepiness, or dizziness. Although there is transfer of naloxone to the fetus there was no obvious side effect. Maternal analgesia was not influenced by the use of naloxone. Maternal beta-endorphin levels decreased significantly with the onset of analgesia and returned to control levels following delivery, irrespective of whether the mothers were given naloxone or not.

Marx et al (1986) studied the effect of epidural analgesia with 2% 2-chloroprocaine on umbilical blood flow velocity waves which confirmed that there was an increase in umbilical artery vascular resistance when the mother lay supine. Following epidural blockade vascular resistance fell indicating an increase in umbilical artery blood flow possibly due to pain relief and inhibition of catecholamine release. It was concluded that the use of epidural analgesia was beneficial provided maternal hypotension did not develop.

MENDELSON'S SYNDROME

Although Mendelson described 46 cases of pulmonary complications during obstetric anaesthesia none of the patients died. This is in marked contrast to the mortality following the inhalation of gastric contents in present day obstetric anaesthesia. MacLennan (1986) has suggested that the severity of the syndrome is due to increased interstitial fluid in the lungs in pregnancy. There are many reasons for this including the administration of fluids as vehicles for drugs prior to epidural analgesia, while oxytocin, opiates and ergometrine affect circulating blood volume by antidiuresis and vasoconstriction. The cardiovascular response to intubation during light anaesthesia may be exaggerated precipitating pulmonary oedema. Drugs to suppress premature labour such as steroids and beta$_2$ sympathomimetic agents may also precipitate cardiac failure (see *Anaesthesia Review 1* pp. 55–64). The hypothesis proposed by MacLennan (1986) is that pulmonary oedema seen in obstetric practice may not necessarily be due to inhalation of gastric contents but may be cardiac in origin, the concept prevailing before the era of Mendelson. The recent Confidential Enquiry into Maternal Deaths (1986) reported that 29 patients died from causes that could be attributed to anaesthesia, of which 22 were directly due to some anaesthetic involvement. Eight patients died from inhalation of gastric contents while problems with endotracheal intubation led to the death of eight patients. In one instance ritodrine was implicated (see below). The efficacy of magnesium trisilicate is doubtful as inhalation of the mixture may cause lung damage while at the same time it only increases the volume of the stomach contents. H$_2$ receptor antagonists reduce acidity.

The report recommends that food and fluids by mouth should be restricted during labour and the stomach should be emptied with an oesophageal tube before induction of anaesthesia. The report concluded with advice about the proper application of cricoid pressure. During intubation the endotracheal tube should be seen to pass through the vocal cords and there should be a recognised drill to deal with patients who are having profuse bleeding. Particular care must be paid to patients who are dark-skinned and who have pre-operative disability including kyphoscoliosis. It also recommended that the use of pancuronium be avoided.

The report emphasises the necessity for proper communication between obstetricians, anaesthetists and all others who look after patients in obstetrics — a feature sometimes difficult to maintain in a busy obstetric unit.

TOCOLYTIC THERAPY

The use of beta sympathomimetic agents (beta-2) has been reported (*Anaesthesia Review 1* and *Review 3*). Hill et al (1985) have suggested the use of long term intravenous ritodrine which is continued until the patients are successfully able to tolerate the drug given orally. In the first 3–4 days of intravenous treatment there are marked cardiovascular and metabolic changes and it is advocated that intravenous tocolytic therapy is safe provided the patients are carefully supervised, which would include fetal and maternal cardiac monitoring. In addition the patients should be weighed regularly, a fluid intake and output chart kept and there are frequent measurements of haemoglobin, haematocrit, plasma glucose and serum potassium. Potassium levels may fall below 2.5 mmol/l. However MacLennan et al (1985) have reported a fatal case of pulmonary oedema following an infusion of intravenous ritodrine. Oxytocin had also been administered. Pulmonary capillary wedge pressure was 14 mmHg. Treatment was with frusemide, diamorphine and propranolol and despite treatment in an intensive care unit the patient died 15 days following admission after a period of cardiac arrest associated with tension pneumothorax.

In a study on animals Gerritse et al (1985) confirmed the antidiuretic effect of ritodrine which markedly reduced urinary output when the dose reached 4 μg/kg. The average dose in patients ranges from 2.5–5 μg/kg. The maternal tachycardia, widening of pulse pressure and vasodilatation, can be reversed with a beta-adrenergic blocking agent such as metoprolol, but it had no effect on the inhibition of urinary output. Gerritse et al (1985) concluded that there were other mechanisms responsible for the decreased urinary output and that when tocolytic therapy ceased there was still a danger of pulmonary oedema which could not necessarily be prevented by beta-adrenergic blockade.

In a controlled study Leveno et al (1986) concluded that although intravenous ritodrine significantly inhibited uterine contractions and delayed the onset of delivery it did not appear to have any effect on the consequences of premature labour. The associated hazards of therapy seem less beneficial than the outcome of treatment especially as Wang-Cheng & Davidson (1986) have reported a case of neutropenia which resolved spontaneously when tocolytic therapy was abandoned.

THYROTOXICOSIS

Although thyrotoxicosis is more common in women the incidence is only 0.2% as there is a tendency for remission during pregnancy. The diagnosis of thyrotoxicosis during pregnancy may be difficult as many of the normal signs of pregnancy including tachycardia and anxiety may be mistaken for thyrotoxicosis. Although thyroxine levels are elevated during normal pregnancy levels above 190 mmol/l are highly suggestive. Treatment may be with propylthiouracil although the drug may cross the placenta resulting in fetal hypothyroidism. Although hypothyroidism may occur in the neonate, of more concern is neonatal thyrotoxicosis. Although theoretically antithyroid drugs may appear in breast milk, breast feeding can be permitted provided the neonate is monitored for thyroid function (Burrow 1985).

The use of beta-adrenergic blocking drugs during pregnancy has been reported to cause fetal bradycardia, hypoglycaemia and impaired response to hypoxia in the developing fetus and neonate and is not advocated as the main agent for the long term management of thyrotoxicosis during pregnancy. However beta-blocking agents and iodides are useful in the rapid control of thyrotoxicosis especially if there is a need for surgical removal of the thyroid. The main indication for surgery is hypersensitivity to antithyroid drugs or in cases where they are ineffectual.

Thyroid crisis may develop and be precipitated by infection, labour or Caesarean section.

CARDIAC DISEASE

The management of patients with severe cardiac disease in pregnancy has been reviewed by Sullivan & Ramanathan (1985). During pregnancy there are increases in blood volume, cardiac output, stroke volume and heart rate while the arterial pressure, total peripheral resistance and pulmonary vascular resistance are decreased. By 8 weeks 50% of the maximum increase in heart rate had already occurred (Clapp 1985). During labour and delivery there are increased haemodynamic loads placed upon the circulation and this is dangerous to women with cardiovascular disease. Pregnancy is well tolerated in patients with mitral regurgitation, aortic regurgitation, atrial septal defect, ventricular septal defect, patent ductus arteriosus (the last three without pulmonary hypertension), pulmonary stenosis and hypertrophic obstructive cardiomyopathy. Pregnancy is badly tolerated in patients with mitral stenosis, aortic stenosis, Eisenmenger's syndrome, pulmonary hypertension, Marfan's syndrome, aortic coarctation, and tetralogy of Fallot (Sullivan & Ramanathan 1985). Patients with prosthetic valves are often treated with warfarin which crosses the placental barrier and heparin should be substituted instead. Epidural anaesthesia has been recommended for patients with cardiovascular disease except in conditions such as aortic stenosis, hypertrophic cardiomyopathy and pulmonary hypertension.

Cardiopulmonary resuscitation

Treatment of cardiac arrest has been considered in *Anaesthesia Review 3* but Lee et al (1986) have drawn attention to the fact that many of the studies on cardiopulmonary resuscitation have been carried out in the non-pregnant and it is easy to forget the anatomical and physiological effects of pregnancy which may influence the outcome of successful resuscitation. These include blood volume and increased cardiac output during pregnancy, the position of the uterus resulting in supine hypotension syndrome, decreased chest compliance, increased oxygen consumption and a tendency towards metabolic acidosis.

Treatment may depend on the viability of the fetus. If the gestation period is less than 25 weeks it is recommended that if cardiopulmonary resuscitation is ineffective despite adequate treatment open chest cardiac massage should be considered. From 25–32 weeks treatment should consist of open chest massage and the need to perform emergency Caesarean section. After 32 weeks emergency Caesarean section should be considered if 2 minutes of continuous resuscitation appears ineffectual.

DIABETES

The care of the pregnant woman with insulin-dependent diabetes has been reviewed by Freinkel et al (1985). Metabolic changes occur mostly in late pregnancy associated with the production of steroids and peptides by the placenta and the growing fuel demands of the fetus. Thus there are increased levels of free fatty acids and ketones and reduced levels of glucose and amino acids when food is not eaten whereas the eating of glucose results in greater and more prolonged levels of plasma glucose and increased triglycerides. When insulin levels are high there appears to be insulin resistance. There are increased complications including toxaemia, hydramnios and neonatal hypoglycaemia. Improvements of monitoring of the diabetes aiming to keep the fasting plasma glucose level at 3.3–5.5 mmol/l has led to a reduction in complications. Postprandial levels should not exceed 7.8 mmol/l and during labour patients should receive 50 g of glucose 6 hourly intravenously and to avoid increased fetal insulin secretion the blood sugar is measured every 1 to 2 hours and insulin given as necessary. Insulin requirements drop dramatically following delivery.

METABOLISM

Ketonuria

Ketonuria may develop during prolonged labour and traditionally high dose infusions of glucose have been administered. Morton et al (1985) suggested that normal saline should be used if patients are dehydrated and only 10 g/h dextrose should be given (physiological requirement). Dextrose infusions (5% or 10%) led to maternal hyperglycaemia and increased plasma levels of insulin with increases in blood lactate and pyruvate. 10% dextrose resulted in increased serum osmolality. Hartmann's solution increased blood lactate and pyruvate concentrations. 10% dextrose also led to a base deficit (venous sample).

On the other hand Evans et al (1986) measured blood glucose, sodium, lactate and beta-hydroxybutyrate during two different fluid regimes prior to epidural analgesia for pain relief during labour. One group of patients had Hartmann's solution and the other had dextrose in half normal saline. The dextrose-saline solution caused small but significant rises in blood glucose and sodium but within the range of values for pregnancy. Hartmann's solution led to a rise in maternal serum beta-hydroxybutyrate suggesting some degree of maternal ketosis. Neither regime had any significant effect on the neonatal blood glucose or sodium.

Sodium excretion

There have been few studies on the sodium excretion in human pregnancy, most of the studies suggesting that 3 mmol of sodium is retained daily. In a study by Brown & Gallery (1986) on a week's dietary sodium loading or deprivation in the second and third trimesters it was found that the plasma arginine vasopressin (AVP) rose only in the second trimester following sodium loading. Plasma sodium concentration and blood pressure were unaltered but the plasma volume only increased slightly. Brown & Gallery (1986) were only able to conclude that AVP increases in the second trimester of pregnancy to assist in the sodium excretion following dietary sodium loading. (See Ch. 6, under Endocrine Response.)

Urinary function

Urinary retention is said to be common following the use of epidural opioids although Bailey & Sangwan (1986) found that it occurred more frequently after the caudal administration of bupivacaine (0.5%) compared with diamorphine. Evron et al (1985) compared epidural methadone and morphine for pain relief for post-Caesarean section. The patients were given 20 ml bupivacaine (0.5%) epidurally for the operative procedure and thereafter at the end of the operation 4 mg methadone or 4 mg morphine in 6 ml saline. The incidence of difficulty in micturition and the need for catheterisation were less in the methadone group and the interval between inject-tion of methadone and the onset of micturition was less. Methadone is more lipid-soluble than morphine with a more rapid onset of action but of shorter duration than morphine.

EPILEPSY

The use of sodium valproate in pregnancy has not been recommended because of the potential dangers of causing fetal malformations. It appears to act by increasing the concentration in the brain of gamma-aminobutyric acid (GABA). GABA lowers ACTH levels but during pregnancy Hatjis et al (1985) were unable to demonstrate any fall in ACTH or cortisol in maternal or umbilical cord blood in pregnant patients receiving sodium valproate.

HEPATITIS

Viral hepatitis has been subdivided into groups A, B, D and two types of non-A, non-B. Hepatitis A appears to pose little risk to the fetus whereas women who contract hepatitis B in the third trimester of pregnancy may more readily transmit the virus to the fetus. The non-A, non-B hepatitis appear to be similar to the hepatitis B while hepatitis D is also closely associated with hepatitis B. The administration of immunoglobulin to infants whose mothers have antigenic evidence of hepatitis B has been recommended (see Snydman 1985).

LIVER FAILURE

Acute fatty liver with jaundice, encephalopathy, disseminated intravascular coagulation was often fatal. Early diagnosis and prompt management with immediate termination of pregnancy and correction of clotting abnormali-ties have dramatically altered the prognosis (Kaplan 1985).

ASTHMA

The treatment of asthma in pregnancy has been reviewed by Chung & Barnes (1987) who recommend prompt treatment to avoid maternal hypox-aemia which might in turn have detrimental effects on the fetus which has only a reserve supply of oxygen for 2 minutes. Chung & Barnes (1987) referred to a series of 1000 patients with asthma and during pregnancy asthma was unaffected in 50%. In 29% of patients the asthma improved while in 21% it became worse. Only 1% of pregnant women suffer from asthma.

If beta adrenoceptor agonists are required they should be given in aerosol form. Terbutaline and salbutamol have been advocated but adrenaline, isoprenaline and ephedrine should be avoided. Although theophylline is less effective than beta-2 agonists their effects are complementary. However theophylline crosses the placenta and also appears in the maternal milk so that tachycardia and irritability have been reported in the neonate. The use of prednisone and prednisolone may be necessary. Beclomethasone aerosol has not increased the incidence of congenital malformations. Sodium cromoglycate also appears to be reasonably safe. It is important to prevent attacks of wheezing and status asthmaticus with the drugs already mentioned as the effects on the fetus appear to have been exaggerated.

SURGERY

There has been a natural reluctance to perform surgical operations during pregnancy for incidental conditions. In a study of women undergoing incidental surgery during pregnancy compared with patients during pregnancy not undergoing surgery there was no significant difference in congenital abnormalities between the groups. However the risk of spontaneous abortion rose in those having surgery under general anaesthesia in the first or second trimesters, in particular for obstetric or gynaecological procedures (Duncan et al 1986). It was concluded that it would be prudent to avoid operations and anaesthesia if at all possible during pregnancy.

COCAINE

Cocaine is widely used even by pregnant women in the United States and in a study by Chasnoff et al (1985) it was found that there was a higher incidence of spontaneous abortion. This may be due to the fact that cocaine inhibits the uptake of noradrenaline giving rise to vasoconstriction of the placenta with a decrease in fetal blood flow. In some women following intravenous self-injection of cocaine the onset of labour was associated with abruptio placentae. Neurobehaviour studies showed that infants of cocaine-addicted mothers fared less well than control groups and also in mothers on methadone.

The abuse of cocaine also leads to an increased incidence of myocardial infarction, ventricular tachycardia and fibrillation, myocarditis and even sudden death (Isner et al 1986).

HAMMAN'S SYNDROME

Hamman's syndrome is a rare complication in obstetrics with subcutaneous emphysema and pneumomediastinum. Reeder (1986) described a case which also included pneumothorax and reviewed 170 cases in the literature. Most of the cases were primiparous and the duration of labour was within accepted normal limits.

REFERENCES

Bailey P M, Sangwan S 1986 Caudal analgesia for perianal surgery. Anaesthesia 41: 499–504

Barron W M, Mujais S K, Zinaman M, Bravo E L, Lindheimer M D 1986 Plasma catecholamine responses to physiologic stimuli in normal human pregnancy. American Journal of Obstetrics and Gynecology 154: 80–84

Brown M A, Gallery E D M 1986 Sodium excretion in human pregnancy. A role for arginine vasopressin. American Journal of Obstetrics and Gynecology 154: 914–919

Burrow G N 1985 Current concepts. The management of thyrotoxicosis in pregnancy. New England Journal of Medicine 313: 562–565

Chasnoff I J, Burns W J, Schnoll S H, Burns K A 1985 Cocaine use in pregnancy. New England Journal of Medicine 313: 666–669

Chung K F, Barnes P J 1987 Treatment of asthma. British Medical Journal 294: 103–105

Clapp J F 1985 Maternal heart rate in pregnancy. American Journal of Obstetrics and Gynecology 152: 659–660

Confidential Enquiry into Maternal Deaths in England and Wales 1979–1981 (1986). HMSO, London

Dailey, P A, Brookshire G L, Shnider S M et al 1985 The effects of naloxone associated with the intrathecal use of morphine in labor. Anaesthesia and Analgesia 64: 658–666

De Swiet M 1985 Antihypertensive drugs in pregnancy. British Medical Journal 291: 365–366

Duncan P G, Pope W D B, Cohen M M, Greer N 1986 Fetal risk of anesthesia and surgery during pregnancy. Anesthesiology 64: 790–794

Evans S E, Crawford J S, Stevens I D, Durbin G M, Daya H 1986 Fluid therapy for induced labour under epidural analgesia: biochemical consequences for mother and infant. British Journal of Obstetrics and Gynaecology 93: 329–333

Evron S, Samueloff A, Simon A, Drenger B, Magora F 1985 Urinary function during epidural analgesia with methadone and morphine in post-cesarean section patients. Pain 23: 135–144

Freinkel N, Dooley S L, Metzger B E 1985 Current concepts. Care of the pregnant woman with insulin-dependent diabetes mellitus. New England Journal of Medicine 313: 96–101

Gallery E D M, Ross M R, Gyory A Z 1985 Antihypertensive treatment in pregnancy: analysis of different responses to oxprenolol and methyldopa. British Medical Journal 291: 563–566

Gerritse R, Pinas I M, Reuwer P J H, Haspels A A, Charbon G A, Beijer H J M 1985 Antidiuretic effect of ritodrine with and without beta-adrenergic blockade. Archives of Internal Pharmacodynamics 278: 107–113

Hatjis C, Rose J C, Pippitt C, Swain M 1985 Effect of treatment with sodium valproate on plasma adrenocorticotropic hormone and cortisol concentrations in pregnancy. American Journal of Obstetrics and Gynecology 152: 315–316

Hill W C, Katz M, Kitzmiller J L, Gill P J 1985 Continuous long-term intravenous beta-sympathomimetic tocolysis. American Journal of Obstetrics and Gynecology 152: 271–274

Holst N, Jenssen T G, Burhol P G, Jorde R, Maltau J M 1986 Plasma vasoactive intestinal polypeptide, insulin, gastric inhibitory polypeptide and blood glucose in late pregnancy and during and after delivery. American Journal of Obstetrics and Gynecology 155: 126–131

Isner J M, Estes N A M, Thompson P D et al 1986 Acute cardiac events temporally related to cocaine abuse. New England Journal of Medicine 315: 1438–1443

Jones C R, McCullouch J, Butters L, Hamilton C A, Rubin P C, Reid J L 1985 Plasma catecholamines and modes of delivery. The relation between catecholamine levels and in-vitro platelet aggregation and adrenoreceptor radioligand binding characteristics. British Journal of Obstetrics and Gynaecology 92: 593–599

Jouppila P, Kirkinen P, Koivula A, Ylikorkala O 1986 Labetalol does not alter the placental and fetal blood flow or maternal prostanoids in pre-eclampsia. British Journal of Obstetrics and Gynaecology 93: 543–547

Kaplan M M 1985 Current concepts. Acute fatty liver of pregnancy. New England Journal of Medicine 313: 367–370

Kofinas G D, Kofinas A D, Tavakoli F M 1985 Maternal and fetal beta-endorphin release in response to the stress of labor and delivery. American Journal of Obstetrics and Gynecology 152: 56–59

Lee R V, Rodgers B D, White L M, Harvey R C 1986 Cardiopulmonary resuscitation of pregnant women. American Journal of Medicine 81: 311–318

Leveno K J, Klein V R, Guzick D S, Young D C, Hankins C D V, Williams M L 1986 Single-centre randomised trial of ritodrine hydrochloride for preterm labour. Lancet 1: 1293–1295

Lindheimer M D, Katz A I 1985 Current concepts: hypertension in pregnancy. New England Journal of Medicine 313: 675–680

MacLennan F 1986 Maternal mortality from Mendelson's syndrome. An explanation? Lancet 1: 587–589

MacLennan F, Thomson M A R, Rankin R, Terry P B, Adey G D 1985 Fatal pulmonary oedema associated with the use of ritodrine in pregnancy. Case report. British Journal of Obstetrics and Gynaecology 92: 703–705

MacPherson M, Broughton Pipkin F, Rutter N 1986 The effect of maternal labetalol on the newborn infant. British Journal of Obstetrics and Gynaecology 93: 539–542

Marx G F, Patel S, Berman J A, Farmakides G, Schulman H 1986 Umbilical blood flow velocity waveforms in different maternal positions and with epidural analgesia. Obstetrics and Gynecology 68: 61–63

Moore T R, Key T C, Reisner L S, Resnik R 1985 Evaluation of the use of continuous lumbar epidural anesthesia for hypertensive pregnant women in labor. American Journal of Obstetrics and Gynecology 152: 404–412

Morton K E, Jackson M C, Gillmer M D G 1985 A comparison of the effects of four intravenous solutions for the treatment of ketonuria during labour. British Journal of Obstetrics and Gynaecology 92: 473–479

Neumark J, Hammerle A F, Biegelmayer C 1985 Effects of epidural analgesia on plasma catecholamines and cortisol in parturition. Acta Anaesthesiologica Scandinavica 29: 555–559

Reeder S R 1986 Subcutaneous emphysema, pneumomediastinum and pneumothorax in labor and delivery. American Journal of Obstetrics and Gynecology 154: 487–489

Richards A M, Moodley J, Graham D I, Bullock M R R 1986 Active management of the unconscious eclamptic patient. British Journal of Obstetrics and Gynaecology 93: 554–562

Snydman D R 1985 Current concepts: hepatitis in pregnancy. New England Journal of Medicine 313: 1398–1401

Sullivan J M, Ramanathan K B 1985 Current concepts: management of medical problems in pregnancy — severe cardiac disease. New England Journal of Medicine 313: 304–309

Vleugels M P, Eling W M, Rolland R, De Graaf R 1986 Cortisol levels in human pregnancy in relation to parity and age. American Journal of Obstetrics and Gynecology 155: 118–121

Wallenburg H C S, Dekker G A, Makovitz J W, Rotmans P 1986 Low-dose aspirin prevents pregnancy-induced hypertension and pre-eclampsia in angiotensin-sensitive primigravidae. Lancet 1: 1–3

Wang-Cheng R, Davidson B J 1986 Ritodrine-induced neutropenia. American Journal of Obstetrics and Gynecology 154: 924–925

Whittaker P G, Gerrard J, Lind T 1985 Catecholamine responses to changes in posture during human pregnancy. British Journal of Obstetrics and Gynaecology 92: 586–592

Sites of action of opiates in production of analgesia

A. INTRODUCTION

Classic observations indicate that opiates can produce a powerful modulation of the response of the organism to a strong, aversive stimulus. The pharmacological characteristics of these drug effects (e.g. structure-activity relationship stereospecificity, selective antagonism by agents such as naloxone and the phenomenon of tolerance with cross tolerance between structurally related members) clearly suggest that these opioids exert their effect upon specific membrane receptors. Important issues are (1) the location of these receptors in the brain, i.e. with which CNS structures are these receptors associated, and (2) the probable mechanism by which these receptors selectively modulate the nature of nociceptive processing. This paper will briefly address these two issues.

B. LOCATION OF CNS ACTION OF OPIOIDS

1. Methodology

A direct approach to the issue of site(s) of action of a drug in the brain may be derived from studies in which agents are administered into circumscribed regions of the neuraxis. For examination of the supraspinal action of a drug, local administration may be accomplished by the use of stereotaxically implanted stainless-steel guide cannulae. These guides are permanently affixed to the skull and after several postoperative days may be used to direct the insertion of smaller (typically 28–32 gauge) injection cannulae into the unanaesthetized animal. Solutions in volume of 0.5 μl or less may be administered and the local effects of agents assessed on the nociceptive threshold. Issues such as volume, diffusion and concentration have been discussed elsewhere (Yaksh & Rudy 1978), and it appears that such an approach can be used to assess reliably the effect of an agent on a circumscribed volume of tissue. Consideration of the probable action of drugs on spinal function have been assessed using catheters chronically placed in the intrathecal space (Yaksh & Rudy 1976, 1977). Given that the goal is to ascertain the role of different sites in the 'analgesic' actions of an opioid, the bioassay is the behavioural response of the unanaesthetized animal to a strong, unconditioned physical stimulus which would otherwise evoke escape behaviour. The use of chronically placed catheters permits such injections to be made without trauma in the unanaesthetized animal without any intervention during the test. The measured behaviours most frequently employed are broadly defined as spinal and supraspinally mediated, e.g. tail flick and skin twitch for the latter, and hot plate stimulus evoked vocalization and shock titration threshold for the former. It is important to note that, in all of these measures, the animal has the absolute ability to escape the stimulus. A second point is that the word analgesia implies a selective obtundation of the response otherwise evoked by a noxious stimulus. Such specificity is difficult to ascertain in the animal model, but the occurrence of a powerful effect on the organized behaviour evoked by an unconditioned stimulus without changes in the ability of the animal to respond or a general suppression of behaviour is the minimal criterion necessary to imply the theoretical construct of analgesia.

2. Micro-injection mapping of opioid-sensitive sites

Using these approaches, the brains of several species have been mapped for their sensitivity to the effects of opioid drugs. In brief, morphine administered into a number of specific brain regions will evoke significant increases in the response latency of the animal to a noxious stimulus without prominent effects on gross behavioural function, e.g as assessed by catalepsy (immobility/rigidity) or evident seizures. Table 18.1 presents a summary of principal sites in brain where sensitivity has been found in the rat.

Consideration of the listed regions emphasizes the fact that the vast majority of brain sites examined with intracerebral injections of opiates show no effect with regard to nociceptive end-points. Thus, direct application into cortex, or into the striatum in general has minimal effect on nociceptive behaviour in primates (Pert & Yaksh 1974) and rat (Yaksh et al 1976, but see Jurna & Heinz 1979). The latter appears in contrast to the high levels of opioid binding sites observed in this region (Wamsley 1983). This emphasizes the fact that the location of receptors by binding does not define the physiological role of the CNS structures with which they are associated. A second consideration is the generality of these findings with regard to species. Though the distribution of sites has been most widely assessed in the rodent, similar micro-injection studies have been carried out in the mouse (Criswell 1976), rabbit (Tsou & Jang, 1964, Teschemacher et al 1973), cat (Ossipov et al 1984), dog (Wettstein et al 1982) and primate (Pert & Yaksh 1974, 1975) and the relevance of the mesencephalic (periaqueductal) sites has been uniformly demonstrated. Though intraparenchymal studies have not been carried out in man, the intraventricular administration of several opioids including morphine (Leavens et al 1982,

Table 18.1 Effects of intracerebrally administered morphine on nociceptive and non-nociceptive aspects of behaviour in the rat

	Antinociception				
	Spinal reflex (tail flick)	Supraspinal (hot plate)	Catalepsy	Seizures	References
Diencephalon					
Medial thalamus	$-^\star$	–	2	2	1,3
Lateral thalamus	–	–	2	2	1,3
Amygdala (corticomedial)	–	2	–	–	2
Mesencephalon					
Peri-aqueductal grey	1	1	2	–	3,7,8,9,10
Mesencephalic reticular function	3	3	2	–	4
Medulla					
Medial medulla (raphe magnus)	3	1–2	–	–	6,10
Lateral medulla (n. gigantocellularis)	3	1–2	–	–	5,10
Spinal cord	1	1	–	–	11,12

*Dose range of morphine sulphate required to produce a maximum effect. 1 = 1–5 μg; 2 = 5–15 μg; 3 = >15 μg;
 – = inactive.
References:
  1 = Walker & Yaksh (1986)
  2 = Rodgers (1977)
  3 = Yaksh et al (1976)
  4 = Haighler et al (1978)
  5 = Takagi et al (1977), Kuraishi et al (1978), Ossipov et al (1986)
  6 = Takagi et al (1976), Dickenson et al (1979)
  7 = Jacquet & Lajtha (1976)
  8 = Sharpe et al (1974)
  9 = Lewis & Gebhart (1977)
 10 = Jensen & Yaksh (1986a)
 11 = Yaksh & Rudy (1977)
 12 = Yaksh & Rudy (1976)

Lenzi et al 1985) and β-endorphin (Foley et al 1979) in terminal cancer patients has been shown to produce a powerful analgesia.

Spinal administration studies have been carried out in a wide variety of species including mouse (Hylden & Wilcox 1983), cat (Yaksh 1978a, Yaksh et al 1986) and primate (Yaksh 1978b, Yaksh & Reddy 1981, Yaksh 1983), and a powerful analgesia has been routinely reported. Similarly, spinal (intrathecal or epidural) administration has been shown to increase the nociceptive threshold and diminish the pain report in a variety of human studies (see Cousins & Mather 1984, Yaksh & Noueihed 1985).

C. FUNCTIONAL CHARACTERISTICS OF THE EFFECTS OF FOCALLY ADMINISTERED OPIATES

The principal consideration is the effect of opiates on nociceptive processing. Evidence that these opioid-linked systems in brain can modulate pain transmission is further emphasized by the fact that the effects of locally administered opioids can alter the response in a wide variety of nociceptive measures including reflex (e.g. hind paw withdrawal (Tsou & Jang 1964), tail flick (Yaksh et al 1976)), simple non-reflex (hot plate (Sharpe et al 1974, Yaksh et al 1976), tail pinch (Takagi et al 1978), formalin-induced paw lick (Kuraishi et al 1983), writhing (Jensen & Yaksh 1986c), shock-evoked jump response (Rodgers 1977)) and in complex behavioural paradigms (shock titration (Pert & Yaksh 1974)). Table 18.1 also indicates that at many of the sites at which morphine produces a change in the response to a strong stimulus it also evokes complex effects on behaviour. Thus, in the thalamus, opioids may produce a syndrome of changes in the pain response, catalepsy and prominent alterations in the EEG. These effects appear to be associated most prominently with the δ-opioid receptor (see below). When such global events occur, one must exercise care in interpreting the failure to respond to a given noxious stimulus, e.g. whether it is a selective modulation of the afferent pain message or a block of the ability to emit the response. Thus, in addition to the effects on supraspinally organized pain behaviour, opioids administered into many brain stem sites will alter spinal nociceptive reflexes, suggesting the activation of bulbospinal pathways which mediate nociceptive reflexes. Though it is often assumed that such inhibition reflects a concurrent inhibition of the afferent limb of the pain pathway, the possibility of an alteration in the efferent activation of the motor reflex alone cannot be uniquely excluded.

Alternatively, it is important to note that doses which produce a significant effect on the nociceptive end-points are frequently not associated with a general suppression of all responses. Thus, in rats for example, in a variety of brain stem sites such as the peri-aqueductal grey (PAG) or the medulla, significant changes in the response to noxious stimuli can be achieved prior to a general behavioural suppression as measured by a tendency to immobility (catalepsy). Opiates, acting on other brain regions, may produce changes in the response to strong stimuli, but only at doses which produce evidence of a broader dysfunction. Thus, a simple interpretation of the significance of the change in nociceptive end-points is not permitted.

D. PHARMACOLOGY OF CENTRAL OPIOID RECEPTORS ASSOCIATED WITH ANALGESIA

In the preceding sections, it was indicated that opioids with an action limited to certain brain regions and the spinal cord would yield a significant analgesia. An important issue relates to whether the local action of the drug is mediated by an opioid receptor, and if so by which of the several opioid receptors known to exist is the effect mediated?

Assessment of this question hinges upon the establishment of the pharmacological profile associated with observed effects produced by the intracerebrally administered agents.

With regard to the general question of the role of opioid receptors, the antinociceptive effects produced by intracerebral morphine listed in Table 18.1 have been shown to be dose dependent, mimicked by other opioid alkaloids (such as methadone, levorphanol, sufentanil), uniformly antagonized by naloxone and where examined stereospecific (see Yaksh 1984a,b for references). In spinal cord, comparable studies have similarly revealed that over a range of doses, the antinociceptive effects possess a characteristically opioid pharmacology (see Yaksh & Noueihed 1985). These minimal criteria early established that the focal action of opiates on these brain regions and in spinal cord were exerting their effects by an opioid receptor.

Current thinking emphasizes that there may be several subclasses of opioid receptors. The focal injection procedures allow us to consider whether the receptors in the several regions which alter nociceptive processing are the same or distinguishable.

Table 18.2 briefly summarizes the pharmacological profile of several proposed subclasses of opioid receptors.

Based on these characteristics the pharmacology of sites in several regions of the neuraxis have begun to be examined in detail in experiments where selective agonists are administered.

Table 18.3 presents a summary of experiments examining the pharmacology of sites in the mesencephalic peri-aqueductal grey and after spinal intrathecal injection.

Though considerably more work remains to be done, the first order analysis of the results in Table 18.3 is that within the PAG, sites exist with affinity for μ-type agents (morphine, sufentanil, DAGO) and κ-type agents (U50488H). The purported μ_1-receptor agonist meptazinol (Dray et al 1986) is weakly active, suggesting that the type of μ sites relevant to the phenomenon may be reflected by this subclass. Significantly, the ligand DSLET is active but DPDPE is not. Though both are thought to have high affinity for the δ-receptor (Clark et al 1986, Itzhak et al 1986); they differ in that

Table 18.2 Pharmacological profile of several proposed subclasses of opioid receptors

	Agonists	Antagonists
μ	Sufentanil, morphine, DAGO	*β-FNA, naloxone
μ_1	Meptazinol	*Naloxonazine, naloxone
δ	DADL, DSLET, DPDPE	ICI-864, +naloxone
κ	U50488H	?, +naloxone
ε	β-Endorphin	?, naloxone

*Non-equilibrium, non-competitive antagonists. See Ward et al (1982) and Ling et al (1986).
+Naloxone has approximately 0.1 × the affinity for the δ and κ sites as compared to the μ site.
? = well defined selective antagonist is not available.
  β-FNA = β-funalnaltrexamine
  DADL = D-Ala^2-D-Leu^5-enkephalin
  DAGO = D-Ala^2-MePhe^4,Gly-ol^5-enkephalin
  DPDPE = D-pencillamine^2-D-penicillamine^5-enkephalin
  DSTLE = D-Ser^2-Thr^6-leucine enkephalin
  U50488H = (trans-3,4-dichloro-N-methyl-N-[2–1 (1-pyrrolindinyl)cyclohexyl]) benzeneacetamide
          = N, N-diallyl-Tyr-Aib-Aib-Phe-Leu-OH

Table 18.3   Effect in the rat on the hot plate response latency of receptor selective opioid ligands administered into the peri-aqueductal grey and spinal cord

Site	Ordering of activity on the hot plate test
*Peri-aqueductal grey	Sufentanil > β-endorphin > morphine ⩾ DAGO > meptazinol = U50488H ≫ DPDPE = 0
*Medial medulla	Sufentanil ⩾ DSLET ⩾ DADL > morphine
+Spinal cord	β-Endorphin ⩾ sufentanil > DAGO ⩾ DSLET ⩾ DPDPE ≫ meptazinol = U50488H = O

*Data from Jensen & Yaksh (1986c) and Al-Rodhan & Yaksh (in preparation). All drugs delivered in volumes of 0.5 μl.
  +Data from Yaksh & Henry (1978), Yaksh et al (1986), Schmauss & Yaksh (1983) and Mjanger & Yaksh (unpublished). All drugs delivered in volumes of 10 μl.

DSLET in contrast to DPDPE has a higher affinity for the μ_1 sites (Clark et al 1986, Itzhak & Pasternak 1986). Indeed, in recent studies we have observed that the effect of μ agonists and DSLET are readily antagonized by the μ-specific non-equilibrium antagonist, β-FNA, further supporting a probable role of a μ-receptor site.

In spinal cord, strong evidence exists to indicate the presence of μ and δ sites (see Tung & Yaksh 1982, Yaksh 1983, Russel et al 1987, Mjanger & Yaksh in preparation). Unlike in the PAG, μ_1 and κ agonists are without effect on the HP response (Schmauss & Yaksh 1983, Mjanger & Yaksh unpublished observations).

Though the data are as yet incomplete, it clearly appears that the nature of the receptor pharmacology of the several sites can be distinguished. The profile of activity in other regions, e.g. the amygdala and the medial medulla is at best only partially characterized (see Jensen & Yaksh 1986c).

E. MECHANISMS WHEREBY OPIOIDS ACTING IN THE SEVERAL BRAIN REGIONS MODULATE NOCICEPTIVE TRANSMISSION

Given the anatomical diversity of substrates where opiates may act to modulate the nociceptive response, it appears unlikely that the mechanisms underlying the effects observed following injection into the several brain regions could be the same. In the following sections, we will briefly consider several probable circuits involving the brain and spinal cord.

1. Brain stem

Currently, we believe that there are four mechanisms whereby opiates acting in the PAG may alter nociceptive transmission: indirect bulbospinal inhibition; indirect brain stem–brain stem inhibition; direct inhibition of brain stem transmission; and forebrain projections.

a. Bulbospinal projections

Early studies with systemic opiates pointed to the probable bulbospinal pathways on the inhibition of spinal cord reflexes (see Yaksh 1985 for references). This was confirmed in a large number of subsequent peri-aqueductal/periventricular micro-injection studies (Tsou & Jang 1964, see also Yaksh & Rudy 1978). More recently, mesencephalic micro-injection of opiates has been shown to inhibit activity in dorsal horn nociceptors (Gebhart et al 1984). These effects coincide with the reports of extensive work by Swedish investigators that bulbospinal monoamine pathways, when activated, could prominently modulate activity in flexor reflex afferents (Anden et al 1966). Several lines of evidence may be accrued to support the likelihood that PAG and medullary opioid receptor linked systems do activate such bulbospinal pathways and thereby directly regulate spinal cord nociceptive processing.

(i) Brain stem opiates result in an increase in spinal cord turnover or release of serotonin and noradrenaline (Takagi et al 1979, Tyce & Yaksh 1981).

(ii) The effects of PAG morphine on nociceptive responses are closely mimicked by the local administration of serotoninergic or adrenergic agonists. Thus, locally applied noradrenaline and 5-HT wlll block activity in dorsal horn nociceptors (Headley et al 1978) and the intrathecal administration of these amines will result in a powerful and functionally specific analgesia (Yaksh & Wilson 1979, Kuraishi et al 1979, Reddy et al 1980). The effects of the noradrenergic agonists appear, by virtue of their pharmacology to act via an α_2-receptor (see Yaksh 1985).

(iii) The effects of PAG opioids on spinal reflexes are antagonized by the spinal administration of adrenergic and serotoninergic receptor antagonists (Yaksh 1979, Jensen & Yaksh 1986b). Importantly, the pharmacology of the spinal receptor sites acted upon by the endogenously released noradrenaline is the same as that for the intrathecally administered drug (e.g. an α_2- but not an α_1- or β-receptor; Camarata & Yaksh 1985).

(iv) Finally, that the antinociceptive effects of PAG opiates reflects the 'activation' of a bulbospinal system is emphasized by the fact that the effects are mimicked by the intracerebral administration of excitatory amino acids (glutamate; Jensen & Yaksh 1984) or by electrical stimulation and the spinal pharmacology of this stimulation cannot be distinguished from that of the opiates (Satoh et al 1983, Jensen & Yaksh 1984, Hammond & Yaksh 1984).

Given that PAG projections to the spinal cord are sparse and are not monoaminergic, early studies emphasized the probability that excitatory projections to more caudal bulbar aminergic nuclei represented the intermediary link (see Yaksh & Rudy 1978).

In spite of the persuasive evidence for the significance of bulbospinal pathways, they alone do not appear uniquely able or necessary to explain the observed effects. Thus, perhaps most interesting is that while the spinal administration of monoamine antagonists may reverse the inhibition of spinal reflexes produced by PAG opiates, it has only transient or limited effects on the supraspinally organized response to the nociceptive stimulus (e.g. as measured on the HP response). Although several alternatives may be entertained, we feel this dissociation between spinal and supraspinally organized responses is real. While it may also mean that bulbospinal inhibition plays a small role in modulating supraspinal transmission (e.g. that it only affects spinal motor reflexes), we consider it more likely that these results emphasize the presence of additional supraspinal mechanisms which modulate the response of the animal to aversive stimuli.

b. Indirect brain stem–brain stem inhibition

The role of spino-reticulo-thalamic properties in pain transmission has been long postulated (Bowsher et al 1968). Mohrland & Gebhart (1980) have shown that stimulation in the PAG will result in an inhibition in n. gigantocellular neurons. Thus, it is conceivable that a 'local' descending inhibition may be relevant.

c. Direct inhibition of brain stem transmission

It is clear that many of the regions in which opiates act (e.g. the medial medulla or the PAG) receive input from spinobulbar fibres or collaterals from spino-diencephalic fibres (Bowsher et al 1968). Though indirect, the fact that spinobulbar cell bodies possess opioid receptors (see below) and given the probability that receptors are transported to distal cell terminals (Atweh et al 1978), it is probable that spinobulbar fibres also have opioid receptors on their bulbar terminals. We speculate that local opioids may block afferent activity into the bulbar core.

d. Forebrain projections

While there is little direct evidence supporting the hypothesis that rostral projections are affected by a bulbar action of opiates or that such rostral projections may be relevant to pain transmission, it should be noted that early studies examining the effect of various lesions on morphine analgesia focused on raphe dorsalis, a serotonin-containing nucleus which projects rostrally (see Messing & Lytle 1977), the possibility exists that opiates may activate systems relevant to the emotional context of the pain message and may employ these systems as a substrate (Xuan et al 1986).

2. Forebrain sites

Though the mechanisms in the brain stem are only incompletely appreciated, forebrain systems are less understood. The effects of opioids in the amygdala reflect this. As noted in Table 18.1, amygdalar injections do not alter spinal reflex function. Thus, consistent with the anatomy, the mechanism probably does not relate to any spinopetal interactions. Alternatively, the amygdala has long been associated with various aspects of emotion and the well appreciated efforts of systemic morphine in the emotional-effective component of pain may be related to an effect on such systems. Similarly, it should be stressed that other portions of the limbic forebrain systems related to emotion may be involved and the failure to detect their relevance to pain, particularly in chronic circumstances, may be the result of insensitive experimental test paradigms. It should also be stressed that a bilateral action of the drug may be necessary for the opioid effect on pain behaviour to be manifested. This may be the case for such systems which modulate the affective aspects of the behavioural response (e.g. compare Rodgers (1977) to Yaksh et al (1976)).

3. Spinal cord

The application of opiates to the spinal surface or directly into tissue by local microtechniques yields a powerful, pharmacologically specific and functionally selective inhibition of activity evoked in wide dynamic range or nociceptive specific neurons evoked by Aδ/C fibre stimulation (see Yaksh & Noueihed 1985). Within the spinal cord, ample evidence exists to suggest that opioids may act to alter nociceptive transmission selectively, by an action both presynaptic on or postsynaptic to the primary afferent.

Evidence for a presynaptic action is based on: (a) the observation that opioid binding in the dorsal horn is largely within the substantia gelatinosa and is significantly, but not totally diminished by rhizotomy or by treatment with a small primary afferent neurotoxin capsaicin (LaMotte et al 1976, Gamse et al 1979) and (b) that opiates will reduce the stimulation-evoked secretion of substance P, a small primary afferent peptide neurotransmitter (Yaksh et al 1980, Pang & Vasko 1986, Go & Yaksh 1987).

That spinal opiates may also act postsynaptically on primary afferents is emphasized (a) by the partial effects of rhizotomy in opioid binding and (b) by the ability of opiates to diminish the response evoked by iontophoretically applied glutamate (Zieglgansberger & Bayerl 1976).

Though opiate binding is found in the dorsal roots (Fields et al 1980), it does not appear that such a site plays a role in the actions of intrathecal opiates in the adult animals. Thus recording in situ from DRG cells revealed no effect of opiates (Williams & Zieglgansberger 1981).

F. INTERACTION BETWEEN BRAIN AND SPINAL OPIOID SENSITIVE SYSTEMS IN THE PRODUCTION OF ANALGESIA

Given the multiple sites of potential action revealed by micro-injection studies, it is reasonable to query how they may interact. Indeed, when an opiate is given systemically, all of the systems are concurrently affected. Several lines of evidence may be considered. First, when opioids are given systemically, it is possible to produce a dose-dependent rightward shift in the systemic morphine dose-response curve by administering an opioid antagonist either in the cerebral ventricles or in the spinal cord (see Yaksh & Rudy 1978). Given that opiates acting in circumscribed brain regions can produce analgesia, the ability to produce shifts in the systemic dose–response curves with local naloxone appears thus contradictory, e.g. the effect of the systemic drug collapses when receptors in either the brain or cord are blocked. Yaksh & Rudy (1978) proposed that this phenomenon might be explained by presuming a synergistic interaction between brain stem and spinal cord opioid-sensitive systems. Such a synergistic interaction would theoretically be revealed by the results, cited above, of the opioid antagonist experiments and by studies in which the dose–response interaction between intraventricular and intrathecal morphine was examined. In such studies it was indeed confirmed that there was a synergistic interaction between brain stem and spinal opioid sensitive systems (Yeung & Rudy 1980). A corollary of this hypothesis would be that if the bulbospinal pathway mediates the effects of brain stem morphine on spinal processing then there should also be a synergistic interaction between spinal morphine and spinal α_2 agonists. This has indeed been demonstrated (Yaksh & Reddy 1981, Monasky & Yaksh 1986, Wigdor & Wilcox 1987). We believe that the substrate for this interaction is reflected by the observation that the slope of the stimulus intensity – cell response curve of spinal neurons is reduced both by bulbospinal stimulation (Gebhart et al 1984) and by spinal opiates (Yaksh 1978b). Such an interaction between manipulations which alter the gain of the system would indeed be expected to show a non-linear (non-additive) functional interaction.

G. EFFECTS ON AUTONOMIC ASPECTS OF PAIN PROCESSING

The above discussion regarding the mechanisms whereby opiates alter pain processing have been closely directed at various aspects of the behavioural response to strong stimuli. It is, however, also clear that the responses to pain are manifested by a wide range of systems. The observation that opiates reduce the MACBAR (minimum aveolar concentration required to block the adrenergic response) is a probable manifestation in modulating the response to $A\delta/C$ fibre evoked stimulation which otherwise activates autonomic outflow. Thus, spinal opiates will diminish the blood pressure response (Go & Yaksh 1987) and adrenal catecholamine secretion (Gaumann & Yaksh unpublished observations) associated with high intensity sciatic nerve stimulation. In man, spinal diamorphine has been shown to diminish the surgically evoked autonomic response (Child & Kaufman 1985). As spinally administered opiates have little effect on resting parameters and do not block autonomic reflexes (e.g. valsalva manoeuvre; see Cousins & Mather 1984), this effect must reflect an action on the somatic afferent input to the intermediolateral cell column, e.g. on the dorsal horn projections.

Bulbospinal pathways are known to project into the intermediolateral cell column (Henry & Calaresu 1974). Activation of these pathways by stimulation of the PAG (Sonoda et al 1986) has been shown to inhibit a variety of visceromotor reflexes. It is thus likely that, similar to the bulbospinal effects on somatic reflexes and organized pain behaviour (see above), brain stem opioid receptors may exert a powerful modulation of the autonomic response evoked by strong stimuli. Whether these modulatory effects are directly on the intermediolateral cell column neurons and/or on the afferent drive to these cells is not known.

H. SUMMARY

In short, systemic opioids produce a powerful effect on various aspects of animal behaviour because of their interaction with several specific classes of receptors which are associated with discrete anatomical structures. The physiological effect of these several systems serves to modulate in a complex fashion the processing of the afferent message both by an effect on its spinal coding and by apparent but as yet undefined changes in its effect on supraspinal response functions.

REFERENCES

Anden N-E, Jukes M G M, Lundberg A, Vyklicky L 1966 The effect of DOPA on the spinal cord. Acta Physiologica Scandinavica 67: 373–386
Atweh S F, Murrin L C, Kuhar M J 1978 Presynaptic localization of opiate receptors in the vagal and accessory optic systems: an autoradiographic study. Neuropharmacology 17: 65–71
Bowsher D, Mallart A, Petit D, Albe-Fessard D 1968 A bulbar relay to the centre median. Journal of Neurophysiology 31: 288–300
Camarata P J, Yaksh T L 1985 Characterization of the spinal adrenergic receptors mediating the spinal effects produced by the microinjection of morphine into the periaqueductal gray. Brain Research 336: 133–142
Child C S, Kaufman L 1985 Effect of intrathecal diamorphine on the adrenocortical, hyperglycaemic and cardiovascular responses to major colonic surgery. British Journal of Anaesthesia 57: 389–393
Clark J A, Itzhak Y, Hruby V J, Yamamura H I, Pasternak G W 1986 [D-Pen^2,D-Pen^5] enkephalin (DPDPE): a δ-selective enkephalin with low affinity for μ_1 opiate binding sites. European Journal of Pharmacology 128: 303–304
Cousins M J, Mather L E 1984 Intrathecal and epidural administration of opioids. Anesthesiology 61: 276–310
Criswell H D 1976 Analgesia and hyperreactivity following morphine microinjection into mouse brain. Pharmacology, Biochemistry and Behaviour 4: 23–26
Dickenson A H, Oliveras J-L, Besson J-M 1979 Role of the nucleus raphe magnus in opiate analgesia as studied by the microinjection technique in the rat. Brain Research 170: 95–111
Dray A, Nunan L, Wire W 1986 Meptazinol: unusual in vivo opioid receptor activity at supraspinal and spinal sites. Neuropharmacology 25: 343–349
Fields H L, Emson P C, Leigh B K, Gilbert R F T, Iversen L L 1980 Multiple opiate receptor sites on primary afferent fibres. Nature 284: 351–353
Foley K M, Kourides I A, Inturrisi C E et al 1979 β-Endorphin: analgesic and hormonal effects in humans. Proceedings of the National Academy of Sciences USA 76: 5377–5381
Gamse R, Holzer P, Lembeck F 1979 Indirect evidence for presynaptic location of opiate

receptors in chemosensitive primary sensory neurones. Naunyn-Schmiedeberg's Archives of Pharmacology 308: 281–285

Gebhart G F, Sandkuhler J, Thalhammer J, Zimmerman M 1984 Inhibition in spinal cord of nociceptive information by electrical stimulation and morphine microinjections at identical sites in midbrain of the cat. Journal of Neurophysiology 51: 75–89

Go V L W, Yaksh T L 1987 Release of substance P from the cat spinal cord. Journal of Physiology 391: 141–167

Haighler H J, Spring D D 1978 A comparison of the analgesic and behavioral effects of [D-Ala^2] met-enkephalinamide and morphine in the mesencephalic reticular formation of rats. Life Sciences 23: 1229–1240

Hammond D L, Yaksh T L 1984 Antagonism of stimulation-produced antinociception by intrathecal administration of methysergide or phentolamine. Brain Research 298: 329–337

Headley P M, Duggan A W, Griersmith B T 1978 Selective reduction by noradrenaline and 5-hydroxytryptamine of nociceptive responses of cat dorsal horn neurones. Brain Research 145: 185–189

Henry J L, Calaresu F R, 1974 Pathways from medullary nuclei to spinal cardioacceleratory neurons in the cat. Experimental Brain Research 20: 505–514

Hylden J L K, Wilcox G L 1983 Pharmacological characterization of substance P-induced nociception in mice: modulation by opioid and noradrenergic agonists at the spinal level. Journal of Pharmacology and Experimental Therapeutics 226: 398–404

Itzhak Y, Pasternak G W 1986 Interaction of [D-Ser^2, Leu^5] enkephalin-Thr^6 (DSLET), a relatively selective delta ligand, with mu$_1$ opioid binding sites. Life Sciences 40: 307–311

Jacquet Y F, Lajtha A 1976 The periaqueductal gray: site of morphine analgesia and tolerance as shown by 2-way cross-tolerance between systemic and intracerebral injections. Brain Research 103: 501–513

Jensen T S, Yaksh T L 1984 Spinal monoamine and opiate system pathways mediate the antinociceptive effects produced by glutamate at brainstem sites. Brain Research 321: 287–297

Jensen T S, Yaksh T L 1986a I. Comparison of antinociceptive action of morphine in the periaqueductal gray, medial and paramedial medulla in rat. Brain Research 363: 99–113

Jensen T S, Yaksh T L 1986b II. Examination of spinal monoamine receptors through which brain stem opiate-sensitive systems act in the rat. Brain Research 363: 114–127

Jensen T S, Yaksh T L 1986c III. Comparison of the antinociceptive action of mu and delta opioid receptor ligands in the periaqueductal gray matter, medial and paramedial ventral medulla in the rat as studied by the microinjection technique. Brain Research 372: 301–312

Jurna I, Heinz G 1979 Anti-nociceptive effect of morphine, opioid analgesics and haloperidol injected into the caudate nucleus of the rat. Naunyn-Schmiedeberg's Archives of Pharmacology 309: 145–151

Kuraishi Y, Fukui K, Shiomi H, Akaike A, Takagi H 1978 Microinjection of opioids into the nucleus reticularis gigantocellularis of the rat: analgesia and increase in the normetanephrine level in the spinal cord. Biochemical Pharmacology 27: 2756–2758

Kuraishi Y, Harada Y, Aratani S, Satoh S, Takagi H 1983 Separate involvement of the spinal noradrenergic and serotonergic systems in morphine analgesia: the differences in the mechanical and thermal algesic tests. Brain Research 273: 245–252

Kuraishi Y, Harada Y, Takagi H 1979 Noradrenaline regulation of pain transmission in the spinal cord mediated by α-adrenoceptors. Brain Research 174: 333–336

LaMotte C, Pert C B, Snyder S H 1976 Opiate receptor binding in primate spinal cord: distribution and changes after dorsal root section. Brain Research 112: 407–412

Leavens M E, Hill C S Jr, Cech D A, Weyland J B, Weston J S 1982 Intrathecal and intraventricular morphine for pain in cancer patients: initial study. Journal of Neurosurgery 56: 241–245

Lenzi A, Galli G, Gandolfini M, Marini G 1985 Intraventricular morphine in paraneoplastic painful syndrome of the cervicofacial region: experience in thirty-eight cases. Neurosurgery 17: 6–11

Lewis V A, Gebhart G F 1977 Evaluation of the periaqueductal central gray (PAG) as a morphine specific locus of action and examination of morphine-induced and stimulation-produced analgesia at coincident PAG loci. Brain Research 124: 283–303

Ling G S F, Simantov R, Clark J A, Pasternak G W 1986 Naloxonazine actions in vivo. European Journal of Pharmacology 129: 33–38

Messing R B, Lytle L D 1977 Serotonin containing neurons: their possible role in pain and analgesia. Pain 4: 1–21

Mohrland S, Gebhart G 1980 Effects of focal electrical stimulation and morphine microinjection in the periaqueductal gray of the rat mesencephalon on neuronal activity in the medullary reticular formation. Brain Research 201: 23–37

Monasky M S, Yaksh T L 1986 Synergistic interaction of intrathecal morphine and an α_2-agonist (ST-91) on antinociception in the rat. Society for Neuroscience Abstracts 12: 1016

Ossipov M H, Gebhart G F 1986 Opioid, cholinergic and α-adrenergic influences on the modulation of nociception from the lateral reticular nucleus of the rat. Brain Research 384: 282–393

Ossipov M H, Goldstein F J, Malseed R T 1984 Feline analgesia following central administration of opioids. Neuropharmacology 23: 925–929

Pang I H, Vasko M R 1986 Morphine and norepinephrine, but not 5-hydroxytryptamine and γ-aminobutyric acid inhibit the potassium stimulated release of substance P from rat spinal cord slices. Brain Research 376: 268–279

Pert A, Yaksh T L 1974 Sites of morphine induced analgesia in the primate brain: relation to pain pathways. Brain Research 80: 135–140

Pert A, Yaksh T L 1975 Localization of the antinociceptive action of morphine in primate brain. Pharmacology, Biochemistry and Behaviour 3: 133–138

Reddy S V R, Maderdrut J L, Yaksh T L 1980 Spinal cord pharmacology of adrenergic agonist-mediated antinociception. Journal of Pharmacology and Experimental Therapeutics 213: 525–533

Rodgers R J 1977 Elevation of aversive threshold in rats by intraamygdaloid injection of morphine sulfate. Pharmacology, Biochemistry and Behaviour 6: 385–390

Russel R D, Leslie J D, Su Y F, Watkins W D, Chang K J 1987 Continuous intrathecal opioid analgesia: tolerance and cross tolerance of mu and delta spinal opioid receptors. Journal of Pharmacology and Experimental Therapeutics 240: 150–158

Satoh M, Oku R, Akaike A 1983 Analgesia produced by microinjection of L-glutamate into the rostral ventromedial bulbar nuclei of the rat and its inhibition by intrathecal α-adrenergic blocking agents. Brain Research 261: 361–364

Schmauss C, Yaksh T L 1983 In vivo studies on spinal opiate receptor systems mediating antinociception. II. Pharmacological profiles suggesting a differential association of mu, delta and kappa receptors with visceral chemical and cutaneous thermal stimuli in the rat. Journal of Pharmacology and Experimental Therapeutics 228: 1–12

Sharpe L G, Garnett J E, Cicero T J 1974 Analgesia and hyperreactivity produced by intracranial microinjections of morphine into the periaqueductal gray matter of the rat. Behavioral Biology 11: 303–313

Sonoda H, Ikenoue K, Yokota T 1986 Periaqueductal gray inhibition of viscerointercostal and galvanic skin reflexes. Brain Research 369: 91–102

Takagi H, Doi T, Akaike A 1976 Microinjection of morphine into the medial part of the bulbar reticular formation in rabbit and rat: inhibitory effects on lamina V cells of spinal dorsal horn and behavioral analgesia. In Archer S, Kosterlitz H W (eds) Opiates and endogenous opioid peptides. Elsevier/North-Holland Biomedical Press, Amsterdam pp 191–198

Takagi H, Satoh M, Akaike A, Shibata T, Kuraishi Y 1977 The nucleus reticularis gigantocellularis of the medulla oblongata is a highly sensitive site in the production of morphine analgesia in the rat. European Journal of Pharmacology 45: 91–92

Takagi H, Satoh M, Akaike A, Shibata T, Yajima H, Ogawa H 1978 Analgesia by enkephalins injected into the nucleus reticularis gigantocellularis of rat medulla oblongata. European Journal of Pharmacology 49: 113–116

Takagi H, Shiomi H, Kuraishi Y, Fukui K, Ueda H 1979 Pain and the bulbospinal noradrenergic system: pain-induced increase in normetanephrine content in the spinal cord and its modification by morphine. European Journal of Pharmacology 54: 99–107

Teschemacher H J, Schubert P, Herz A 1973 Autoradiographic studies concerning the supraspinal site of the antinociceptive action of morphine when inhibiting the hindleg flexor reflex in rabbits. Neuropharmacology 12: 123–131

Tsou K, Jang C S 1964 Studies on the site of analgesic action of morphine by intracerebral microinjection. Scientia sinica 13: 1099–1109

Tung A S, Yaksh T L 1982 In vivo evidence for multiple opiate receptors mediating analgesia in the rat spinal cord. Brain Research 247: 75–83

Tyce G M, Yaksh T L 1981 Monoamine release from cat spinal cord by somatic stimuli: an intrinsic modulatory system. Journal of Physiology (London) 314: 513–529

Walker G E, Yaksh T L 1986 Studies on the effects of intrathalamically injected DADL and morphine on nociceptive thresholds and electroencephalographic activity: A thalamic δ receptor syndrome. Brain Research 383: 1–14

Wamsley J K 1983 Opioid receptors: autoradiography. Pharmacological Reviews 35: 69–83

Ward S J, Portoghese P S, Takemori A E 1982 Pharmacological characterization in vivo of the novel opiate. β-funaltrexamine. Journal of Pharmacology and Experimental Therapeutics 220: 494–498

Wettstein J G, Kamerling S G, Martin W R 1982 Effects of microinjections of opioids into and electrical stimulation (ES) of the canine periaqueductal gray (PAG) on EEG electrogenesis (EEG), heart rate (HR), pupil diameter (PD), behavior and analgesia. Neuroscience Abstracts 8: 229

Wigdor S, Wilcox G L 1987 Central and systemic morphine antinociception in the mouse: contribution of descending serotonergic and noradrenergic pathways. Journal of Pharmacology and Experimental Therapeutics: (in press)

Williams J, Zieglgansberger W 1981 Mature spinal ganglion cells are not sensitive to opiate receptor mediated actions. Neuroscience Letters 21: 211–216

Xuan Y T, Shi Y S, Zhou Z F, Han J S 1986 Studies on the mesolimbic loop of antinociception. II. A serotonin-enkephalin interaction in the nucleus accumbens. Neuroscience 19: 403–409

Yaksh T L 1978a Inhibition by etorphine of the discharge of dorsal horn neurons: effects upon the neuronal response to both high- and low-threshold sensory input in the decerebrate spinal cat. Experimental Neurology 60: 23–40

Yaksh T L 1978b Analgesic actions of intrathecal opiates in cat and primate. Brain Research 153: 205–210

Yaksh T L 1979 Direct evidence that spinal serotonin and noradrenaline terminals mediate the spinal antinociceptive effects of morphine in the periaqueductal gray. Brain Research 160: 180–185

Yaksh T L 1983 In vivo studies on spinal opiate receptor systems mediating antinociception. I. Mu and delta receptor profiles in the primate. Journal of Pharmacology and Experimental Therapeutics 226: 303–316

Yaksh T L 1984a Multiple opioid receptor systems in brain and spinal cord: part 1. European Journal of Anaesthesiology 1: 171–199

Yaksh T L 1984b Multiple opioid receptor systems in brain and spinal cord: part 2. European Journal of Anaesthesiology 1: 201–243

Yaksh T L 1985 Pharmacology of spinal adrenergic systems which modulate spinal nociceptive processing. Pharmacology, Biochemistry and Behaviour 22: 845–858

Yaksh T L, Henry J L 1978 Antinociceptive effects of intrathecally administered human β-endorphin in the rat and cat. Canadian Journal of Physiology and Pharmacology 56: 754–760

Yaksh T L, Jessell T M, Gamse R, Mudge A W, Leeman S E 1980 Intrathecal morphine inhibits substance P release from mammalian spinal cord in vivo. Nature 286: 155–156

Yaksh T L Noueihed R 1985 The physiology and pharmacology of spinal opiates. Annual Review of Pharmacology and Toxicology 25: 433–462

Yaksh T L, Noueihed R Y, Durant P A C 1986 Studies of the pharmacology and pathology of intrathecally administered 4-anilinopiperidine analogues and morphine in rat and cat. Anaesthesiology 64: 54–66

Yaksh T L, Reddy S V R 1981 Studies in the primate on the analgesic effects associated with intrathecal actions of opiate, α-adrenergic agonists and baclofen. Anesthesiology 54: 451–467

Yaksh T L, Rudy T A 1976 Analgesia mediated by a direct spinal action of narcotics. Science 192: 1357–1358

Yaksh T L, Rudy T A 1977 Studies on the direct spinal action of narcotics in the production of analgesia in the rat. Journal of Pharmacology and Experimental Therapeutics 202: 411–428

Yaksh T L, Rudy T A 1978 Narcotic analgesics: CNS sites and mechanisms of action as revealed by intracerebral injection techniques. Pain 4: 299–359

Yaksh T L, Wilson P R 1979 Spinal serotonin terminal system mediates antinociception. Journal of Pharmacology and Experimental Therapeutics 208: 446–453

Yaksh T L, Yeung J C, Rudy T A 1976 Systemic examination in the rat of brain sites sensitive to the direct application of morphine: observation of differential effect within the periaqueductal gray. Brain Research 114: 83–103

Yeung J C, Rudy T A 1980 Multiplicative interaction between narcotic agonisms expressed at spinal and supraspinal sites of antinociceptive action as revealed by concurrent intrathecal and intracerebroventricular injections of morphine. Journal of Pharmacology and Experimental Therapeutics 215: 633–642

Zieglgansberger W, Bayerl H 1976 The mechanisms of inhibition of neuronal activity by opiates in the spinal cord of the cat. Brain Research 115: 111–128

Aspects of spinal anaesthesia

The local anaesthetic properties of cocaine were first utilised in 1884 by Koller in Vienna (Koller 1884). The following year Corning, a North American neurologist, administered cocaine 'spinally' (Corning 1885) and it is probable that he unintentionally and unknowingly produced the first spinal anaesthetic. It was not until 1898, and after Quincke had demonstrated the feasibility of lumbar puncture as a diagnostic aid (Quincke 1891), that Bier, working in the same hospital, introduced spinal anaesthesia into surgical practice (Bier 1899). The technique was subsequently popularised by Tuffier (1899) in France and Barker (1907, 1908a,b) in England. Labat (1922) and Sise (1928, 1935) were responsible for much of the early enthusiasm in North America.

The value of spinal anaesthesia was immediately appreciated because of the superior muscle relaxation achieved in comparison to the techniques of general anaesthesia available in the early part of the century. Later, the capability of providing hypotension, with reduction in surgical blood loss during major surgery was exploited as an additional advantage (Griffiths & Gillies 1948). However, the introduction of curare into clinical practice (Griffith & Johnson 1942) enabled the particular bonus of spinal anaesthesia — muscle relaxation — to be produced by other means. The parallel development of anaesthesia as a specialty with practitioners skilled in the arts of airway management and control of ventilation hastened the decline in the popularity of spinal anaesthesia.

The publication of a review entitled 'The grave spinal cord paralyses caused by spinal anesthesia' by Kennedy et al (1950), was a further setback to the enthusiasm of those using the technique at that time. Kennedy et al totally condemned spinal anaesthesia, concluding their review with the statement:

> From a neurological point of view we give the opinion that spinal anesthesia should be rigidly reserved for those patients unable to accept a local or general anaesthetic. Paralysis below the waist is too large a price for a patient to pay in order that the surgeon should have a fine relaxed field of operation.

Such was the authority of this opinion that many gave up using the technique altogether.

In the UK another major setback befell spinal anaesthesia when the Woolley and Roe case was heard in the High Court in London in 1953 (Cope 1954). In 1947 these two patients received spinal anaesthetics for relatively minor surgery during the same operating list and both subsequently developed adhesive arachnoiditis. The court's conclusion was that this was due to leakage of phenol, used for sterilisation, into the ampoules through fine cracks in the glass. Chemical sterilisation of ampoules has not been recommended since then, nor has the use of unlabelled ampoules.

The condemnation of spinal anaesthesia by Kennedy et al was refuted by the publication of subsequent reviews of large numbers of cases without a single major problem (e.g. Dripps & Vandam 1954), but the damage to the technique's reputation had been done. In addition, the many developments in anaesthesia that followed the Second World War (quite apart from those mentioned above), led to the belief that every clinical problem could be overcome with some variation on the basic theme of general anaesthesia. The passage of time demonstrated that this was not so and a number of other factors contributed to a resurgence of interest in spinal anaesthesia.

Firstly, the development of obstetric epidural services has made a new generation of anaesthetists aware of the benefits of regional techniques, notably their ability to control postoperative pain. Secondly, research on the physiological effects of surgery under general or regional anaesthesia showed that the latter was better at preventing the hormonal and metabolic changes that may occur (Kehlet 1984). The implication was that both mortality and morbidity after surgery could be reduced.

A study by MacLaren et al (1978) claiming that spinal anaesthesia was associated with a lower incidence of postoperative mortality than general anaesthesia for the surgical treatment of fractures of the neck of the femur was not substantiated on longer term follow-up. However, there was a significant short term gain as shown by a lower initial mortality and reductions in postoperative confusion and nursing workload (McKenzie et al 1980, 1984, Valentin et al 1986). A study in elderly patients undergoing lower limb amputation showed no difference in mortality between spinal and general anaesthesia, but the early return of oral fluid intake was a distinct advantage in the spinal group (Mann & Bissett 1983). The reduction in the incidence of deep vein thrombosis in patients receiving spinal anaesthesia for total hip replacement (Sculco & Ranawat 1975) is also noteworthy.

INDICATIONS

It is logical at least to consider spinal anaesthesia for *any* surgery to the lower limbs, perineum or lower abdomen. Profound analgesia, muscle relaxation and a reduction in bleeding are produced rapidly by the injection of a small dose of a single drug. The proper use of the technique should mean that the systemic effect on the patient is significantly less than a general anaesthetic, so that the elderly patient with cardiorespiratory disease is particularly likely to benefit. Epidural block is the regional alternative to spinal, but it is more difficult and time-consuming to perform, its onset is slightly slower and the dose of drug required is larger so that the risk of systemic drug toxicity is greater. The duration of an epidural may be more readily extended with a catheter technique.

The majority of British patients expect to be asleep during surgery that is anything but very minor in character. In the prepared patient sleep may be obtained easily and safely with intravenous sedation (McClure et al 1983). The effect on protective reflexes may be minimised by careful dosage, but for major (particularly abdominal) surgery the combination of a spinal with a light inhalational anaesthetic, administered through a face-mask or endotracheal tube, may have much to offer. In the less well prepared patient, preservation of consciousness and the airway is a distinct advantage. Careful explanation of the reasons and the use of distraction techniques will work with many patients, but cautious intravenous titration of opioids or the inhalation of 50% nitrous oxide in oxygen may also be employed.

In obstetrics, regional techniques have distinct advantages for operative delivery for they allow the mother to enjoy the birth of her child and preserve her airway, so minimising the risks of failed intubation and the acid aspiration syndrome. *In skilled hands* spinal anaesthesia may have distinct advantages for the 'distressed' fetus (Marx et al 1984), enabling anaesthesia to be established rapidly and with minimal systemic drug effect. That it is again being promoted for Caesarean section is perhaps the best indicator yet of the 'renaissance' that spinal anaesthesia is undergoing (Atkinson & Lee 1985), but recent publications have also suggested it for outpatient surgery (Flaatten & Raeder 1985), acute war injuries (Bion 1984) and even patients with chronic spinal cord lesions (Barker et al 1985).

CONTRA-INDICATIONS

It is probably reasonable to state that there are no absolute contra-indications to any technique of anaesthesia, but when considering a spinal anaesthetic a number of factors should be taken into account (particularly by the inexperienced) when making a decision. One absolute rule is that spinal anaesthesia should *not* be used as a way of circumventing some inconvenient contra-indication to general anaesthesia such as an upper respiratory tract infection.

Infection

Pyogenic infection at, or close to, the site of lumbar puncture is certainly a clear contra-indication to use of spinal anaesthesia, for the risks of a catastrophic meningeal infection are unacceptable. Infection distant to the site of injection is a more questionable problem, for blood-borne bacteria may reach the needle site and produce an abscess in the small haematoma caused by the needle. In the young, fit patient who is toxic due to an abscess, a spinal anaesthetic for its drainage is unwise. In the elderly patient with intercurrent disease and requiring amputation of an ischaemic foot which has become infected, but has been treated with antibiotics, a spinal anaesthetic is the method of choice. Between these extremes is a whole range of patients needing careful assessment of risk.

Coagulation disorders

In patients with abnormal coagulation, the risk is that the insertion of a needle will cause a significant epidural or subarachnoid haematoma, with resultant pressure on the cauda equina or spinal cord. Major coagulation disorders and anticoagulant therapy have, until recently been considered to be clear contra-indications to any major regional anaesthetic technique. Recently Odoom & Sih (1983) published details of a series of 950 patients on anticoagulant therapy who received epidural catheters without complication. There must be some risk involved, but at least this experience allows the accepted views to be questioned. The use of a fine (i.e. 26 G) lumbar puncture needle by an experienced anaesthetist in a patient who has received subcutaneous heparin therapy as prophylaxis against thrombo-embolic complications is considered acceptable. Most practitioners are still very conservative about using larger needles or catheters in such patients, let alone those who have more overt changes in coagulation or platelet dysfunction.

Neurological disease

Concern about spinal anaesthesia in patients with neurological disease relates to the reports mentioned earlier and to the fact that some of the early local anaesthetic drugs may have been somewhat irritant. With modern drugs there is little to suggest that any harm will come to the patient with a neurological condition, but it has been suggested that regional anaesthesia should only be employed in such patients when a clear indication exists (Charlton 1986). It is wise to document the extent of any deficit prior to anaesthesia, so that the patient does not ascribe any deterioration to the anaesthetic.

The acute abdomen

Superficially, patients presenting for emergency abdominal surgery may seem suitable for spinal anaesthesia, but there are a number of good reasons why it should not be used. The patient may have a very considerable fluid deficit and will require resuscitation before any form of anaesthesia is administered. However, maintenance of the circulation may still depend on intact circulatory reflexes and severe hypotension, intractable to treatment, may occur if spinal anaesthesia is employed. The profound sympathetic nerve block that causes this also leads to bowel wall contraction and an increased risk of rupture and soiling of the peritoneum with faecal material. Finally there is nearly always some doubt about the extent and duration of the projected surgery so that the block may turn out to be inadequate.

Patient reluctance

The majority of patients who express concern about receiving a spinal anaesthetic are really anxious about being conscious during the operation. We find it better not to use terms such as 'spinal injection' and 'lumbar puncture' with patients whose previous experience (personal or apocryphal) may have been of an inexpert attempt at lumbar puncture performed by an inexperienced houseman using a large needle! We simply tell patients that they will receive an injection to 'freeze' the lower half of the body and indicate that a second injection will put them to sleep. If they want more information, they are given it (especially about the advantages), but very few are concerned to know more once they have been reassured that they will be unaware during the procedure.

MODE AND SITE OF ACTION

Spinal anaesthesia is normally performed by puncture of the dura and arachnoid mater in the lumbar region, and local anaesthetic is introduced directly into the cerebrospinal fluid (CSF) surrounding the nerve roots and spinal cord. The solution will spread longitudinally through the CSF and the drug will be taken up by the neuronal tissues. Whether an effective concentration results in a particular nerve will depend on the accessibility, lipid content and blood flow of the particular tissue (Greene 1983). The nerve roots, especially of the cauda equina, are easily accessible and will be exposed over a considerable surface area (assuming that solution spreads to a particular root — see below).

Factors affecting spread

The most important determinants of a spinal anaesthetic are the factors which affect spread of solution through the CSF. Greene (1985) has enumerated 25 of these and recent controlled clinical trials, using loss of sensation to pinprick to define spread, have indicated the clinically important factors. This work has been reviewed (Greene 1985, Wildsmith & Rocco 1985) and may be summarised as follows.

1. Solution baricity

Using 0.5% amethocaine, Brown et al (1980) found that baricity had a major effect on the spread of analgesia. The solution was injected at the third lumbar interspace in patients placed in the lateral horizontal position and turned supine immediately afterwards. The hyperbaric solution resulted in a mean block to T5 and isobaric to T10 (Fig. 19.1). The hypobaric solutions gave a mean level of T11, but the blocks were patchy and of poor quality.

Mean duration was longer with an isobaric than with a hyperbaric solution of similar dose. This was presumed to relate to the wider spread of the hyperbaric solution allowing absorption to take place over a greater surface area. Increasing the dose injected from 10 to 15 mg had no effect on the level of spread achieved with any solution (Fig. 19.1), but increased the duration of them all.

Baricity is affected by temperature but the change that takes place between 20 and 37 degrees is very small. The temperature of the injected solution is considered to warm rapidly to body temperature, and therefore is not a factor affecting spread.

EFFECT OF BARICITY AND DOSE

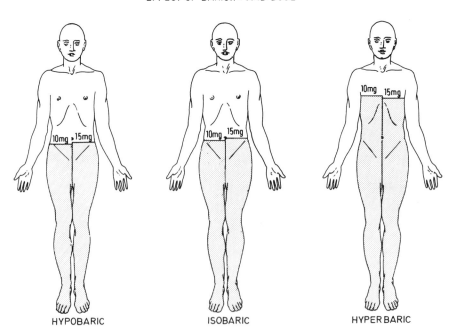

HYPOBARIC   ISOBARIC   HYPERBARIC

Fig. 19.1 To show the *mean* level of block (stippled area) obtained ($n = 10$ in each group) when 10 mg or 15 mg of amethocaine 0.5% were injected in hypobaric, isobaric or hyperbaric solution (data derived from Brown et al (1980))

2. Patient posture

Posture has been used since the time of Barker's (1907, 1908a,b) classic descriptions to aid or restrict spread of injected solution. If a patient is turned supine immediately after injection at the third or fourth lumbar interspace, the solution will be at the apex of the lumbar spinal curve. Gravity will thus cause a hyperbaric solution to spread down from the apex in both sacral and thoracic directions. With a hyperbaric solution it is not necessary to use the Trendelenburg position to ensure spread to mid-thoracic level. Sinclair et al (1982) found that all it did was to increase the variability of height of block and to increase the incidence of blocks extending into the cervical region. Accentuation of the lumbar curve in pregnancy may explain in part the increased spread seen when spinal anaesthesia is performed with a hyperbaric solution for Caesarean section. Conversely, flexion of the hips in the supine position reduces the lumbar curve and has been shown to reduce the spread of hyperbaric solutions (Smith 1968).

A major reason for using posture to control the spread of hyperbaric solutions is to try and restrict spread to the lower limbs and perineum. Wildsmith et al (1981) investigated the effect of maintaining both the lateral and sitting positions for 5 minutes after the injection of hyperbaric or isobaric solutions of amethocaine. They concluded that if posture is to be used to control the spread of a hyperbaric solution, then the posture must be maintained for considerably longer than is often practised. They also found that posture had no effect at all on the spread of a truly isobaric solution, which they recommended for use when a block restricted to the legs or perineum is required.

3. Volume and rate of injection

Increasing the volume of a spinal anesthetic injection usually increases the dose of drug injected, so a study was devised in which a standard dose of amethocaine was dissolved in 1, 2 or 4 ml of isobaric solution (McClure et al 1982). There was very little difference in mean spread with the different volumes, but the larger the volume injected, the greater was the range of blocks — i.e. predictability was reduced (Fig. 19.2). Slowing the rate of injection of 4 ml reduced the range of blocks produced (Fig. 19.2) and made the solution more predictable again. It was concluded that the most predictable spinal blocks might be produced by injecting a low volume solution at a slow rate.

4. Patient characteristics

Many anaesthetists relate the dose of local anaesthetic that they use for a spinal anaesthetic to the patient's height or weight. While restricted spread

SPREAD OF 10mg AMETHOCAINE CRYSTALS DISSOLVED IN SALINE

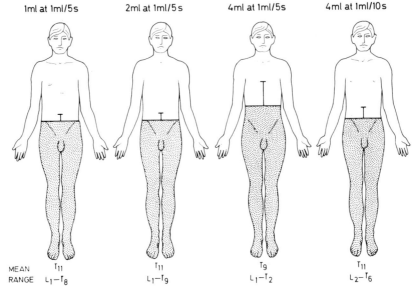

Fig. 19.2 To show the mean level (stippled area) of block, its SD (bars) and the range of blocks obtained ($n = 10$ in each group) when amethocaine 10 mg was injected in 1 ml, 2 ml or 4 ml of isobaric solution. Injection was at 0.2 ml s^{-1} except in the fourth group in which it was 0.1 ml s^{-1} (reproduced from McClure et al (1982) with permission)

is sometimes seen in the very thin patient, and the opposite in the obese, many studies have found that spread correlates very poorly with patient size, certainly within the adult range. For instance, McCulloch & Little-wood (1986) have shown that there is some increase in spread in the obese patient, but the range of blocks is so wide (Fig. 19.3**A**) that this is of very little predictive help. Level of block was totally unrelated to patient height (Fig. 19.3**B**). Similarly, some correlation has been shown between patient age and spread (Cameron et al 1981, Pitkanen et al 1984), but again the range of blocks seen in any particular age group is still too wide for the information to be of any practical help.

5. *Effect of clinical interactions*

The results of the studies outlined above have indicated how the major factors affect the spread of local anaesthetic solution after intrathecal injection. However, it is important to appreciate that these studies were performed in healthy patients under very carefully controlled conditions. In the routine clinical situation variations in technique, differences in solution composition and individual patient factors (e.g. distortion of the spine with age) may individually or together result in different effects on spread.

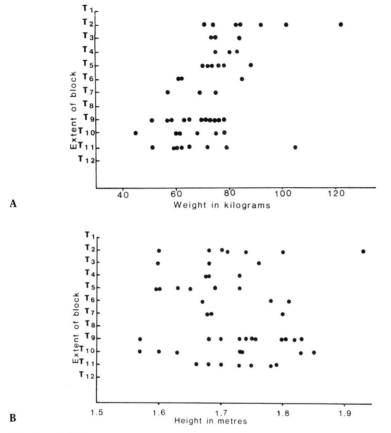

Fig. 19.3 Relationship between level of block and **A** weight or **B** height in 50 patients given 4 ml bupivacaine 0.5% (reproduced from McCulloch & Littlewood (1986) with permission)

For instance, Axelsson et al (1984) studied the spread of plain bupivacaine 0.5% (a slightly hypobaric solution) in patients who were sitting for 2 minutes after injection and then placed in the lithotomy position. They found that cephalad spread was proportional to the logarithm of the volume injected. Again, Chambers et al (1982b) found that volume had no effect on the spread of hyperbaric 0.5% bupivacaine, but that there was an effect on the spread of hyperbaric 0.75% bupivacaine. Others (Axelsson et al 1982, Sundnes et al 1982) have in fact demonstrated some relationship between volume injected and the spread of hyperbaric 0.5% bupivacaine.

Such contradictory results may be due to a number of factors, including simple chance. It is important to remember that any technique of spinal anaesthesia results in a range of blocks, even when it is applied consistently by a single practitioner. Therefore it is not surprising that there should be some variation between the results of studies in which there may be subtle, seemingly irrelevant variations in technique, drug composition and patient characteristics.

Factors affecting duration

Studies investigating the duration of spinal blockade vary considerably in their definitions of duration and this has made interpretation difficult (Chambers et al 1981a). In addition, the patient who has undergone an abdominal operation under spinal anaesthesia has little interest in the duration of block in the feet, which is thus of little clinical relevance. However, recent work has shown that the main determinants of duration are the drug used (Moore 1980, Cummings et al 1984, Skretting et al 1984, Marstrand et al 1985, McKeown et al 1986) and the dose injected (Brown et al 1980, Wildsmith et al 1981, Chambers 1982).

It is common practice, especially in North America, to add vasoconstrictors to spinal anaesthetic solutions. The assumption is that the efficacy and the duration will be increased because of delayed vascular absorption. Recent controlled studies have shown that *no* clinically significant prolongation of effect is produced by the addition of adrenaline to lignocaine, bupivacaine or amethocaine (Chambers et al 1981a, 1982a, Armstrong et al 1983). Phenylephrine does produce a significant prolongation in the duration of amethocaine, but a more marked effect may be produced simply by increasing the dose of local anaesthetic that is injected. This also avoids the (at least theoretical) risk of decreasing spinal cord blood flow by vasoconstriction.

DRUGS AND RECOMMENDATIONS

Virtually every local anaesthetic that has been produced has been used for spinal anaesthesia. Given solutions *equipotent* in concentration and of the *same baricity*, the only variation to be expected in clinical effect is in duration of action, although there is some evidence that there may be subtle differences. For instance, amethocaine is said to be associated with a greater incidence of tourniquet discomfort than bupivacaine (Rocco et al 1984). Generally, clinical decisions will very much depend on what is readily available and that is governed mainly by commercial factors. In recent times both mepivacaine and cinchocaine have been withdrawn on this basis alone. It is to be hoped that the current increase in interest in spinal anaesthesia will result in more preparations becoming available.

The ideal spinal anaesthetic preparation should contain no preservatives since these may damage the nerve fibres which only acquire a protective layer of perineurium after passing through the dura mater. The preparation should be in a form which enables the anaesthetist to adjust its baricity (by adding water, saline or dextrose) prior to use, but still produce a relatively small volume to inject. In North America amethocaine (tetracaine,

Pontocaine, Sterling-Winthrop) is available as a 1% (isobaric) solution and a crystalline preparation, both of which meet these requirements. At the time of writing, these preparations are very difficult to obtain in the UK.

The only solution specifically marketed for intrathecal use in the UK is bupivacaine 0.5% dissolved in dextrose 8% (bupivacaine 0.75% in dextrose 8.25% is also available in North America). In clinical use this is very similar to hyperbaric amethocaine and is becoming very popular, although it does have a very high dextrose concentration. The readily available alternatives are solutions of local anaesthetics produced primarily for other uses. The plain solution of bupivacaine 0.5% is used widely, but has two slight drawbacks. It is slightly hypobaric at 37°C and has to be injected in relatively large volumes (3–4 ml) to ensure an adequate dose. The net effect is that plain bupivacaine, while producing the same mean spread as isobaric amethocaine, produces a much wider range of blocks (McClure et al 1982, Pitkanen et al 1984) which are unpredictable (Logan et al 1986).

The spread of plain solutions is also influenced by posture, perhaps reflecting the slight hypobaricity of this agent. Tuominen et al (1982) found that the spread of 3 ml bupivacaine 0.75% was significantly greater in patients kept sitting for 2 minutes after injection. Russell (1984) has postulated that it was alterations in epidural venous pressure displacing CSF rostrally that caused the increased spread seen when patients who had received plain bupivacaine 0.5% were moved from the lateral to the supine position. In an earlier study, Russell (1983) also demonstrated an increased spread in pregnant women moved from the lateral to the supine position after the intrathecal injection of plain bupivacaine 0.5%. However, failure to achieve adequate anaesthesia for Caesarean section in three out of 33 patients is further testimony to the unpredictability of plain bupivacaine. Whenever considering a method of spinal anaesthesia it is at least as important to know the range of blocks likely to be produced as it is to know the mean effect.

Hyperbaric bupivacaine 0.5% has the advantage that the block spreads to the low or mid-thoracic region in a patient turned supine immediately after injection in the lateral horizontal position (Chambers et al 1981b, Moller et al 1984). The hyperbaric solution of bupivacaine 0.75% was found to cause excessive spread and its use was abandoned by Chambers et al (1982b). When using bupivacaine for spinal anaesthesia, the hyperbaric preparation may be used with some confidence to produce a block to the mid to low thoracic segment. Like all hyperbaric solutions, it can be used reliably for surgery below the level of the umbilicus. The glucose-free solution should be reserved for surgery of the perineum and distal part of the lower limbs since blocks extending no higher than L2 are seen fairly frequently. Plain amethocaine (a truly isobaric solution) can be used with confidence for any procedure on the lower limb, yet has a much lower incidence of excessively high blocks than plain bupivacaine.

Bupivacaine and amethocaine have one disadvantage in common — they are both relatively long acting local anaesthetics. Their durations may be manipulated to some extent by varying the dose, but for many procedures a shorter acting agent would be better. In some countries a hyperbaric preparation of lignocaine is available (Xylocaine, Astra), and can be obtained in Britain by special order if required. As with bupivacaine the plain solution of lignocaine 2% may be used for spinal anaesthesia, but also produces a wide range of blocks (McKeown et al 1986).

A hyperbaric solution injected into a patient placed supine immediately thereafter will almost certainly produce a block to the mid-thoracic dermatomes which will be adequate for any procedure for which spinal anaesthesia is likely to be deemed appropriate. Some patients will become hypotensive, but far fewer than many anaesthetists would believe. For those that do, treatment is simple and effective. Plain solutions may be used when it is certain that only a restricted block is required and confidence in the particular preparation has been acquired. In the case of plain bupivacaine the very unpredictable nature of the solution must be appreciated.

Patient management and complications

Adequate premedication is perhaps more appropriate before a regional block than before a general anaesthetic. Vasovagal attacks are particularly common after lumbar puncture in the apprehensive patient and the resulting hypotension should be distinguished from that due to the block itself. The full facilities of a properly equipped anaesthetic room must be available and venous access should be secured before the block is started. It is the authors' preference to perform the block with the patient sedated, but conscious and in control of the airway. After institution of the block intravenous sedation (increments of benzodiazepine or an infusion of chlormethiazole) or light general anaesthesia is given depending on the patient's condition and the type and duration of surgery.

Hypotension

This is the most common complication. Once vagal overactivity has been excluded, this can usually be attributed to blockade of the sympathetic outflow, but the possibility of hypovolaemia secondary to haemorrhage must never be forgotten. As a general rule, the higher the block the more likely is hypotension to occur. Blocks above T5 are most likely to be associated with significant hypotension because the cardiac nerves will be affected.

Figure 19.4 relates the change in systolic blood pressure seen in a large series of patients to the level of block. Treatment was instituted on clinical grounds of apparent peripheral circulatory inadequacy. All the patients who were so treated had decreases in blood pressure in excess of 30% of control and this would seem to be an important figure to keep in mind. Many

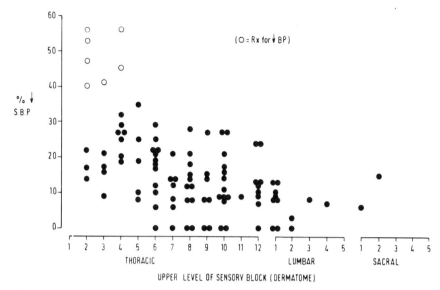

Fig. 19.4 Relationship between upper level of sensory block and per cent decrease in systolic blood pressure in 100 patients given amethocaine in a variety of solutions (data derived from Brown et al (1980) and Wildsmith et al (1981)). No prophylactic treatment was given and the open circles indicate the seven patients who required treatment with atropine or ephedrine because of clinical circulatory inadequacy

anaesthetists give prophylactic treatment for hypotension routinely, but it must be noted that hypotension is not inevitable even in patients blocked to the upper thoracic segments. Because of this we prefer to monitor our patients carefully and administer treatment as needed. Any patient who has had a spinal anaesthetic should be kept in a slight Trendelenburg tilt to ensure that venous return is preserved.

The commonest form of prophylactic treatment for hypotension is pre-load with an electrolyte solution. This will reduce the incidence of hypotension, but does not guarantee that it will not occur (Clark et al 1976). In addition such pre-loading with fluid can have adverse effects. In a patient with poor cardiac function, pulmonary oedema may be produced. It may also lead to a high incidence of urinary retention because the bladder overdistends with the fluid while its nerve supply is still blocked. Because of these various problems we prefer to use vasoconstrictors, although we would again emphasise that any degree of hypovolaemia must be treated energetically.

The choice of drug for the treatment of hypotension due to spinal anaesthesia is best related to the patient's heart rate. If it is below 60, atropine is given i.v. in increments of 0.3 mg. If the heart rate is between 60 and 90 increments of ephedrine 3 mg (a mixed α/β-agonist) are given and if it is above 90, a pure α-agonist such as methoxamine 1–2 mg or phenylephrine 0.1–0.2 mg is used. If it is found that repeated doses are needed a larger dose may be given i.m. or by i.v. infusion to maintain the circulation. Pure α-agonists should not be used in obstetrics because they will decrease placental blood flow.

Headache

Headache subsequent to spinal anaesthesia is generally accepted as being due to leakage of CSF through the puncture hole in the dura mater. The reduction in CSF volume causes the weight of the brain to stretch its dural attachments and this is why the headache is related to posture. Headache in the postoperative period is not uncommon and it is important to obtain a history of posture-related headache before assuming that the spinal anaesthetic is the cause. It is a most distressing complication and every possible attempt should be made to minimise its incidence. Young, especially female, patients seem to be most at risk, with the highest incidence in obstetric practice. If it occurs, treatment must be prompt to relieve patient discomfort and prevent further complication, such as intradural haemorrhage (Newrick & Read 1982), which can occur if a dural vessel is stretched to the point where it tears.

A major factor in the aetiology of post-spinal headache is the size of the needle used. An 18 G needle may result in an incidence as high as 37% (Carbaat & van Crevel 1981), whereas a figure of 0.33% has been reported with 26 G needles (Myers & Rosenberg 1962). The smallest possible needle should thus be used, and every care taken to ensure that only one puncture hole is made in the dura. It is also important to align the needle so that the bevel splits the fibres of the dura, which run longitudinally, rather than cuts across them. The latter practice will result in a much higher incidence of headache (Mihic 1985). What does *not* seem to influence the incidence is the long established practice of keeping the patient flat in bed for 24 hours (Carbaat & van Crevel 1981). This merely delays the onset of the condition and should be abandoned if only because it is contrary to the modern trend for early mobilisation after surgery.

Patients should be allowed to sit up and move as the block wears off. If the nursing staff suspect that the patient has a headache this should be reported to the anaesthetist as soon as possible. In the interim, minor analgesics, a high fluid intake (to maximise CSF production) and limited bed rest should be prescribed. If the headache is clearly related to the anaesthetic, it is likely that further measures will be necessary. These have been reviewed (Jones 1974, Crawford 1980), and our preference is for early epidural blood patch because it is simple, quick, effective and allows early mobilisation.

Other complications

Hypotension and headache are the two most important complications of spinal anaesthesia. For the beginner, failure to produce an adequate block is a source of some anxiety. The basic requirements are a sound technique of lumbar puncture and an understanding of how the drug being used is likely to perform. Accurate identification of the subarachnoid space and free aspiration of CSF are essential before any local anaesthetic is injected. If an inadequate block does develop it may be repeated or supplemented with other local blocks, systemic medication, or a general anaesthetic. It should be remembered that it is much easier to manage a block which is a few dermatomes higher than required for surgery than one which is one segment too low.

A great many other complications have been described (Lee et al 1985), but are very rare when spinal anaesthesia is properly performed. Full patient assessment and sensible case selection, a good aseptic technique, proper patient positioning during and after injection, gentle needle insertion, obsessive checking that only the intended local anaesthetic solution is injected and continuing observation throughout the procedure should ensure that spinal anaesthesia is both successful and complication free.

REFERENCES

Armstrong I R, Littlewood D G, Chambers W A 1983 Spinal anesthesia with tetracaine — effect of added vasoconstrictors. Anesthesia and Analgesia 62: 793–795
Atkinson R S, Lee J A 1985 Editorial: spinal anaesthesia and day case surgery. Anaesthesia 40: 1059–1060
Axelsson K H, Edstrom H H, Widman G B 1982 Spinal anaesthesia with hyperbaric 0.5% bupivacaine — effects of volume. Acta Anaesthesiologica Scandinavica 26: 439–445
Axelsson K H, Edstrom H H, Widman G B 1984 Spinal anaesthesia with glucose free 0.5% bupivacaine — effects of different volumes. British Journal of Anaesthesia 56: 271–278
Barker A E 1907 Clinical experiences with spinal analgesia in 100 cases. British Medical Journal 1: 665
Barker A E 1908a A second report on clinical experiences with spinal analgesia. British Medical Journal 1: 264
Barker A E 1908b A third report on clinical experiences with spinal analgesia. British Medical Journal 2: 453
Barker I, Alderson J, Lydon M, Franks C I 1985 Cardiovascular effects of spinal subarachnoid anaesthesia. A study in patients with chronic spinal cord injuries. Anaesthesia 40: 533–536
Bier A 1899 Versuche uber cocainisierung uber ruchenmarkes. Deutsche Zeitschrift für Chirurgie 51: 362–369
Bion J F 1984 Isobaric bupivacaine for spinal anaesthesia in acute war injuries. Anaesthesia 39: 554–559
Brown D T, Wildsmith J A W, Covino B G, Scott D B 1980 Effect of baricity on spinal anaesthesia with amethocaine. British Journal of Anaesthesia 52: 589–596
Cameron A E, Arnold R W, Ghoris M W, Jamieson V 1981 Spinal analgesia using bupivacaine 0.5% plain. Variations in the extent of block with patient age. Anaesthesia 36: 318–322
Carbaat P A T, van Crevel H 1981 Lumbar puncture headache: controlled study on the preventive effect of 24 hours bed-rest. Lancet 2: 1133–1135
Chambers W A, Littlewood D G, Logan M R, Scott D B 1981a Effect of added epinephrine on spinal anesthesia with lidocaine. Anesthesia and Analgesia 60: 417–420
Chambers W A, Edstrom H H, Scott D B 1981b Effect of baricity on spinal anaesthesia with bupivacaine. British Journal of Anaesthesia 53: 279–282

Chambers W A, Littlewood D G, Scott D B 1982a Spinal anesthesia with hyperbaric bupivacaine: effect of added vasoconstrictors. Anesthesia and Analgesia 61: 49–52

Chambers W A, Littlewood D G, Edstrom H H, Scott D B 1982b Spinal anaesthesia with hyperbaric bupivacaine: effects of concentration and volume administered. British Journal of Anaesthesia 54: 75–80

Chambers W A 1982 Editorial: intrathecal bupivacaine. British Journal of Anaesthesia 54: 799–801

Charlton J E 1987 The management of regional anaesthesia. In Wildsmith J A W, Armitage E N (eds) Principles and practice of regional anaesthesia. Churchill Livingstone, Edinburgh, Ch 4

Clark R B, Thomson D S, Thomson C H 1976 Prevention of spinal hypotension associated with Caesarean section. Anesthesiology 45: 679–674

Cope R W 1954 The Woolley and Roe case. Woolley and Roe versus the Ministry of Health and others. Anaesthesia 9: 248–270

Corning J L 1885 Spinal anaesthesia and local medication of the cord. New York State Journal of Medicine 42: 483–485

Crawford J S 1980 Experiences with epidural blood patch. Anaesthesia 35: 513–515

Cummings G C, Bambes D B, Edstrom H H, Rubin A P 1984 Subarachnoid blockade with bupivacaine. A comparison with cinchocaine. British Journal of Anaesthesia 56: 573–579

Dripps R D, Vandam L D 1954 Long term follow-up of patients who received 10,098 spinal anesthetics. 1. Failure to discover major neurological sequelae. Journal of the American Medical Association 156: 1486

Flaatten H, Raeder J 1985 Spinal anaesthesia for outpatient surgery. Anaesthesia 40: 1108–1111

Greene N M 1983 Review: uptake and elimination of local anesthetics during spinal anesthesia. Anesthesia and Analgesia 62: 1013–1024

Greene N M 1985 Distribution of local anaesthetic solutions within the subarachnoid space. Anesthesia and Analgesia 64: 715–730

Griffith H R, Johnson C E 1942 The use of curare in general anesthesia. Anesthesiology 3: 418

Griffiths H W C, Gillies J 1948 Thoraco-lumbar splanchninectomy and sympathectomy: anaesthetic procedure. Anaesthesia 3: 134–141

Jones R J 1974 The role of recumbency in the prevention and treatment of post spinal headache. Anesthesia and Analgesia 53: 788–796

Kehlet H 1984 Stress-free anaesthesia: regional anaesthesia. In Scott D B, McClure J H, Wildsmith J A W (eds) Regional anaesthesia 1884–1984. ICM AB Sodertalje, pp 159–162

Kennedy F, Effron A S, Perry G 1950 The grave spinal cord paralyses caused by spinal anesthesia. Surgery, Gynecology and Obstetrics 91: 385–398

Koller C 1884 On the use of cocaine for producing anaesthesia of the eye. Lancet 2: 990

Labat G 1922 Regional anesthesia. Its technique and clinical applications. Saunders Philadelphia

Lee J A, Atkinson R S, Watt M J 1985 Lumbar puncture and spinal analgesia (5th edn) Churchill Livingstone, Edinburgh

Logan M R, McClure J H, Wildsmith J A W 1986 Plain bupivacaine — an unpredictable spinal anaesthetic agent. British Journal of Anaesthesia 58: 292–296

McClure J H, Brown D T, Wildsmith J A W 1982 Effect of injected volume and speed of injection on the spread of spinal anaesthesia with isobaric amethocaine. British Journal of Anaesthesia 54: 917–920

McClure J H, Brown D T, Wildsmith J A W 1983 Comparison of the intravenous administration of midazolam and diazepam as sedation during spinal anaesthesia. British Journal of Anaesthesia 55: 1089–1093

McCulloch W J D, Littlewood D G 1986 Influence of obesity on spinal analgesia with isobaric 0.5% bupivacaine. British Journal of Anaesthesia 58: 610–614

McKenzie P J, Wishart H Y, Dewar K M S, Gray I, Smith G 1980 Comparison of the effects of spinal anaesthesia and general anaesthesia on postoperative oxygenation and perioperative mortality. British Journal of Anaesthesia 52: 49–54

McKenzie P J, Wishart H Y, Smith G 1984 Long term outcome after repair of fractured neck of femur. British Journal of Anaesthesia 56: 581–585

McKeown D W, Stewart K, Littlewood D G, Wildsmith J A W 1986 Spinal anesthesia with plain solutions of lidocaine 2% and bupivacaine 0.5%. Regional Anesthesia 11: 68–71

MacLaren A D, Stockwell M C, Reid V T 1978 Anaesthetic techniques for surgical correction of fractured neck of femur. A comparative study of spinal and general anaesthesia in the elderly. Anaesthesia 33: 10–14

Mann R A M, Bisset W I K 1983 Anaesthesia for lower limb amputation. A comparison of spinal analgesia and general anaesthesia in the elderly. Anaesthesia 38: 1185–1191

Marstrand T, Sorensen M, Andersen S 1985 Spinal anaesthesia with 0.75% bupivacaine and 0.5% amethocaine in 5% glucose. British Journal of Anaesthesia 57: 971–975

Marx G F, Luykx W M, Cohen S 1984 Fetal-neonatal status following Caesarean section for fetal distress. British Journal of Anaesthesia 56: 1009–1013

Mihic D N 1985 Postspinal headache and relationship of needle bevel to longitudinal dural fibres. Regional Anesthesia 10: 76–81

Moller I W, Fernandes A, Edstrom H H 1984 Subarachnoid anaesthesia with 0.5% bupivacaine: effects of density. British Journal of Anaesthesia 56: 1191–1195

Moore D C 1980 Spinal anesthesia: bupivacaine compared with tetracaine. Anesthesia and Analgesia 59: 743–750

Myers L, Rosenberg M 1962 The use of the 26 gauge spinal needle. A survey. Anesthesia and Analgesia 41: 509–515

Newrick P, Read D 1982 Subdural haematoma as a complication of spinal anaesthetic. British Medical Journal 285: 341–342

Odoom J A, Sih I L 1983 Epidural analgesia and anticoagulant therapy. Experience with one thousand cases of continuous epidurals. Anaesthesia 38: 254–259

Pitkanen M, Haapaniemi L, Touminen M, Rosenberg P H 1984 Influence of age on spinal anaesthesia with isobaric 0.5% bupivacaine. British Journal of Anaesthesia 56: 279–284

Quinke H I 1891 Lumbalpunction des hydrocephalus. Berliner Klinische Wochenschrift 38: 929

Rocco A G, Conception M A, Sheskey M C, Murray E, Edstrom H H, Covino B G 1984 A double-blind evaluation of intrathecal bupivacaine without glucose and a standard solution of hyperbaric tetracaine. Regional Anesthesia 9: 1–7

Russell I F 1983 Spinal anaesthesia for Caesarean section. The use of 0.5% bupivacaine. British Journal of Anaesthesia 55: 309–314

Russell I F, 1984 Posture and isobaric subarachnoid anaesthesia — the influence on spread of spinal anaesthesia with isobaric 0.5% bupivacaine plain. Anaesthesia 39: 865–867

Sculco C J, Ranawat C 1975 The use of spinal anesthesia for total hip replacement arthroplasty. Journal of Bone and Joint Surgery 57A: 173–177

Sinclair C J, Scott D B, Edstrom H H 1982 Effect of the Trendelenberg position on spinal anaesthesia with hyperbaric bupivacaine. British Journal of Anaesthesiology 54: 497–500

Sise L F 1928 A device for facilitating the use of fine gauge lumbar puncture needles. Journal of the American Medical Association 91: 1186

Sise L F 1935 Pontocaine-glucose solution for spinal anesthesia. Surgical Clinics of North America 55: 1501–1504

Skretting P, Vaagenes P, Sundnes K O, Edstrom H H, Lind B 1984 Subarachnoid anaesthesia: comparison of hyperbaric solutions of bupivacaine and amethocaine. British Journal of Anaesthesia 56: 155–159

Smith T C 1968 The lumbar spine and subarachnoid block. Anesthesiology 29: 60–64

Sundnes K O, Vaagenes P, Skretting P, Lind P, Edstrom H H 1982 Spinal anaesthesia with hyperbaric bupivacaine. Effects of volume of solution. British Journal of Anaesthesia 54: 69–74

Tuffier T 1899 Analgesie chirurgicale per l'injection sous arachnoidienne lombaire de cocaine. Comptes Rendus Paris 51: 882

Tuominen M, Kalso E, Rosenberg P H 1982 Effects of posture on the spread of spinal anaesthesia with isobaric 0.75% or 0.5% bupivacaine. British Journal of Anaesthesia 54: 313–318

Valentin N, Lomholt B, Jensen J S, Hejgaard N, Kremer S 1986 Spinal or general anaesthesia for surgery of the fractured hip. A prospective study of mortality in 578 patients. British Journal of Anaesthesia 58: 284–291

Wildsmith J A W, McClure J H, Brown D T, Scott D B 1981 Effects of posture of the spread of isobaric and hyperbaric amethocaine. British Journal of Anaesthesia 53: 273–278

Wildsmith J A W, Rocco A G 1985 Current concepts in spinal anaesthesia. Regional Anesthesia 10: 119–124

Pain

INTRATHECAL OPIOIDS

The use of intrathecal opioids was discussed in *Anaesthesia Review 4*. There is also an extensive review of the use of epidural opioid analgesia by Staren & Cullen (1986). This discusses the anatomy, physiology and pharmacology of drugs used for epidural analgesia, the effects on pulmonary and cardio-vascular function and a note suggesting that the risks of epidural techniques in the presence of low dose heparin have been exaggerated. The merits and potential hazards of epidural morphine are considered in detail concluding that the technique is of great value but the patient needs to be closely supervised.

In the Wellcome Foundation lecture Kosterlitz (1985) drew attention to the similarity between acetylcholine and the opioid peptides. Acetylcholine is destroyed by cholinesterase and acts at more than one site e.g. the muscarinic and nicotinic receptors. The opioid peptides are destroyed by peptidases with the exception of beta-endorphin and dynorphin A. The enkephalins and beta-endorphin act at mu and delta receptor sites while the dynorphins selectively affect the kappa receptors. There are 10 opioid fragments which arise from endogenous precursors; some of these have non-opioid actions.

The further complexity of endogenous opioids has been reviewed by Bicknell (1985) drawing attention to their effect on the release of gonado-trophins and oxytocin. Gonadotrophin release is due to an action on the epsilon receptors (Grossman et al 1986). Apparently oxytocin and vaso-pressin neurones can synthesise and store opioid peptides. The kappa opioid agonist tifluadom, U50488 and ethyleketocyclazocine induced a diuresis which can be antagonised by naloxone, in rats. Apparently kappa opioid agonists act centrally by suppressing the release of AVP but there appears to be a peripheral mechanism involving the adrenal medulla (Black-burn et al 1986).

CARDIOVASCULAR SYSTEM

The cardiovascular actions of morphine and endogenous opioid peptides have been reviewed by Johnson et al (1985) drawing attention to the distribution of the various receptors and the similarity between ACTH, beta-endorphin and the enkephalins which are derived from pro-opiocortin in the pituitary. The mechanism of action of morphine on the cardiovascular system may be direct on receptors, secondary due to altered activity in the autonomic nervous system or the release of histamine or 5-hydroxytryptamine. Central mu opioid receptors impair baroreceptor control of sympathetic and cardiovascular function (Gordon 1986). Beta-endorphin causes hypotension which is reversed by naloxone. The effects in man are variable and it has been reported that there may be an initial tachycardia followed by bradycardia and some degree of hypotension. Naloxone has little effect on blood pressure in normal subjects but appears to have a pressor effect in patients with prolonged hypotension associated with sepsis. It has also been suggested that endogenous opioids are involved in the fall in blood pressure that occurs during sleep.

CATECHOLAMINES

Bromage et al (1983) found the addition of adrenaline to epidural morphine resulted in a more rapid onset of analgesia which was more intense while the duration of action was more prolonged. Rechtine et al (1984) were unable to confirm the value of adding adrenaline. However the use of a selective neurotoxin administered intrathecally to animals depleted noradrenaline in the spinal cord resulting in diminished analgesia (Zhong et al 1985).

Nordberg et al (1986) assessed the influence of adrenaline on extradural morphine (2 mg in 10 ml saline) and 50 μg adrenaline were added to the solution in half the patients. CSF samples were collected from the space below the epidural injection site. Following the plain morphine injection the peak morphine concentrations in the CSF were 20 times those in the plasma. During the elimination phase the CSF concentration exceeded that in the plasma by about 150 times. The CSF concentrations of morphine were not markedly affected by adrenaline. Duration of analgesia was related to the amount of morphine in the CSF. Glynn et al (1986) have postulated that adrenergic mechanisms at spinal level may be involved in the de-afferentation pain following spinal cord injury. Epidural clonidine (150 μg in 5 ml saline) provided pain relief in some of their patients.

RESPIRATION

There have been extensive studies on the effects of endogenous opioids, especially the enkephalins and beta-endorphins as well as exogenous opioid drugs. In animal studies opioids and naloxone have been given by the intracisternal or intraventricular route. Clinical studies in neonates have shown that respiration is influenced by endogenous opioids (Santiago &

Edelman 1985). It is singularly disappointing to realise that under normal conditions endogenous opioids have little effect on the control of breathing in the unanaesthetised adult but during general anaesthesia or in response to surgical stimulation endogenous opioids may be released.

Studies in man have shown an inverse relationship between plasma levels of beta-endorphin and the respiratory response to hypercapnia. In patients who were pretreated with naloxone there was an increase in plasma endorphin levels (Weinberger et al 1985). In contrast Rochat et al (1985) found that plasma levels of beta-endorphin and met-enkephalin did not correlate with the respiratory response to either hypercapnia or hypoxia.

Endogenous opioids appear to have a tonic effect in the neonate which might explain improvements in ventilation or the reduction of the duration of apnoea following the administration of naloxone. The effect of endogenous opioids in the neonate only appears to last a few days.

SPINAL OPIOIDS — CENTRAL OR PERIPHERAL ACTION

The distribution of spinal opioids in the CNS is still debated. In animal studies Gustafsson et al (1985) compared morphine with pethidine and found that the hydrophilic morphine persisted for a longer period in the spinal cord compared with pethidine which is lipophilic. The pethidine is rapidly taken up by nerve tissues, systemically absorbed and eliminated leaving little to spread centrally in the CSF. In contrast the onset of penetration of the brain by morphine was slow, remaining there for a much longer period and would account for the pattern of respiratory depression seen clinically. Other animal studies by Gregory et al (1985) found that intrathecal morphine ascends in the subarachnoid space and is absorbed into the spinal cord and medulla, reaching a maximum at 6 hours when respiration is markedly depressed.

In studies in man with cancer pain 10 mg of morphine in 10 ml of saline was introduced via a lumbar epidural catheter. Within 5 minutes there was a peak concentration in the plasma but it took 60 minutes for morphine to be detected in significant concentrations in the cervical (C7–T1 space) CSF; the peak concentration occurred after 3 hours. This would suggest that the late onset of respiratory depression is due to the passive flow of morphine in the the CSF towards the brain stem (Gourlay et al 1985).

Max et al (1985) studied epidural morphine, methadone and beta-endorphin and found that all three drugs reached peak levels in the lumbar CSF within 30 minutes which were 50 to 1300 times higher than the concentration in the plasma. The rate of removal of the drug from the CSF was related to the lipid solubility with methadone declining more rapidly than morphine or beta-endorphin. Following intrathecal morphine or methadone high levels of morphine were detected as early as 1 hour after injection but methadone levels were lower or undetectable. Max et al (1985) concluded that the analgesia produced by intrathecal or epidural morphine acted at spinal and supraspinal sites and that the technique was of little value in the management of terminal cancer pain.

Studies in man by Kotob et al (1986) have compared plasma and CSF levels of morphine following the intrathecal injection of 1 mg of morphine or heroin. (Heroin is rapidly transformed into morphine in the plasma.) Significant concentrations of morphine were seen in the plasma following heroin, reaching a peak at 10 minutes, whereas intrathecal morphine took 216 minutes. The elimination half-life of heroin from the CSF was 43 minutes as opposed to morphine which was 73 minutes. This emphasises the safety of heroin and because of its lipophilic properties heroin would be eliminated from the CSF quicker into the bloodstream and less drug would be available to be transmitted to the brain.

Willer et al (1985) still maintained that the relief of pain with epidural morphine is at spinal level despite the increased concentrations reported in the brain and medulla (see above). A feature overlooked is that topically applied morphine or fentanyl does not block nerve conduction in afferent fibres, especially the A beta, A delta and C fibres (Yuje et al 1985).

Although measurements have been made of plasma and CSF levels of morphine in its intrathecal use, similar measurements have been made following intramuscular morphine. Following 10 mg of intramuscular morphine the peak CSF level was reached 3 hours later, levels being only slightly lower than that of the plasma. After epidural morphine the CSF levels are 100 times greater than those found following the intramuscular injection (Nordberg et al 1985).

There is an obvious place for the development of selective kappa agonists for relief of pain without causing respiratory depression. This has been shown to be possible in animals with a kappa agonist u-50,448H (Castillo et al 1986).

POSTOPERATIVE PAIN RELIEF

The use of intrathecal morphine for postoperative pain relief following spinal surgery has been reported by O'Neill et al (1985). The patients who were given 1 mg morphine in 2 ml saline intrathecally had better postoperative pain relief than those given intramuscular papaveretum and there was also a reduction in the need for additional postoperative analgesia. The only troublesome complication was pruritus.

Cullen et al (1985) compared the use of epidural morphine (0.1 mg/ml), epidural bupivacaine (0.1%) and a mixture of epidural morphine and bupivacaine. The solutions were given by epidural catheter at the rate of 3 ml/h if the patients were over 60 years of age and less than 66 inches in height. Otherwise the dose rate was 4 ml/h. Pain relief was monitored for 72 hours and those patients given the combination of morphine and bupivacaine had superior pain relief. Pruritus again was the only troublesome complication. In another study during major abdominal surgery epidural analgesia was achieved during surgery with etidocaine and postoperatively with bupivacaine (0.5%) and morphine. 10 ml bupivacaine was administered 3 hours after the skin incision and thereafter 5 ml every 4 hours during the first 24 hours. 4 mg epidural morphine was given 3 hours following the skin incision and given 12 hourly for 72 hours (Hjortso et al 1985). Despite the excellent postoperative pain relief there was no significant reduction in postoperative morbidity or mortality. The incidence of postoperative pneumonia, cardiac arrhythmias, wound complications, deep vein thrombosis, postoperative weight loss and fatigue was similar to that following general anaesthesia with fentanyl and intramuscular opiates.

Downing et al (1985) found that 0.8 mg of intrathecal morphine reduced the requirement of papaveretum in the first 48 hours following cholecystectomy but there was no significant difference in analgesic requirements by 72 hours. It is probable that the requirement between 48 and 72 hours was equal to that of the control group because patients now felt pain for the first time and hence required their full complement of analgesia.

Larsen et al (1986) found that 5 mg of epidural morphine in 10 ml saline given via epidural catheter failed to improve on the analgesia produced in another group of patients given subcutaneous nicomorphine on demand (synthetic equi-analgesic morphine-like drug). Postoperatively there was a decrease in FVC, FEV_1, peak expiratory flow rate and also a fall in PaO_2 in both groups of patients.

Peri-anal surgery

Epidural opioids appear to be successful in producing prolonged postoperative analgesia for anorectal surgery. Gurel et al (1986) studied the use of 20 ml of 2% epidural prilocaine followed by 3 mg of morphine in 3 ml saline or 3 ml saline (control group) and found that all the patients given only prilocaine required additional postoperative analgesia. 25% of those patients receiving epidural morphine required no additional postoperative analgesia. However, urinary retention was a troublesome side effect in the morphine group.

Bailey & Sangwan (1986) compared the use of 20 ml 0.5% bupivacaine and 2.5 mg diamorphine in 10 ml saline for providing pain relief following peri-anal surgery. The patients were all anaesthetised with thiopentone, nitrous oxide and oxygen, one group of patients having bupivacaine caudally and another diamorphine also by the caudal route. Bupivacaine produced better analgesia for the first 8 hours than the control group whereas diamorphine was effective for 24 hours. 60% of the diamorphine group required no analgesia in the first 24 hours compared with 30% for the bupivacaine group. Urinary retention occurred only in the bupivacaine group.

Intravenous morphine and epidural bupivacaine

Lund et al (1985) found that 10 mg of intravenous morphine enhanced the spread of analgesia during epidural bupivacaine infusion given for the relief of postoperative pain. In a study of eight patients who underwent abdominal surgery under epidural bupivacaine (0.5%) under general anaesthesia bupivacaine was infused continuously at the rate of 8 ml/h following an initial test dose and bolus dose. Postoperative pain was assessed by pinprick or by pain score. When analgesia regressed by more than five segments the administration of 10 mg of intravenous morphine led to increased pain relief and a return to the initial level of analgesia. This synergistic effect of systemic morphine on epidural analgesia with bupivacaine may be due to morphine stimulating descending inhibitory pain fibres.

Epidural morphine and epidural bupivacaine

Hjortso et al (1986) have shown that epidural morphine enhances the action of epidural bupivacaine in providing postoperative pain relief following major abdominal surgery. Despite receiving bupivacaine (0.5%) at the rate of 8 ml/h only one patient out of ten was completely pain free 16 hours after skin incision whereas all patients who had in addition, epidural morphine (initial bolus of 4 mg in 10 ml saline followed by 0.5 mg/h) were completely pain-free. The explanation for this effect may be similar to that seen after intravenous morphine and epidural bupivacaine (see above) or due to a direct effect on the spinal cord.

PETHIDINE

Intramuscular pethidine (1 mg/kg) was compared to 20 or 60 mg of extradural pethidine for pain relief following total hip replacement. The operation was conducted under epidural mepivacaine (with adrenaline) and the analgesia was administered in the postoperative period. There was little difference in pain time between all groups while the time to peak, plasma clearance and terminal half-lives were not significantly different. This confirms that pethidine, a lipophilic agent, has a short duration when administered epidurally (Gustafsson et al 1986).

In another study Cozian et al (1986) described the effects of spinal pethidine in elderly men having prostatectomy. The patients were given 1 mg/kg of pethidine in 1 ml of 30% dextrose; no other drugs were administered and premedication consisted of 10 mg of diazepam. The mean onset time for analgesia to reach the level of T12 was 7 minutes with a maximum spread of analgesia taking 14 minutes. The highest level reached was T8 and analgesia lasted 2 hours although perineal analgesia was still present after 4 hours. The onset of motor block occurred after 5 minutes lasting approximately 2 hours. The onset of the sympathetic blockade occurred after 5 minutes lasting for $1\frac{1}{2}$ hours and was approximately 2 segments higher than the sensory block. Although clinically there was no obvious depression of ventilation the arterial PCO_2 rose and the arterial oxygen and pH fell. The mean arterial pressure decreased significantly as did the right atrial pressure, the pulmonary arterial pressure and the pulmonary capillary wedge pressure. The changes in the mean arterial pressure were related to the alterations in the systemic vascular index. The levels of plasma adrenaline, noradrenaline, plasma renin activity, plasma aldosterone and histamine did not change significantly. There was some correlation between noradrenaline levels due to changes in mean arterial pressure and the systemic vascular resistance index. The significance of these findings are discussed and it is of interest to note that operations on the perineum, in this case transurethral resection of the prostate, intrathecal pethidine provided adequate analgesia for the whole of the operation and the spinal blockade affected not only sensation but the motor and sympathetic nerves. This may have been due to the local anaesthetic action usually ascribed to pethidine. Pruritis of the face and itching of the body were the main complications.

In a study of over 100 patients undergoing perineal surgery Acalovschi et al (1986) reported the successful use of pethidine for the production of saddle blockade. They used a 5% solution of pethidine hydrochloride (100 mg in 2 ml) given intrathecally with the patient in a sitting position. Sensory blockade, which was limited to the innervation corresponding to S2–5 segments, reached its maximum spread within 4–8 minutes and was followed by motor blockade 1–2 minutes later. There were no respiratory or cardiovascular complications and postoperative analgesia lasted for 5 hours.

PAIN RELIEF FOR TERMINAL CANCER

Slattery & Boas (1985) outlined the need for achieving and maintaining adequate blood concentrations of drugs in the management of pain of terminal cancer. They discussed the place of oral opiates, controlled release opiates as well as the sublingual administration of buprenorphine. They also considered intravenous administration by continuous infusion, or that which can be patient controlled. They also referred to intrathecal and epidural administration of the opioids and considered that epidural morphine in a dose of 5 to 7 mg with 1:200 000 adrenaline, provided a more rapid onset and a prolongation of analgesia. Intrathecal beta-endorphin and dynorphin produced pain relief that was effective for $4\frac{1}{2}$ and 7 hours respectively in the treatment of chronic pain (Wen et al 1985).

The need for repeated intrathecal or epidural injections has led to the development of reservoirs which may be located subcutaneously and which can be punctured repeatedly to supplement drugs as necessary (Obbens et al 1985). The commonest complications included intracranial haemorrhage, reservoir malfunction and meningitis.

Cherry et al (1986) reported a case where epidural morphine failed to provide expected pain relief in a patient with carcinoma of the prostate. Secondary deposits in the vertebrae caused compression of the subarachnoid space preventing the spread of morphine in the cerebrospinal fluid. CSF samples drawn from C7–T1 interspace revealed the absence of morphine although the expected level following 10 mg of morphine in 10 ml saline given extradurally was approximately 500 ng/ml.

COMPLICATIONS

Tissue reactions to epidural opioids has been assumed to be insignificant. In a study in goats Larson et al (1986) showed that saline caused minimal changes around the catheter including the formation of the fibrous membrane, scattered fat necrosis, small cell infiltration and occasional haemorrhages. However after morphine the changes were more severe including a diffuse inflammatory reaction, fat cell necrosis, and chronic inflammatory reaction in the vicinity of the catheter. Larson et al (1986) suggested in fact that the so-called tolerance to morphine when given repeatedly may be due to the formation of the fibrous membrane around the catheter preventing the drug reaching the site of action. Yaksh et al (1986) postulated that high dose spinal morphine may produce non-opiate receptor effects which antagonise the analgesic actions of morphine. Other factors may be involved such as stress which can induce analgesia (Drugan et al 1985).

SUBCUTANEOUS MORPHINE

Jones & Hanks (1986) have described a portable infusion pump for the prolonged subcutaneous administration of opioid analgesics in patients with advanced cancer. The pump, Act-a-Pump (Pharmacia), was primed with diamorphine and it was found that patients seldom required more than 500 mg per day (2 ml). The pump could be used continuously for over a month and it was found that although doubts have been cast on the stability of diamorphine in aqueous solution the concentrations of monoacetylmorphine and morphine, the main breakdown products, were less than 1% of the final concentration of the parent drug.

MORPHINE INTOXICATION

In renal failure it has been widely assumed that morphine cannot be excreted and its accumulation leads to side effects such as respiratory failure. However Osborne et al (1986) have demonstrated the signs of morphine intoxication in the absence of raised plasma levels. Respiratory depression was due to one of the metabolites, morphine-6-glucuronide, which is not excreted in renal failure and concluded that in renal failure morphine was excreted but the active metabolite was not. Using gas chromatography — mass spectrometry Woolner et al (1986) have confirmed that renal failure does not impair the elimination of morphine.

DENTAL PAIN

In a double-blind cross-over study following oral surgery under local analgesia Olstad & Skjelbred (1986) compared the analgesic effect of steroids and paracetamol. A total of 84 mg of methylprednisolone was given starting 2 hours after surgery with 24 mg and thereafter in decreasing doses for 4 days. After the other operation paracetamol 1 g was given at 2, 6 and 9 hours after surgery and then 500 mg four times daily for 2 days. There was no significant difference in the pain scores, except that at 3 and 4 hours after operation there was better pain relief with paracetamol but thereafter analagesia was equal in both groups. On the third postoperative day there was less swelling in the patients who received methylprednisolone.

REFERENCES

Acalovschi I, Ene V, Lorinczi E, Nicolaus F 1986 Saddle block with pethidine for perineal operations. British Journal of Anaesthesia 58: 1012–1016
Bailey P M, Sangwan S 1986 Caudal analgesia for perianal surgery. Anaesthesia 41: 499–504
Bicknell R J 1985 Endogenous opioid peptides and hypothalamic neuroendocrine neurones. Journal of Endocrinology 107: 437–446
Blackburn T P, Borkowski K R, Friend J, Rance M J 1986 On the mechanisms of kappa opioid induced diuresis. British Journal of Pharmacology 89: 593–598
Bromage P R, Camporesi E M, Durant P A, Nielsen C H 1983 Influence of epinephrine as an adjunct to epidural morphine. Anesthesiology 58: 257–262
Castillo R, Kissin I, Bradley E L 1986 Selective kappa opioid agonist for spinal analgesia without the risk of respiratory depression. Anesthesia and Analgesia 65: 350–354
Cherry D A, Gourlay G K, Cousins M J 1986 Epidural mass associated with lack of efficacy of epidural morphine and undetectable CSF morphine concentrations. Pain 25: 69–73
Cozian A, Pinaud M, Lepage J Y, Lhoste F, Souron R 1986 Effects of meperidine spinal anesthesia on hemodynamics, plasma catecholamines, angiotensin 1, aldosterone and histamine concentrations in elderly men. Anesthesiology 64: 815–819
Cullen M L, Saren E D, El-Ganzouri A, Logas W G, Ivankovich A D, Economou S G 1985 Continuous epidural infusion for analgesia after major abdominal operations. A randomized, prospective, double-blind study. Surgery 98: 718–728
Downing R, Davis I, Black J, Windsor C W O 1985 When do patients given intrathecal morphine need postoperative systemic opiates? Annals of the Royal College of Surgeons of England 67: 251–253
Drugan R C, Ader D N, Maier S F 1985 Shock controllability and the nature of stress-induced analgesia. Behavioral Neuroscience 99: 791–801
Glynn C J, Jamous M A, Teddy P J, Moore R A, Lloyd J W 1986 Role of spinal noradrenergic system in transmission of pain in patients with spinal cord injury. Lancet 2: 1249–1250
Gordon F J 1986 Central opioid receptors and baroreflex control of sympathetic and cardiovascular function. Journal of Pharmacology and Experimental Therapeutics 237: 428–436

Gourlay G K, Cherry D A, Cousins M J 1985 Cephaled migration of morphine in CSF following lumbar epidural administration in patients with cancer pain. Pain 23: 317–326

Gregory M A, Brock-Utne J G, Bux S, Downing J W 1985 Morphine concentration in brain and spinal cord after subarachnoid morphine injection in baboons. Anesthesia and Analgesia 64: 929–932

Grossman A, Moult P J A, Cunnah D, Besser M 1986 Different opioid mechanisms are involved in the modulation of ACTH and gonadotrophin release in man. Neuroendocrinology 42: 357–360

Gurel A, Unal N, Elevli M, Eren A 1986 Epidural morphine for postoperative pain relief in anorectal surgery. Anesthesia and Analgesia 65: 499–502

Gustafsson L L, Post C, Edvardsen B, Ramsay C H 1985 Distribution of morphine and meperidine after intrathecal administration in rat and mouse. Anesthesiology 63: 483–489

Gustafsson L L, Johannisson J, Garle M 1986 Extradural and parenteral pethidine as analgesia after total hip replacement: effects and kinetics. A controlled clinical study. European Journal of Clinical Pharmacology 29: 529–534

Hjortso N C, Neumann P, Frosig F et al 1985 A controlled study on the effect of epidural analgesia with local anaesthetics and morphine on morbidity after abdominal surgery. Acta Anaesthesiologica Scandinavica 29: 790–796

Hjortso N C, Lund C, Mogensen T, Bigler D, Kehlet H 1986 Epidural morphine improves pain relief and maintains sensory analgesia during continuous epidural bupivacaine after abdominal surgery. Anesthesia and Analgesia 65: 1033–1036

Johnson M W, Mitch W E, Wilcox C S 1985 The cardiovascular actions of morphine and the endogenous opioid peptides. Progress in Cardiovascular Diseases 27: 435–450

Jones V A, Hanks G W 1986 New portable infusion pump for prolonged subcutaneous administration of opioid analgesics in patients with advanced cancer. British Medical Journal 292: 1496

Kosterlitz H W 1985 The Wellcome Foundation Lecture 1982 — Opioid peptides and their receptors. Proceedings of the Royal Society of London 225: 27–40

Kotob H I M, Hand C W, Moore R A et al 1986 Intrathecal morphine and heroin in humans. Six-hour drug levels in spinal fluid and plasma. Anesthesia and Analgesia 65: 718–722

Larsen V H, Christensen P, Brinklov M M, Axelsen F 1986 Postoperative pain relief and respiratory performance after thoracotomy: a controlled trial comparing the effect of epidural morphine and subcutaneous nicomorphine. Danish Medical Bulletin 33: 161–164

Larson J-J, Svendsen O, Andersen H B 1986 Microscopic epidural lesions in goats given repeated epidural injections of morphine: use of a modified autopsy procedure. Acta Pharmacologica et Toxicologica 58: 5–10

Lund C, Hjortso N-C, Mogensen T, Kehlet H 1985 Systemic morphine enhances spread of sensory analgesia during postoperative epidural bupivacaine infusion. Lancet 2: 1156–1157

Max M B, Inturrisi C E, Kaiko R F, Grabinski P Y, Li C H, Foley K M 1985 Epidural and intrathecal opiates: cerebrospinal fluid and plasma profiles in patients with chronic cancer pain. Clinical Pharmacology andd Therapeutics 38: 631–641

Nordberg G, Borg L, Hedner T, Mellstrand T 1985 CSF and plasma pharmacokinetics of intramuscular morphine. European Journal of Clinical Pharmacology 27: 677–681

Nordberg G, Mellstrand T, Borg L, Hedner T 1986 Extradural morphine: influence of adrenaline admixture. British Journal of Anaesthesia 58: 598–604

Obbens E A M T, Leavens M E, Beal J W, Lee Y-Y 1985 Ommaya reservoirs in 387 cancer patients. A 15-year experience. Neurology 35: 1274–1278

Olstad O A, Skjelbred P 1986 Comparison of the analgesic effect of a corticosteroid and paracetamol in patients with pain after oral surgery. British Journal of Clinical Pharmacology 22: 437–442

O'Neill, P, Knickenberg C, Bogahalanda S, Booth A E 1985 Use of intrathecal morphine for postoperative pain relief following lumbar spine surgery. Journal of Neurosurgery 63: 413–416

Osborne R J, Joel S P, Slevin M L 1986 Morphine intoxication in renal failure. The role of morphine-6-glucuronide. British Medical Journal 292: 1548–1549

Rechtine G R, Reinerts C M, Bohlman H H 1984 The use of epidural morphine to decrease postoperative pain in patients undergoing lumbar laminectomy. Journal of Bone and Joint Surgery 66: 113–116

Rochat T, Junod A F, Gaillard R C 1985 Circulating endogenous opioids and ventilatory response to CO_2 and hypoxia. Respiration Physiology 61: 85–93

Santiago T V, Edelman N H 1985 Opioids and breathing. Journal of Applied Physiology 59: 1675–1685

Slattery P J, Boas R A 1985 Newer methods of delivery of opiates for relief of pain. Drugs 30: 539–551

Staren E D, Cullen M L 1986 Epidural catheter analgesia for the management of postoperative pain. Surgery, Gynecology and Obstetrics 162: 389–404

Weinberger S E, Steinbrook R A, Carr D B et al 1985 Endogenous opioids and ventilatory responses to hypercapnia in normal humans. Journal of Applied Physiology 58: 1415–1420

Wen H L, Meha Z D, Ong B H, Ho W K K, Wen D Y K 1985 Intrathecal administration of beta-endorphin and dynorphin-(1-13) for the treatment of intractable pain. Life Sciences 37: 1213–1220

Willer J-C, Bergeret S, Gaudy J-H 1985 Epidural morphine strongly depresses nociceptive flexion reflexes in patients with postoperative pain. Anesthesiology 63: 675–680

Woolner D F, Winter D, Frendin T J, Begg E J, Lynn K L, Wright G J 1986 Renal failure does not impair the metabolism of morphine. British Journal of Clinical Pharmacology 22: 55–69

Yaksh T L, Harty G J, Onofrio B M 1986 High doses of spinal morphine produce a nonopiate receptor-mediated hyperesthesia: clinical and theoretic implications. Anesthesiology 64: 590–597

Yuge O, Matsumoto M, Kitahata L M, Collins J G, Senami M 1985 Direct opioid application to peripheral nerves does not alter compound action potentials. Anesthesia and Analgesia 64: 667–671

Zhong F-X, Ji, X-Q, Tsou K 1985 Intrathecal DSP4 selectively depletes spinal noradrenaline and attenuates morphine analgesia. European Journal of Pharmacology 116: 327–330

Update (1)

ABDOMINAL ANAESTHESIA

Colonic blood flow

Colonic blood flow especially to the mucosa is the critical factor in determining the successful outcome of the intestinal anastomosis (see *Anaesthesia
Review 3*). Banks et al (1985) presented a summary of a symposium on
vasoactive agents which affect the mesenteric circulation. H_1 and H_2
receptors are involved in the dilatation of mesenteric and renal
circulations. Histamine may be involved in the dilatation. There
are also vasodilator responses of the bowel to foods and in particular
to chyme. The physiological role of serotonin (5-HT), substance P and
motilin is still uncertain. Phenoxybenzamine, propranolol, atropine, indomethacin and H_1 and H_2 receptor blockers did not affect the hyperaemic
response of substance P on the gut. Increases in splanchnic vascular resistance are initially compensated by increased oxygen extraction but this
mechanism fails when there is an extensive decrease in blood flow. Bowel
damage is noted initially in the mucosa with the muscle layer being spared.
Noradrenaline, adrenaline and dopamine cause vasoconstriction of the
precapillary resistance vessels in the splanchnic area with a reduction in
flow. Alpha-adrenergic agonists also cause constriction in the postcapillary
capacitance vessels. Vasopressin and angiotensin II are vasoconstrictors
resulting in a decrease in mesenteric blood flow. Prostaglandins and leukotrienes produce vasoconstriction while prostaglandin inhibitors such as
indomethacin and aspirin also decrease resting levels of blood flow. 5-HT
in high doses and digoxin also increase splanchnic vascular resistance.
   Banks et al (1985) discussed the effects of anaesthesia, surgery, stress
response and gastrointestinal haemorrhage on the splanchnic circulation.
Thiopentone and nitrous oxide have little effect but halothane and spinal
anaesthesia, by producing a fall of cardiac output, reduce splanchnic blood
flow without affecting vascular resistance. Cyclopropane and methoxyflurane increase splanchnic resistance. Haemorrhage, pain, acidosis and
hypothermia also increase splanchnic resistance while hypotension from
hypovolaemia or cardiogenic shock resulted in a decrease of both the

splanchnic vascular resistance and the total peripheral resistance. During hypotension the rise in splanchnic vascular resistance may be up to 13 times greater than that seen in the peripheral circulation and may be associated with an increase of angiotensin II and increased plasma renin activity. This effect does not appear to be related to noradrenaline but vasopressin appears to be involved. The treatment of gastrointestinal haemorrhage by infusion of vasoconstrictors such as vasopressin may lead to coronary vasoconstriction as well but the use of prostaglandin ($PGF_{2\text{-alpha}}$) appears to be a more promising agent. The effect of vasodilators on the mesenteric circulation is complex as drugs may affect the precapillary and postcapillary vessels and studies have included effects on capillary filtration, osmotic pressure in the splanchnic vessels and tissue oxygen tensions.

From animal experiments Foster et al (1985a) re-affirmed the dangers of poor tissue perfusion in the elderly and in low rectal anastomosis which can lead to a leakage rate which is often as high as 13%. They advocated the use of isoxsuprine (Duvadilan) an alpha-adrenergic antagonist and a beta-adrenergic agonist which also reduces blood viscosity and which resulted in improved circulation in ischaemic rat colon. Blood flow was measured using laser Doppler techniques.

Gerstmann et al (1985) advocated a non-invasive method of measuring intestinal ischaemia by measuring the change in pulmonary clearance of helium instilled into the colon. Oxygen tension in the colon fell significantly following 10% blood loss (Foster et al 1985b). Tissue oxygen tension was lower when interrupted stitches were used. If the tissue oxygen tension in the anastomotic area was above 7.3 kPa (55 mmHg) the leak rate was 10% whereas it was 100% if the tension was less than 3.3 kPa (25 mmHg) (Shandall et al 1985). During hyperventilation there was an increase in intestinal vascular resistance induced by 'the stress response'. There was a decreased response during hypoventilation and this may be associated with the peripheral vasodilator effects of CO_2 (Winso et al 1985).

Intestinal anastomosis

Mechanical factors affecting anastomosis involve the loss of collagen in the first 3 postoperative days. In a recent study (Jonsson et al 1986) it was found that the strength of the bowel wall at a distance of 3.5 mm from the anastomosis was not reduced and this was related to the collagen content. Previous reported studies of any weakness appear to be limited to the suture line.

Anaesthetic agents

Tverskoy et al (1985) found that isoflurane increased splanchnic vascular resistance decreasing blood flow. This effect was abolished by phentolamine suggesting that the vascular effect had been produced by circulating catecholamines. However Ostman et al (1986) found that the reflex vasocon-striction in the renal and intestinal blood flow in response to surgical stimulation could be suppressed by isoflurane in a dose-dependent manner. If the results of these animal experiments can be applied to man 1.5 MAC of isoflurane may help to maintain the renal and intestinal circulation during operative procedures.

Drugs

Morphine slightly increased the lower oesophageal sphincter pressure but it significantly inhibited the relaxation of the sphincter, the effect being maximal 30 minutes after injection (Dowlatshahi et al 1985). In other studies of morphine and atropine on motility in the human ileum, Borody et al (1985) showed that morphine initially stimulated ileal flow while atro-pine was ineffectual. Atropine reduced the occurrence of sporadic pressure waves in the ileum but morphine had no effect. Atropine reduced the transit time of food from mouth to ileum but morphine had no action. Naloxone had no effect on motility or flow when administered by itself but it did reverse the stimulation actions of morphine and atropine. Studies of drugs on the distal colon have shown that preparations of drugs in capsules or pellets have a transit time of 4 hours (Hardy et al 1985).

Patients with asthma who were under treatment with atropine exhibited prolonged gastric emptying time (Botts et al 1985).

Physiology

In animal studies Dettmar et al (1986) found that the colon was under the influence of a mechanism which is non-adrenergic and non-cholinergic. Stimulation of prejunctional alpha$_2$-adrenoceptors reduced inhibition while postjunctional alpha$_1$-adrenoceptors were inhibitory. Motility studies on the rectosigmoid colon in man have demonstrated that beta$_2$-adrenoceptor stimulation decreases colonic pressure while beta$_1$-stimulation resulted in changes which were similar to that of the control (Lyrenas et al 1985).

The bowel may reflect the psychological profile of the population. Cortisol levels were greater in patients with high intestinal tone than in those with psychological depression and low tone. Intramuscular clonidine (2.5 μg/kg) reduced diastolic blood pressure and plasma noradrenaline in those with low intestinal tone, the cortisol level being less than in the control group. It was felt that the use of clonidine might be a reasonable index of sympathetic activity in depressed patients (Lechin et al 1985). The effect of oral clonidine on plasma cortisol in children was consistent with the fall in serum levels associated with diurnal variation (Ellis et al 1986).

The sphincter of Oddi and analgesia

Interest has been shown in an observation made by Mossberg (1964) that drugs like morphine may cause pain, not unlike that of myocardial infarction in patients who have had a cholecystectomy. In animal studies continuous biliary pressure and EMG activity of the sphincter of Oddi and gastrointestinal tract were recorded following morphine, pethidine and pentazocine. The drugs caused intense bursts of spike potentials at the sphincter of Oddi and duodenum but if the gallbladder had previously been removed there was a significant rise in biliary pressure (Coelho et al 1986). The presence of the gallbladder may absorb some of the increased pressure following the use of morphine. This study confirmed recent personal observations that morphine should be avoided not only in patients who have gallstones but also in those who have had a cholecystectomy. The ensuing pain readily responds to intravenous naloxone.

Patients with undefined biliary pain either prior to or after cholecystectomy were given intramuscular morphine 0.12 mg/kg and neostigmine (0.012 mg/kg) and it was found when compared with controls that not only did patients experience pain but there was a rise in serum aspartate aminotransferase (AST) and serum amylase. There appears to be an increased spasm of the sphincter of Oddi in these patients resulting in high biliary pressures: the increase in liver enzyme after the challenge by morphine and neostigmine could be abolished by endoscopic sphincterotomy (Roberts-Thomson & Toouli 1985).

Postoperative ileus

Studies in man with bipolar electrodes placed in the ascending and descending colon during laparotomy showed that the magnitude and duration of the operation did not influence the period of postoperative ileus. The frequencies of electrical activity were analysed. Electrical activity initially occurred randomly with disorganised single bursts of activity during 3 postoperative days after which activity increased and on the 4th postoperative day there were long bursts of continuous activity at a higher velocity than previously recorded which was accompanied by the passage of flatus. There were variations in activity between the right and left colon. Morphine stimulated electrical activity, but this was not propagated. Morphine did not appear to alter the duration of postoperative ileus (Condon et al 1986).

Pain relief following abdominal surgery

There is still a need to improve postoperative analgesia and this is reflected in the number of regimes that have been advocated. Levack et al (1986) proposed the use of postoperative wound perfusion with 10 ml of 0.5% bupivacaine twice daily through an in-dwelling drainage tube for 3 days. Although analgesia, as assessed by visual analogue scoring, was similar in a control group given only saline, the forced vital capacity (FVC) was significantly improved when the patients were given bupivacaine. They also had less postoperative opioid analgesia than the control group. Rimback et al (1986) found the intra-abdominal instillation of bupivacaine (2 ml/kg) shortened the period of postoperative colonic inhibition but did not affect colonic transport. The bupivacaine was dissolved in 300 ml of isotonic saline which was given through a small incision into the peritoneal cavity 10 minutes prior to the main incision. Blood glucose concentrations were lower in the bupivacaine-treated group at 30 minutes, 1 hour and 4 hours after the local anaesthetic had been instilled. The plasma concentrations of bupivacaine were well below toxic levels and it was suggested that the bupivacaine inhibited the inflammatory responses in the bowel and shortened the duration of ileus.

Intravenous fluids

Sjovall et al (1986) studied the effects of absorption of fluids in the human jejunum by mimicking a reduction in circulating blood volume of approximately 600–800 ml by lowering the legs to a dependent position with resulting venous status. There is increased sympathetic activity as is shown by an increased resistance and a reduction in forearm blood flow. There was an increased absorption of fluid, sodium and chloride but not glucose.

Nielsen & Engell (1986) have studied the importance of plasma colloid osmotic pressure in patients undergoing elective abdominal operations. If the colloid pressure fell below 20 mmHg there was an increase in interstitial fluid volume. It was felt that the colloid osmotic pressure should be maintained above 20 mmHg after major abdominal surgery and the positive fluid balance should not exceed 5 litres during the day of operation.

It has been suggested that there is little damage to vessels following total parenteral nutrition when large central veins are used as the route of administration but Mulvihill et al (1985) demonstrated in the rat model damage to the right atrium, pulmonary artery and lung tissue. This might account for the possible pulmonary hypertension occurring in patients on long term parenteral therapy.

Total parenteral nutrition results in an increased oxygen consumption, CO_2 production and minute ventilation and this appears to be the result of the protein component in the infused fluid (Rodriguez et al 1985).

In patients with septicaemia signs of circulatory failure, an elevated blood lactate level appears to be a favourable predictor of response to fluid loading with 6% starch or 5% human albumin as judged by an increase in oxygen delivery and increase in oxygen consumption. When there was no lactateacidaemia, haemodilution resulted in decreased oxygen delivery and oxygen consumption (Haupt et al 1985).

REFERENCES

Banks R O, Gallavan R H, Zinner M J et al 1985 Vasoactive agents in control of the mesenteric circulation. Federation Proceedings 44: 2743–2749

Borody T J, Quigley E M M, Phillips S F et al 1985 Effects of morphine and atropine on motility and transit in the human ileum. Gastroenterology 89: 562–570

Botts L D, Pingleton S K, Schroeder C E, Robinson R G, Hurwitz A 1985 Prolongation of gastric emptying by aerosolized atropine. American Review of Respiratory Disease 131: 725–726

Coelho J C U, Runkel N, Herfarth C, Senninger N, Messmer K 1986 Effect of analgesic drugs on the electromyographic activity of the gastrointestinal tract and sphincter of Oddi and on biliary pressure. Annals of Surgery 204: 53–58

Condon R E, Cowles V E, Schulte W J, Frantzides C T, Mahoney J L, Sarna S K 1986 Resolution of postoperative ileus in humans. Annals of Surgery 203: 574–581

Dettmar P W, Kelly J, MacDonald A 1986 Alpha-adrenoceptors in the rat colon. Proceedings of the British Pharmacological Society (9–11 April) p 178

Dowlatshahi K, Evander A, Walther B, Skinner D B 1985 Influence of morphine on the distal oesophagus and the lower oesophageal sphincter — a manometric study. Gut 26: 802–806

Ellis N F, MacGillivray M H, Voorhess M L 1986 Effects of clonidine on plasma cortisol concentrations. Clinical Pharmacology and Therapeutics 39: 660–663

Foster M E, Brennan S S, Morgan A, Leaper D J 1985a Colonic ischaemic and anastomotic healing. European Surgical Research 71: 133–139

Foster M E, Laycock J R D, Silver I A, Leaper D J 1985b Hypovolaemia and healing in colonic anastomoses. British Journal of Surgery 72: 831–834

Gerstmann D R, Waffarn F, Huxtable R F, Beran A V 1985 A noninvasive method for monitoring intestinal ischemia. Changes in the pulmonary clearance of helium instilled into the colon as an index of colonic blood flow. Pediatric Research 19: 1025–1028

Hardy J G, Wilson C G, Wood E 1985 Drug delivery to the proximal colon. Journal of Pharmacy and Pharmacology 37: 874–877

Haupt M T, Gilbert E M, Carlson R W 1985 Fluid loading increases oxygen consumption in septic patients with lactic acidosis. American Review of Respiratory Disease 131: 912–915

Jonsson K, Kiborn H, Zederfeldt B 1986 Mechanical and biochemical alterations in the intestinal wall adjacent to an anastomosis. American Journal of Surgery 151: 387–390

Lechin F, van der Dijs B, Jakubowicz D et al 1985 Effects of clonidine on blood pressure, noradrenaline, cortisol, growth hormone and prolactin plasma levels in high and low intestinal tone depressed patients. Neuroendocrinology 41: 156–162

Levack I D, Holmes J D, Robertson G S 1986 Abdominal wound perfusion for the relief of postoperative pain. British Journal of Anaesthesia 58: 615–619

Lyrenas E, Abrahamsson H, Dotevall G 1985 Effects of beta-adrenoceptor stimulation on rectosigmoid motility in man. Digestive Diseases and Sciences 30: 536–540

Mossberg S M 1964 Myocardial infarction like syndrome in cholecystectomy patients given narcotics. British Medical Journal 1: 948–950

Mulvihill S J, Takamatsu H, Albert A, Fonkalsrud E W 1985 Pulmonary pathology associated with hypertonic central venous fluid administration. Surgery, Gynecology and Obstetrics 161: 535–540

Nielsen O M, Engell H C 1986 The importance of plasma colloid osmotic pressure for interstitial fluid volume and fluid balance after elective abdominal vascular surgery. Annals of Surgery 203: 25–29

Ostman M, Biber B, Martner J, Reiz S 1986 Influence of isoflurane on renal and intestinal vascular responses to stress. British Journal of Anaesthesia 58: 630–638

Rimback G, Cassuto J, Faxen A, Hogstrom S, Wallin G, Tollesson P O 1986 Effect of intra-abdominal bupivacaine instillation on postoperative colonic motility. Gut 27: 170–175

Roberts-Thomson J C, Toouli J 1985 Abnormal responses to morphine-neostigmine in patients with undefined biliary type pain. Gut 26: 1367–1372

Rodriguez J L, Askanazi J, Weissman C, Hansle T W, Rosenbaum S H, Kinney J M 1985 Ventilatory and metabolic effects of glucose infusions. Chest 88: 512–518

Shandall A, Lowndes R, Young H L 1985 Colonic anastomotic healing and oxygen tension. British Journal of Surgery 72: 606–609

Sjovall H, Abrahamsson H, Westlander G et al 1986 Intestinal fluid and electrolyte transport in man during reduced circulating blood volume. Gut 27: 913–918

Tverskoy M, Gelman S, Fowler K C 1985 Intestinal circulation during inhalation anesthesia. Anesthesiology 62: 462–469

Winso O, Biber B, Martner J 1985 Effects of hyperventilation and hypoventilation on stress-induced intestinal vasoconstriction. Acta Anaesthesiologica Scandinavica 29: 726–732

MUSCLE RELAXANTS

Allergy

Vervloet (1985) has reviewed the literature on the anaphylactoid reactions associated with the use of muscle relaxants. In a French national study of 200 000 general anaesthetics the incidence of a major complication was 1:4500 and despite treatment 6% of this group died. Muscle relaxants appear to be responsible for 50% of adverse reactions during anaesthesia.

The most frequent reactions are tachycardia, cardiovascular collapse, urticaria, but also bronchospasm, diarrhoea and coagulation defects can occur. The incidence of adverse reactions is higher in women. The mechanisms have been discussed by Assem (1984). It appears that the quaternary ammonium ions react with the IgE antibodies with the resultant release of histamine.

Brain injury

Hypoxaemia associated with brain injury may be complicated by increased intracranial pressure and pulmonary oedema. In an animal study Millis et al (1985) suggested that the hypoxaemia was exacerbated in the presence of uncontrolled skeletal muscle activity and that there was an improvement in the arterial PO_2 when the animals were ventilated with a muscle relaxant which also abolished the muscle activity.

Atracurium

Atracurium has been recommended as the muscle relaxant of choice in patients with myasthenia gravis (see *Anaesthesia Review 4*). In a further study, Vacanti et al (1985) found that the response to atracurium was variable but it seemed a reasonable preference in myasthenia because of the rapid rate of recovery. They did however stress the need for monitoring of neuromuscular function.

Atracurium (0.6 mg/kg) leads to an increase in plasma histamine but this had returned to control levels after 4 minutes. Atracurium is less likely to lead to histamine release than tubocurarine. There is a poor correlation between plasma histamine levels and the clinical signs of histamine release; the skin reactions seen after atracurium do not necessarily indicate that plasma histamine levels are increased (Barnes et al 1986).

Atracurium was found to lower the intra-ocular pressure significantly when compared with pancuronium but neither drug suppressed the increase in pressure following the stress of laryngoscopy and intubation (Murphy et al 1985).

Vecuronium

Vecuronium in the dose of 0.1 mg/kg resulted in a slight decrease in intracranial pressure which was associated with a decrease in central venous pressure following muscular relaxation which permits better drainage of cerebral venous blood (Rosa et al 1986). A similar fall in central venous pressure has been reported by Jantzen et al (1986) and this effect appeared to be responsible for the decrease in intra-ocular pressure. Vecuronium appeared to be a suitable neuromuscular blocking agent in patients with perforating eye injuries and for operations in the treatment of glaucoma.

Suxamethonium

Attempts have been made to reduce the rise in intra-ocular pressure which occurs following suxamethonium. Murphy et al (1986) performed a study using intravenous lignocaine (1.5 mg/kg) prior to induction and found that this failed to prevent the rise in intra-ocular pressure either after suxamethonium or even pancuronium. The rise in intra-ocular pressure was associated with the hypertensive response to intubation; the changes following suxamethonium were of less significance.

Atropine

Intravenous atropine in doses ranging from 0.3 to 1 mg may give rise to serum levels of 2–6 ng/ml with an elimination half-life of approximately 4 hours. Atropine is frequently used in nebulized form for bronchodilatation and if the drug is administered 4–6 hourly for 48 hours then serum levels may be greater than 2 ng/ml (Kradjan et al 1985).

Glycopyrronium

Glycopyrronium has been recommended in preference to atropine to suppress the muscarinic actions of 5 mg of neostigmine which has a long duration of action. Salem & Ahearn (1986) found that postoperative bradycardia could be prevented by glucopyrronium but only in a dose of 0.9 mg. The drug was also capable of reducing the volume of postoperative gastric contents but not the pH, thus reducing the risk of possible regurgitation and inhalation of gastric contents (Fry 1986). However in a study of neostigmine-induced colonic activity Child (1984) was unable to demonstrate any significant difference in mean intraluminal pressure or total colonic activity prior to the administration of atropine 1.2 mg or glycopyrronium 0.6 mg.

Neostigmine

The accumulation of acetylcholine causes fade of tetanic contraction by affecting the sodium channels in the region around the end-plates while the resultant sustained fade is due to a reduction in the amount of transmitter released. These results are from studies on mouse diaphragm using neo-stigmine to inhibit acetylcholinesterase (Chang et al 1986). In other animal studies chronic neostigmine treatment reduced the amplitude of miniature end-plate potentials and decreased the depolarization produced by acetyl-choline. Apparently chronic neostigmine treatment causes 'an adaptive reduction in the number of functional acetylcholine receptors at the endplate without otherwise affecting single channel properties' (Gwilt & Wray 1986).

Dantrolene

Dantrolene, which acts directly on skeletal muscle fibres, causes a reduction in inspired and expired ventilation rates (in rats). There are compensatory mechanisms to maintain ventilation and these include increased frequency of discharge of the motor units supplying respiratory muscle, increasing the time during which the motor units are active and an increase in recruitment of motor units (Farquhar et al 1986).

Oral or intravenous dantrolene (4–6 mg/kg/day) reduced the mortality of tetanus markedly in children aged from 4 days to 13 years. Dantrolene appeared to have little effect on respiratory depression either when given alone or administered with other drugs such as phenobarbitone or diazepam (Bernal et al 1986).

Muscular dystrophy

Kelly et al (1986) reported the mechanism of the increased resistance to tubocurarine in dystrophic mice but in clinical practice the dose of non-depolarizing muscle relaxants should be reduced.

REFERENCES

Assem E S K 1984 Allergic responses during anaesthesia: methods of detection. In: L Kaufman (ed) Anaesthesia review 2, Churchill Livingstone, London, pp 49–62
Barnes P K, De Renzy-Martin N, Thomas V J E, Watkins J 1986 Plasma histamine levels following atracurium. Anaesthesia 41: 821–824
Bernal O R A, Bender M A, Lacy M E 1986 Efficacy of dentrolene sodium in management of tetanus in children. Journal of the Royal Society of Medicine 79: 277–281
Chang C C, Hong S J, Ko J-L 1986 Mechanisms of the inhibition by neostigmine of tetanic contraction in the mouse diaphragm. British Journal of Pharmacology 87: 757–762
Child C S 1984 Prevention of neostigmine-induced colonic activity. A comparison of atropine and glucopyrronium. Anaesthesia 39: 1083–1085
Farquhar R, Leslie G C, Part N J 1986 How is ventilation maintained in the presence of the muscle relaxant, dantrolene sodium? A study in the anaesthetised rat. British Journal of Pharmacology 88: 79–86
Fry E N S 1986 Postoperative gastric aspirations reduced by glycopyrrolate during upper abdominal surgery. Journal of the Royal Society of Medicine 79: 334–338
Gwilt M, Wray D 1986 The effect of chronic neostigmine treatment on channel properties at the rat skeletal neuromuscular junction. British Journal of Pharmacology 88: 25–31

Jantzen J-P, Hackett G H, Erdmann K, Earnshaw G 1986 Effect of vecuronium on intraocular pressure. British Journal of Anaesthesia 58: 433–436

Kelly S S, Morgan G P, Smith J W 1986 The origin of (+)– tubocurarine resistance in dystrophic mice. British Journal of Pharmacology 89: 47–53

Kradjan W A, Smallridge R C, Davis R, Verma P 1985 Atropine serum concentrations after multiple inhaled doses of atropine sulfate. Clinical Pharmacology and Therapeutics 38: 12–15

Millis R M, Wood D H, Trouth C O 1985 Amelioration of hypoxemia by neuromuscular blockade following brain injury. Life Sciences 37: 739–747

Murphy D F, Eustace P, Unwin A, Magner J B 1985 Atracurium and intraocular pressure. British Journal of Ophthalmology 69: 673–675

Murphy D F, Eustace P, Unwin A, Magner J B 1986 Intravenous lignocaine pretreatment to prevent intraocular pressure rise following suxamethonium and tracheal intubation. British Journal of Ophthalmology 70: 596–598

Rosa G, Sanfilippa M, Vilardi V, Orfei P, Gasparetto A 1986 Effects of vecuronium bromide on intracranial pressure and cerebral perfusion pressure. British Journal of Anaesthesia 58: 437–440

Salem M G, Ahearn R S 1986 Atropine or glycopyrrolate with neostigmine 5 mg. A comparative dose-response study. Journal of the Royal Society of Medicine 79: 19–24

Vacanti C A, Ali H H, Schweiss J F, Scott R P 1985 The response of myasthenia gravis to atracurium. Anesthesiology 62: 692–694

Vervloet D 1985 Allergy to muscle relaxants and related compounds. Clinical Allergy 15: 501–508

PHAEOCHROMOCYTOMA

The diagnosis, pre-operative preparation and anaesthetic management of phaeochromocytoma have been reviewed by Hull (1986). The clinical presentation is described including the various manifestations of a phaeochromocytoma crisis. These are details of diagnosis and localization of the tumour as well as an account of the adrenergic blocking agents used in the pre-operative preparation and during the course of anaesthesia. Hull's preferred technique includes alfentanil, vecuronium and etomidate followed by nitrous oxide oxygen and enflurane with a continuous infusion of alfentanil.

Phaeochromocytoma may present in unusual patterns. Jones & Durning (1985) described two patients in whom the condition presented as an acute abdomen and pulmonary oedema developed soon after induction of anaesthesia. One patient died before adrenergic blockers could be administered while in the second patient, who also died, abdominal pain was accompanied by sweating, tachycardia, extrasystoles and a moderately raised blood pressure.

Reliance on computed tomography or iodobenzylguanidine may give negative or misleading results in the diagnosis of phaeochromocytoma (Dunn et al 1986).

Delayed recovery may follow the removal of phaeochromocytoma and this may be due to hypoglycaemia. High catecholamine levels inhibit the action of insulin and when the tumour is removed there may be a rise in insulin level. Hypoglycaemia may be augmented by beta-adrenoreceptor blocking agents such as propranolol (Meeke et al 1985).

Stirt et al (1985) reported on the successful use of atracurium in a young girl with a phaeochromocytoma. Atracurium has less autonomic activity compared with pancuronium although the possibility of histamine release should be considered. Atracurium has been used during removal of a tumour in a patient who was symptomless and in whom tests for phaeochromocytoma were negative. Cardiovascular stability occurred throughout the procedure until the tumour (subsequently shown to be a phaeochromocytoma) was removed when profound hypotension occurred. This readily responded to an infusion of noradrenaline (personal series).

In a series of 62 patients Stenstrom et al (1985) commented favourably on the pre-operative use of phenoxybenzamine which resulted in a smooth peri-operative course with a statistically significant reduction in the incidence of excessive blood pressure fluctuations. Pre-operative blood transfusion had no effect on the incidence of hypotension suggesting that it was unrelated to blood volume. However Stentrom & Kutti (1985) found that pre-operative treatment with phenoxybenzamine increased the total blood volume secondary to an increase in plasma volume. This is in contrast to previous studies and may be due to the fact that Stenstrom & Kutti (1985) used larger doses than those previously reported and treatment was continued for 2–3 weeks (see *Anaesthesia Review 1* p. 28).

Although phaeochromocytoma may be associated with thyroid disorders the incidence of hypercalcaemia is unusual. Stewart et al (1985) described a child who had a phaeochromocytoma with hypercalcaemia but there was no evidence to suggest that there was excessive parathyroid hormone secretion. Adrenalectomy promptly reduced the plasma level of calcium, the tumour containing a substance that produced bone re-absorption. The tumour also contained potent adenylate-cyclase-stimulating activity similar to that extracted from tumour associated with the hypercalcaemia of malignancy.

In contrast to the high levels of catecholamines found in phaeochromocytoma Robertson et al (1986) have described a patient with reduced plasma noradrenaline levels (less than 10% of normal). The patient presented with severe orthostatic hypotension and ptosis but with normal autonomic activity. They presented evidence to show that this patient had reduced dopamine-beta-hydroxylase activity.

REFERENCES

Dunn G D, Brown M J, Sapsford R N et al 1986 Functional middle mediastinal paraganglioma (phaemochromocytoma) associated with intercarotid paragangliomas. Lancet 1: 1061–1064
Hull C J 1986 Phaeochromocytoma. Diagnosis, preoperative preparation and anaesthetic management. British Journal of Anaesthesia 58: 1453–1468
Jones D J, Durning P 1985 Phaeochromocytoma presenting as an acute abdomen: report of two cases. British Medical Journal 291: 1267–1268
Meeke R I, O'Keeffe J D, Gaffney J D 1985 Phaeochromocytoma removal and postoperative hypoglycaemia. Anaesthesia 40: 1093–1096
Robertson D, Goldberg M R, Onrot J et al 1986 Isolated failure of autonomic

noradrenergic neurotransmission. Evidence for impaired beta-hydroxylation of dopamine. New England Journal of Medicine 314: 1494–1497

Stenstrom G, Haljamae H, Tisell L E 1985 Influence of pre-operative treatment with phenoxybenzamine on the incidence of adverse cardiovascular reactions during anaesthesia and surgery for phaeochromocytoma. Acta Anaesthesiologica Scandinavica 29: 797–803

Stenstrom G, Kutti J 1985 The blood volume in pheochromocytoma patients before and during treatment with phenoxybenzamine. Acta Medica Scandinavica 218: 381–387

Stewart A F, Hoecker J L, Mallette L E, Segre G V, Amatruda T T, Vignery A 1985 Hypercalcemia in pheochromocytoma. Annals of Internal Medicine 102: 776–779 .

Stirt J A, Brown R E, Ross W T, Althaus J S 1985 Atracurium in a patient with pheochromocytoma. Anesthesia and Analgesia 64: 5478–559

RESUSCITATION

Attempts have been made to involve the public in the principles of management of cardiorespiratory arrest. However there are deficiencies in the training of hospital staff as has recently been shown in the monitoring of the quality of resuscitation after simulated cardiac arrest (Sullivan & Guyatt 1986). Mouth-to-mouth respiration was inadequate: there was confusion regarding the use of defibrillators especially as more than one type were available: suction equipment was ineffectual.

The paraphysiology and neurological complications following cardiopulmonary arrest have been reviewed by Bass (1985). He discussed the brain changes during ischaemia reminding us that cell function is not necessarily restored as soon as the circulation returns. Cardiac arrest may lead to a variety of complications including stroke, encephalopathy, myoclonus, peripheral nerve damage, blindness, amnesia, impairment of intellect, vegetative state and brain death. Attempts to reduce brain metabolism by hypothermia and barbiturates are singularly disappointing in global ischaemia. Seizures in the unconscious are difficult to treat but diazepam followed by dilantin has been recommended. Haemodilution therapy may decrease blood viscosity while the use of calcium blocking agents has its advocates preventing the ions accumulating within the cell. A blood sugar level greater than 16.6 mmol/l (300 mg/dl) signified a poor outcome while the use of bicarbonate has been questioned. Although steroids are often used to treat brain oedema the evidence of its success is scanty.

Longstreth et al (1986) reported blood sugar levels during resuscitation ranging form 2.3–47.5 mmol/l (42–854 mg/dl) and the levels rose during cardiopulmonary resuscitation. Although there appears to be an association between poor neurological recovery and the high blood glucose levels following cardiac arrest it is the prolonged resuscitation that leads to the poor outlook of recovery. Bass (1985) has also discussed in detail the causes of delayed neurological complications following cardiac arrest.

The acid base status during cardiopulmonary resuscitation has been measured by Weil et al (1986) and it was found that the arterial blood does not reflect accurately the acid base state. During cardiac arrest the arterial pH, PCO_2 and bicarbonate were not significantly altered but the mixed venous blood had a low pH and an increased PCO_2. It has been customary to believe that the metabolic acidosis was due to the anaerobic production of lactic acid but Weil et al (1986) concluded that there was also an element of respiratory acidosis which was not detected by arterial blood sampling. They also questioned the need for the administration of bicarbonate.

The use of calcium in the management of cardiac arrest has been debated by Hughes & Ruedy (1986) who concluded that there was no indication for the routine use of calcium solutions in the treatment of ventricular fibrillation or cardiac asystole. They suggested that calcium chloride (5–10 ml of 10% solution) or calcium gluconate (10–20 ml of 10% solution) should be restricted to patients who have had an overdose of calcium blocking agents and those with cardiac arrhythmias resulting from hyperkalaemia and hypocalcaemia. Calcium salts may have a place in the electromechanical dissociation.

Davis (1985) in a follow-up study of patients who had suffered an episode of ventricular fibrillation found there was a high rate of subsequent cardiac arrest. He concluded that tests should be undertaken to assess the efficacy of anti-arrhythmic agents and the need for training relatives of these patients in cardiopulmonary resuscitation.

Koster & Dunning (1985) found that the use of automatic injector to deliver 400 mg of lignocaine intramuscularly (deltoid muscle) was of value to patients suspected of having acute myocardial infarction. It could be administered by paramedical personnel to patients awaiting admission to hospital. The incidence of ventricular fibrillation and ventricular tachycardia was reduced. Side effects were minimal and did not contribute to mortality.

Caldwell et al (1985) described the use of simple mechanical methods of cardioversion by precordial thump or a cough. Conscious patients were encouraged to cough and this terminated ventricular tachycardia. Precordial thumping of the chest was successful in terminating not only ventrical tachycardia but also ventricular fibrillation.

Pearn (1985) has reviewed in detail the management of near-drowning including first aid and hospital management. Prolonged submersion especially with hypothermia is still compatible with complete recovery. If a child gasps within 20 minutes of being rescued then recovery is usually complete. Deterioration after rescue may result from the loss of surfactant or anoxic damage to the alveolar membrane. The intrapulmonary shunt may increase to 75%. Electrolyte changes are transient and were thought at one time to differentiate between drowning in salt or fresh water. The merits and disadvantages of the management of raised intracranial pressure are discussed in detail and there is still debate as to whether active treatment of this complication improves survival.

Barbiturates have been recommended for the possibility of reducing brain damage following global ischaemia. In a study of 262 comatose survivors of cardiac arrest those who received thiopentone (30 mg/kg) did not fair better than those who received the standard intensive care therapy and therefore thiopentone could not be recommended for treatment following cardiac arrest (Brain Resuscitation Clinical Trial I study Group 1986).

REFERENCES

Bass E 1985 Cardiopulmonary arrest. Pathophysiology and neurologic complications. Annals of Internal Medicine 103: 920–927

Brain Resuscitation Clinical Trial I Study Group 1986 Randomized clinical study of thiopental loading in comatose survivors of cardiac arrest. New England Journal of Medicine 314: 397–402

Caldwell G, Millar G, Wuinn E, Vincent R, Chamberlain D A 1985 Simple mechanical methods for cardioversion: defence of the precordial thump and cough version. British Medical Journal 291: 627–630

Davis L 1985 Cardiac arrest: a follow-up study. Medical Journal of Australia 142: 671–672

Hughes W G, Ruedy J R 1986 Should calcium be used in cardiac arrest? American Journal of Medicine 81: 285–296

Koster R W, Dunning A J 1985 Intramuscular lidocaine for prevention of lethal arrhythmias in the prehospitalization phase of acute myocardial infarction. New England Journal of Medicine 313: 1105–1110

Longstreth W T, Diehr P, Cobb L A, Hanson R W, Blair A D 1986 Neurologic outcome and blood glucose levels during out-of-hospital cardiopulmonary resuscitation. Neurology 36: 1186–1191

Pearn J 1985 Regular review: the management of near drowning. British Medical Journal 291: 1447–1452

Sullivan M J J, Guyatt G H 1986 Simulated cardiac arrest for monitoring quality of in-hospital resuscitation. Lancet 2: 618–620

Weil M H, Rackow E C, Trevino R, Grundler W, Falk J L, Griffel M I 1986 Difference in acid-base state between venous and arterial blood during cardiopulmonary resuscitation. New England Journal of Medicine 315: 153–156

BLOOD TRANSFUSION

There are still misgivings about the use of blood substitutes such as the perfluorocarbon 'Fluosol-DA'. Although they are capable of carrying oxygen and carbon dioxide and may be used for resuscitation when blood is not available there has been concern about their retention in the reticulo-endothelial system and activation of complement (see Singer & Goldstone 1985, Leading Article Lancet 1986). There have also been reports of hypotension, pulmonary insufficiency and reduction in white cell count. Stroma-free haemoglobin (solutions containing haemoglobin from haemo-lysed red cells) are being developed but have a short intravascular half-life and a high affinity for oxygen due to a reduction in 2,3-DPG. Solutions containing polymerized haemoglobin and pyridoxylated haemoglobin are being developed but as yet their use has still to be accepted.

It has been suggested that increased blood viscosity may reduce blood flow and hence oxygen transport. The reduced haemoglobin concentration is believed to reduce peripheral resistance and increase blood flow. However

Daniel et al (1986) suggested that compensating mechanisms are less than complete and oxygen transport falls on account of the reduced haemoglobin. To achieve the maximum oxygen transport requires the highest packed cell volume that can be achieved.

There have been reports of relationship between cancer of the colon and blood transfusion and the possibility that recurrence might be related to the administration of blood. Hamblin (1986) has summarized the debate and although further study is necessary, it appears that a factor present in the plasma may be responsible for encouraging metastatic spread. There may thus be a place for the routine use of packed red cells (whose viscosity is such that rapid transfusion is difficult) or red cells suspended in SAM solution.

REFERENCES

Daniel M K, Bennett B, Dawson A A, Rawles J M 1986 Haemoglobin concentration and linear cardiac output, peripheral resistance, and oxygen transport. British Medical Journal 292: 923–926
Hamblin T J 1986 Blood transfusions and cancer: anomalies explained? British Medical Journal 293: 517–518
Leading Article 1986 Blood substitutes. Has the right solution been found? Lancet 1: 717–718
Singer C R J, Goldstone A H 1985 Recent advances in blood transfusion and blood products. Kaufman L (ed) Anaesthesia review 3, Churchill Livingstone, London pp 156–182

SPINAL AND EXTRADURAL ANALGESIA

Shivering frequently occurs following extradural analgesia and this has been frequently observed in obstetric patients receiving bupivacaine. Walmsley et al (1986) noted that bupivacaine injected extradurally at 4°C resulted in almost a 50% incidence of shivering. The injection of the cold solution resulted in the temperature of the extradural space falling to 20°C. They suggested that extradural solutions should be warmed to 37°C before injection.

Wilson et al (1986) noted that obstetric patients given 150 mg of ranitidine by mouth 2 hours before extradural anaesthesia for Caesarean section had higher plasma bupivacaine concentrations than a control group, the difference being significant at 40 minutes although the level was below the toxic level.

Epidural analgesia has been advocated by Reynolds et al (1986) for spinal surgery including laminectomy and cordotomy. They reported excellent reports using bupivacaine or lignocaine. The patients remained conscious and were operated on in the prone position. There were no neurological problems despite the presence of pre-existing neurological deficit

Bigler et al (1986) compared the effects of intrathecal bupivacaine (3 ml — 5% in glucose) with tetracaine (3 ml — 0.5% in glucose). The onset of analgesia took 22 minutes following both drugs but there was a more profound fall in blood pressure following tetracaine. There was also a more pronounced sympathetic blockade confirmed by measurement of plasma noradrenaline and adrenaline. This is probably due to the higher spread centrally of the tetracaine blockade rather than a specific effect on sympathetic nerve fibres.

The neurological complications of spinal analgesia may be due to the lumbar puncture, or to the use of the drug or from contamination of the solution injected. The complications of spinal tap are discussed by Marton & Gean (1986) while the neurological complications following epidural analgesia are outlined by Skouen et al (1985) (see Complications, below).

REFERENCES

Bigler D, Hjorrso N C, Edstrom H, Christensen N J, Kehlet H 1986 Comparative effects of intrathecal bupivacaine on analgesia, cardiovascular function and plasma catecholamines. Acta Anaesthesiologica Scandinavica 30: 199–203
Marton K I, Gean A D 1986 The spinal tap: a new look at an old test. Annals of Internal Medicine 104: 840–848
Reynolds A F, Dauntenhahn D L, Fragraeus L, Pollay M 1986 Safety and efficacy of epidural analgesia in spinal surgery. Annals of Surgery 203: 225–227
Skouen J S, Wainapel S F, Willock M M 1985 Paraplegia following epidural anaesthesia. Acta Neurologica Scandinavica 72: 437–444
Wilson C M, Moore J, Ghaly R G, McClean E, Dundee J W 1986 Plasma bupivacaine concentrations associated with extradural anaesthesia for caesarean section. Influence of pretreatment with ranitidine. British Journal of Anaesthesia 58: 1330P–1331P
Walmsley A J, Giescke A H, Lipton J M 1986 Contribution of extradural temperature to shivering during extradural anaesthesia. British Journal of Anaesthesia 58: 1130–1134

COMPLICATIONS

Allergy

Ethylene oxide

Anaphylaxis may occur during haemodialysis with cardiovascular and respiratory side effects including hypotension, urticaria, wheezing and shortness of breath. Ethylene oxide has been implicated as a possible cause but the dialysis membrane (cuprammonium cellulose) may also be involved (Nicholls 1986).

Muscle relaxants
See above.

Epidural anaesthesia

Paraplegia

A recent case of paraplegia following epidural anaesthesia has been reported by Skouen et al (1985). The patient underwent cystectomy under epidural anaesthesia with 15 ml of 1.5% plain lignocaine. Additional doses of 10 ml of lignocaine 1.5% with adrenaline 1:100 000 were given on three occasions. The patient was also anaesthetized with thiopentone, fentanyl, suxamethonium and the duration of operation was 6 hours. During operation there was a period of hypotension which was thought to be due to retractors and packs which presumably compressed vessels for when these were removed the blood pressure and cardiac output were restored. Postoperative analgesia was achieved with an infusion of 0.2% bupivacaine, 10 ml/h administered via the epidural catheter and controlled by an Imed pump. On the following day when the epidural analgesia was discontinued motor power of the limbs was diminished but sensation was normal. Four months later there was improved motor function but the patient still required crutches for walking. The authors ascribed the cause of the paraplegia to the hypotension developing during operation although the purely motor symptoms were difficult to explain.

Skouen et al (1985) reviewed the literature of paraplegia following epidural anaesthesia and suggested they could be classified into five groups.

Group 1 is associated with dural puncture in which a massive dose of local anaesthetic may be given resulting in respiratory or circulatory depression. Sensory or motor loss postoperatively is usually temporary. If arachnoiditis develops either from contaminants or drugs such as 2-chloroprocaine then paralysis is likely to be permanent.

Group 2 is associated with instillation of a large volume of fluid into the subarachnoid space and may be due to compression of nerves in a narrow spinal canal. Neurological symptoms develop early postoperatively but are unlikely to be permanent.

Group 3. In this group there is ischaemia of the spinal cord following hypotension below 80 mmHg. There may also be pre-operative cardiovascular disease with poor perfusion of the spinal cord. Symptoms develop early but neurological damage is likely to be permanent.

Group 4. Neurological symptoms may be precipitated by epidural haematoma and may occur within a few hours to a few days postoperatively. If recognized early and treated by laminectomy there is usually a full recovery.

Group 5. This consists of a multiplicity of factors associated with compression, ischaemia and neurotoxicity of the local anaesthetic.

Endotracheal intubation

The acute complications of endotracheal intubation have been reported by Rashkin & Davis (1986). They studied 61 patients in intensive care units who had been intubated for more than 3 days and found that re-intubation and prolonged intubation led to a higher incidence of complications which included cuff-leak, pneumonia, stridor, tube malposition, aspiration, pneumothorax and miscellaneous orotracheal problems. The incidence of acute tracheolaryngeal complications, however, was not affected by re-intubation or prolonged intubation. The acute tracheolaryngeal complications included eight cases of oedema of the vocal cords, granuloma, tracheomalacia with necrosis, posterior laryngeal abscess and tracheal ulcer. Repeated intubation in neonates may result in tracheal stenosis (Graham, personal communication).

Although the prolonged high cuff pressure is a factor resulting in mucosal damage to the larynx, Cavo (1985) has shown that this factor may also affect the anterior branch of the recurrent laryngeal nerve just below the posterior end of the vocal cord. Endotracheal tubes should have a mark 1.5 cm above the upper level of the cuff to ensure accurate positioning of the tube — if this were standard practice the incidence of laryngeal paralysis would be considerably reduced (Leading Article Lancet 1986).

In animal models Whited (1985) found that in addition to cuff-pressure injury to the larynx there was also moderate to severe inflammatory oedema of the arytenoids which was only noted 3 days following extubation. There was limitation of vocal cord movement and incomplete adduction of the posterior part of the vocal cords. Whited (1985) claimed that the shaft of the endotracheal tube causes ulceration due to pressure and movement at the point of contact at the crico-arytenoid area and this is not alleviated by inserting a small tube which only allows it to move even more posteriorly into the interarytenoid space. From this study it would seem that the shape of the endotracheal tube needs to be redesigned. The use of sterile silastic tubes, which are claimed to be non-irritant have been found to reduce the incidence of postintubation hoarseness and tracheitis (personal series).

Multicore disease

Some of the features of multicore disease include congenital myopathy, hypotonia and delayed motor development. Koch et al (1985) have suggested that patients with this disease may react abnormally to anaesthesia. A patient aged $2\frac{1}{2}$ years developed congestive cardiac failure which was controlled with digoxin and diuretics. Following cardiac catheterization which demonstrated a large septal defect and mitral regurgitation the child developed a high temperature and died 26 hours later despite efforts at resuscitation. The drugs used during the cardiac catheterization included lignocaine and ketamine and it was suggested that the patient might have had an unusual form of malignant hyperpyrexia but most of the features of this were absent. The hyperthermia could be accounted for by sepsis or pulmonary infection in a hypotonic child.

REFERENCES

Cavo J W 1985 True vocal cord paralysis following intubation. Laryngoscope 95: 1352–1359
Graham Personal communication
Koch B M, Bertorini T E, Eng G D, Boehm R 1985 Severe multicore disease associated with reaction to anesthesia. Archives of Neurology 42: 1204–1206

Leading Article 1986 Laryngeal paralysis after endotracheal intubation. Lancet 1: 536–537
Nicholls A 1986 Ethylene oxide and anaphylaxis during haemodialysis. British Medical
    Journal 292: 1221–1222
Rashkin M C, Davis T 1986 Acute complications of endotracheal intubation. Relationship
    to reintubation, route, urgency and duration. Chest 89: 165–167
Skouen J S, Wainapel S F, Willock M M 1985 Paraplegia following epidural anesthesia.
    Acta Neurologica Scandinavica 72: 437–443
Whited R E 1985 A study of post-intubation laryngeal dysfunction. Laryngoscope
    95: 727–729

PAEDIATRICS

Respiration

The use of dry powdered surfactant administered via an endotracheal tube in babies with surfactant deficiency has proved singularly disappointing and compared with controls there was no difference in ventilator pressure or use of oxygen therapy. In the first 2 years of life morbidity and mortality were unaltered (Wilkinson 1985). In contrast Merritt et al (1986) using human surfactant obtained from amniotic fluid found that the prophylactic administration by endotracheal tube at birth of infants between 24–29 weeks prevented the respiratory distress syndrome or reduced its severity. There were fewer deaths, fewer cases of bronchopulmonary complications such as interstitial emphysema and pneumothorax as well as reduced period of intensive care.

Tarnow-Mordi et al (1986) have drawn attention to the inadequacy of humidification of inspired gases during artificial ventilation of the newborn. The physiological humidity of inspired air at body temperature in the mid-trachea is 44 mg H_2O/l and it was found from a questionnaire submitted to neonatal units in the British Isles that most babies were ventilated well below the minimum humidity recommended by the British Standards Institution (33 mg H_2O/l). Inadequate humidity could result in secretions becoming more viscous and ciliary activity and mucus flow being reduced.

Attempts at weaning from ventilators in infants is notoriously difficult but Mehta et al (1986) have designed a patient-triggered system which uses the SLE ventilator and the Graseby monitor. The system may be used for synchronized ventilation, that is for those infants who are breathing spontaneously but require ventilatory assistance, or alarm-triggered, that is for infants who are breathing adequately on CPAP but who are liable to apnoeic attacks. The apparatus was used successfully on nine infants but further studies are required to assess incidence of pneumothorax in acute hyaline membrane disease.

Southall et al (1985) described episodes of severe hypoxaemia in awake infants following noxious stimuli. The arterial PO_2 fell below 20 mmHg within 20 seconds resulting in unconsciousness and even convulsions. Inspiratory flow was absent with continuation of expiration. Phosphatidyl-choline was reduced in the tracheal aspirate which would affect surface tension. Continuous positive airway pressure (CPAP) increased the level of phosphatidylcholine.

Neonatal breathing patterns have been discussed by Johnson (1985) and in another study by Guilleminault et al (1986) infants classified as 'near-miss sudden infant death syndrome' (SIDS) had mixed and obstructive sleep apnoea. Other members of the family had obstructive sleep apnoea. X-rays have shown that the upper airways behind the base of the tongue are reduced in size and this may be a familial factor resulting in apnoea in infancy (see also Thawley 1985).

In a study of the regional ventilation in infants and small children Davies et al (1985) found that the distribution of ventilation was away from the dependent lung which is the reverse of that which occurs in adults. This may be due to differences in lung mechanics and diaphragmatic action. Thus young children with unilateral lung disease should be positioned with the normal lung uppermost.

Klein & Reynolds (1986) studied upper airway obstruction which occurred during sleep in children aged between 2 weeks and 45 months. They found that warm humidified air passed through a thin nasal pharyngeal tube at the rate of 2–10 l/min relieved the obstruction immediately. The work of breathing decreased and transcutaneous oxygen tension improved. The authors claim that the method is simple but the gas needs to be humidified and warmed to prevent drying up of secretions.

Cardiovascular system

Colley et al (1986) described the use of a sensor which can detect fetal heart sounds when placed on the mother's abdomen. It can also detect fetal breathing and results correlated well with those obtained from ultrasound. When the fetus was breathing there was a significant increase in variability of both systolic and diastolic times when compared with fetal non-breathing periods.

There has been a reappraisal of the technique of external cardiac massage. At present external cardiac compression is applied over the middle third of the sternum. However in a recent radiographic study taken of infants' thoraces it was shown that the centre of the heart lay behind the lower third of the sternum and in view of this finding it is suggested that external cardiac compression should be applied over the lower rather than the middle third of the sternum (Phillips & Zideman 1986).

REFERENCES

Colley N, Talbert D G, Abraham N G, Davies W L, Fayers P, Southall D P 1986 The fetal phonogram. A measurement of fetal activity. Lancet 1: 931–935
Davies H, Kitchman R, Gordon I, Helms P 1985 Regional ventilation in infancy: reversal of adult pattern. New England Journal of Medicine 313: 1626–1628

Guilleminault C, Heldt G, Powell N, Riley R 1986 Small upper airway in near-miss sudden infant death syndrome infants and their families. Lancet 1: 402–407

Johnson P 1985 Prolonged expiratory apnoea and implications for control of breathing. Lancet 2: 877–879

Klein M, Reynolds L G 1986 Relief of sleep-related oropharyngeal airway obstruction by continuous insufflation of the pharynx. Lancet 1: 935–939

Mehta A, Wright B M, Callan K, Stacey T E 1986 Patient-triggered ventilation in the newborn. Lancet 2: 17–19

Merritt T, Hallman M, Bloom B T et al 1986 Prophylactic treatment of very premature infants with human surfactant. New England Journal of Medicine 315: 785–790

Phillips G W L, Zideman D A 1986 Relation of infant heart to sternum: its significance in cardiopulmonary resuscitation. Lancet 1: 1024

Southall D P, Johnson P, Salmons S et al 1985 Prolonged expiratory apnoea: a disorder resulting in episodes of severe arterial hypoxaemia in infants and young children. Lancet 2: 571–577

Tarnow-Mordi W O, Fletcher M, Sutton P, Wilkinson A R 1986 Evidence of inadequate humidification of inspired gas during artificial ventilation of newborn babies in the British Isles. Lancet 2: 909–910

Thawley S E 1985 Sleep apnea disorders — symposium. Medical Clinics of North America 69: 1123–1358

Wilkinson A 1985 Two controlled trials of dry artificial surfactant: early effects and later outcome in babies with surfactant deficiency. Lancet 2: 287–291

Update (2)

GENERAL ANAESTHESIA

The mechanism of action of general anaesthesia is still not completely understood although interest has now focused on the calcium ion. Dolin & Little (1986) studied the effects of calcium-channel antagonists and found that they increased the potency of general anaesthesia. The drugs did not produce anaesthesia per se and did not affect concentrations of the anaesthetic agents either. On the other hand high pressure (70–130 atmospheres absolute) decreased the potency of althesin and methohexitone but to different degrees suggesting that the drugs act at different molecular sites (Halsey et al 1986).

With the advent of modern techniques depth of anaesthesia has become more difficult to gauge and the incidence of awareness appears to be increasing especially in obstetric anaesthesia. Analysis of the frequency and amplitude of the EEG has been singularly disappointing but auditory evoked potentials although of value in assessing depth of anaesthesia with volatile agents has proved again disappointing with intravenous drugs. Monitoring the contractility of the lower oesophagus is a new technique introduced for monitoring and may hold promise (Leading Article Lancet 1986).

The clinical pharmacokinetics of the new induction and analgesic agents are discussed in detail by Davis & Cook (1986). In addition the importance of plasma binding of drugs during anaesthesia has been outlined by Wood (1986) drawing attention not only to anaesthetic agents but also to drugs which might be used for patient treatment, the influence of age, pregnancy, hepatic disease, burns, myocardial infarction as well as the effects of surgery.

Thiopentone

Many recently introduced intravenous agents have been withdrawn because of possible toxic or allergic side effects. These include propanidid, althesin and minaxolone. Thiopentone continues to be the most frequently used

induction agent and interest has recently been awakened in its administration as the primary anaesthetic agent as a continuous infusion (Crankshaw et al 1985). An initial bolus dose was given based on lean body mass
to achieve a plasma concentration of 15 or 20 μg/ml. Plasma thiopentone
concentrations were maintained between 10 and 20 μg/ml during infusion
given in stages or in an exponential regime of infusion. The mean recovery
time was 111 minutes and the plasma clearance correlating with lean body
mass and to some extent with total body weight.

Etomidate

Etomidate is a short acting non-barbiturate induction agent producing
central depressant effects like GABA. Etomidate also has a local anaesthetic
on peripheral nerves but in concentrations much greater than that likely to
be produced in clinical anaesthesia (Benoit et al 1987). It produces pain if
injected into small veins but its major advantage is that it is said to produce
less cardiovascular depression. It is 75% protein bound, is metabolized in
the liver and has a short duration of action. Prolonged infusion with etomidate caused suppression of plasma cortisol and it is now contra-indicated
for intensive care use (Fellows et al 1983, Wagner et al 1984). Wanscher
et al (1985) found that etomidate completely blocked the adrenocortical
response to corticotrophin stimulation for at least 24 hours after surgery and
felt that the drug was contra-indicated for induction and maintenance of
anaesthesia. Fellows et al (1985) noted in patients having operation for
repair of inguinal hernia that etomidate suppressed the circulating levels of
cortisol at 90 and 120 minutes following induction and there was also an
elevation of plasma ACTH at 240 and 360 minutes. The effect of etomidate
on cortisol was transitory and there was no depression of the cardiovascular
system. At 90 minutes following induction there was also suppression of
circulating testosterone levels suggesting that etomidate acted not only at
the 11-beta-hydroxylase point but also at the 17-alpha-hydroxylase enzyme.
Boidin et al (1986) showed that an infusion of ascorbic acid (1000 mg)
restored the serum cortisol levels during etomidate infusion. They
concluded that etomidate interacts with cytochrome P450 which is involved
in ascorbic acid metabolism rather than corticosteroid synthesis.

De Coster et al (1985) noted that plasma aldosterone levels remained
within the normal range with etomidate but there was a twofold increase
if thiopentone was used as the induction agent. Bailey (1987) noted that
etomidate produced a 20% decrease in cortisol levels following induction
with etomidate and this lasted for at least 5 hours postoperatively. Mehta
et al (1985) also noted that plasma cortisol levels were suppressed with an
increase in ACTH and suggested that suppression of the endocrine response
to surgery is deemed to be beneficial. Moore et al (1985), using an etomidate infusion in patients undergoing hysterectomy, endorsed this view
adding that there were no adverse clinical sequelae attributable to the

suppression of cortisol. Gartner et al (1986) treated a patient with hyper-cortisolism due to ectopic ACTH production with an infusion of etomidate.

Propofol (Diprivan)

Another non-barbiturate recently introduced is propofol which is rapidly redistributed and metabolized so that repeated doses may be given without cumulative effects. The drug was initially introduced in cremophor EL but is now presented in soya bean oil and purified egg phosphatide. The recommended dose is 2.5 mg/kg. The main side effects appear to be pain on injection and depression of cardiac output in the elderly (Healy et al 1985).

REFERENCES

Bailey P M 1987 In press
Benoit E, Carratu M R, Dubois J M, Mitolo-Chieppa D, Preziusi P 1987
   Electrophysiological studies of the effects of the general anaesthetic etomidate on frog
   myelinated nerve fibre. British Journal of Pharmacology 90: 7–14
Boidin M P, Erdmann W E, Faithfull N S 1986 The role of ascorbic acid in etomidate
   toxicity. European Journal of Anaesthesiology 3: 417–422
Crankshaw D P, Edwards N E, Blackman G L, Boyd M D, Chan H N J, Morgan D J
   1985 Evaluation of infusion regimens for thiopentone as a primary anaesthetic agent.
   European Journal of Clinical Pharmacology 28: 543–552
Davis P J, Cook D R 1986 Clinical pharmacokinetics of the newer intravenous anaesthetic
   agents. Clinical Pharmacokinetics 11: 18–35
De Coster R, Helmers J H, Noorduin H 1985 Effects of etomidate on cortisol biosynthesis:
   site of action after induction of anaesthesia. Acta Endocrinologica 110: 526–531
Dolin S J, Little H J 1986 Augmentation by calcium channel antagonists of general
   anaesthetic potency in mice. British Journal of Pharmacology 88: 909–914
Fellows I W, Bastow M D, Byrne A J, Allison S P 1983 Adrenocorticol suppression in
   multiple injured patients: a complication of etomidate treatment. British Medical Journal
   287: 1835–1837
Fellows I W, Yeoman P M, Selby C, Byrne A J 1985 The effect of anaesthetic induction
   with etomidate on the endocrine response to surgical trauma. European Journal of
   Anaesthesiology 2: 285–290
Gartner R, Albrecht M, Muller O A 1986 Effect of etomidate on hypercortisolism due to
   ectopic ACTH production. Lancet 1: 275
Halsey M J, Wardley-Smith B, Wood S 1986 Pressure reversal of alphaxalone/alphadolone
   and methohexitone in tadpoles; evidence for different molecular sites for general
   anaesthesia. British Journal of Pharmacology 89: 299–305
Healy T E J (joint editor) 1985 Propofol (Diprivan). A new intravenous anaesthetic.
   Postgraduate Medical Journal 61 (suppl 3). Macmillan Press, London
Leading Article 1986 The depth of anaesthesia. Lancet 2: 553–554
Mehta M P, Dillman J B, Sherman B M, Ghoneim M M, Lemke J H 1985 Etomidate
   anesthesia inhibits the cortisol response to surgical stress. Acta Anaesthesiologica
   Scandinavica 29: 486–489
Moore R A, Allen M C, Wood P J, Rees L L H, Sear J W 1985 Perioperative endocrine
   effects of etomidate. Anaesthesia 40: 124–130
Wagner R L, White P F, Kan P B, Rosenthal M H, Feldman D 1984 Inhibition of adrenal
   steroidogenesis by the anaesthetic etomidate. New England Journal of Medicine
   310: 1415–1421
Wanscher M, Tonnesen E, Huttel M, Larsen K 1985 Etomidate infusion and
   adrenocortical function. Acta Anaesthesiologica Scandinavica 29: 483–485
Wood M 1986 Plasma drug binding: implications for anesthesiologists. Anesthesia and
   Analgesia 65: 786–804

ANAESTHETIC PROBLEMS

Paediatric radiotherapy

The difficulties of anaesthetizing and monitoring small children for radio-therapy have been outlined by Casey et al (1986). Initially ketamine was thought to be the ideal agent but the administration of the drug became stressful for the patients, the parents and even the anaesthetist. A more satisfactory technique involved the use of inhalational agents such as cyclo-propane and oxygen followed by nitrous oxide, oxygen and enflurane. Anaesthesia was maintained by insufflation via an oropharyngeal airway. During irradiation the child was observed from outside the treatment room with monitoring using an infra-red carbon dioxide analyzer which detected not only hypoventilation but also respiratory obstruction.

Ankylosing spondylitis

The pulmonary, neurological and cardiovascular complications of anky-losing spondylitis are hazards which may confront the anaesthetist. Fusion of the cervical vertebrae presents great difficulty with intubation and indi-rect laryngoscopy predicts the probability of problems. Fusion of the joints involved in the chest wall leads to ventilatory difficulties of a restrictive nature. Wittman & Ring (1986) described the management of patients at operation using thiopentone, nitrous oxide, oxygen and halothane without intubation for total hip replacement. The use of epidural or spinal block may be contra-indicated because of possible ossification of intraspinous liga-ments, or there may even be fractured vertebrae. Consideration should also be given to the possibility of the cardiorespiratory complications of spinal or epidural blockade in the situation where rapid intubation may be imposs-ible. Alternative methods of intubation are described including awake intubation, fibreoptic laryngoscopy and the use of percutaneous trans-tracheal jet ventilation.

Dental anaesthesia

Hamilton-Farrell & Nightingale (1986) investigated the cause of cardiac dysrhythmias seen during dental surgery under general anaesthesia. Although dysrhythmias were more common in the patients breathing spon-taneously with halothane compared with a group of patients who were ventilated to normocapnia, there appeared to be no correlation between the PCO_2, blood halothane levels and the appearance of dysrhythmias.

Fractured femur — use of methylmethacrylate cement

There have been numerous reports of cardiovascular instability during the use of bone cement during hip replacement for fractured femur. Svartling et al (1986) wondered whether the type of anaesthesia might have an influence on blood pressure during the procedure. Spinal analgesia with bupivacaine led to a fall in blood pressure with unaltered levels of plasma cortisol whereas under general anaesthesia with thiopentone, fentanyl, pancuronium, nitrous oxide and oxygen there was a rise in arterial blood pressure and plasma cortisol. The arterial oxygen fell in both groups of patients following the application of cement and was thought to be due to micro-embolism and pulmonary vasoconstriction. The stimulus of the cement application and impaction of the hip prosthesis is blocked by spinal analgesia leading to hypotension whereas the aftermath of endocrine stimulation under general anaesthesia served to keep the blood pressure elevated. In the elderly the use of spinal analgesia therefore may be less advantageous.

REFERENCES

Casey W F, Price V, Smith H S 1986 Anaesthesia and monitoring for paediatric radiotherapy. Journal of the Royal Society of Medicine 79: 454–456
Hamilton-Farrell, Nightingale J J 1986 Cardiac dysrhythmias, carbon dioxide tension and blood halothane concentrations during dental anaesthesia. British Journal of Clinical Pharmacology 22: 212P–213P
Svartling N, Lehtinen A-M, Tarkkanen L 1986 The effect of anaesthesia on changes in blood pressure and plasma cortisol levels induced by cementation with methylmetacrylate. Acta Anaesthesiologica Scandinavica 30: 247–252
Wittmann F W, Ring P A 1986 Anaesthesia for hip replacement in ankylosing spondylitis. Journal of the Royal Society of Medicine 79: 457–459

BENZODIAZEPINE

Wyllie et al (1986) have studied the effects of nitrazepam when used as an anticonvulsant in small children. In a controlled study they showed that nitrazepam delayed cricopharyngeal relaxation which allowed pharyngeal contents to reach the upper oesophagus before the upper oesophageal sphincter relaxed with the result that food was aspirated into the tracheobronchial tract. Secretions may also overflow from the mouth.

Withdrawal symptoms have been reported following the long term use of benzodiazepines including tinnitus, involuntary movements and confusion. Symptoms occurred earlier in patients who were being treated with short acting benzodiazepines (Busto et al 1986) but were likely to last for up to 4 weeks.

Roncari et al (1986) studied the pharmacokinetics of a benzodiazepine antagonist, Ro 15-1788 and found that following oral administration of 200 mg the drug was rapidly absorbed reaching a peak between 20 and 90 minutes. When 20 mg was given intravenously the drug was rapidly metabolized by the liver. The benzodiazepine antagonist has been used to shorten the recovery time following the use of intravenous midazolam for minor surgical procedures (Wolff et al 1986).

REFERENCES

Busto U, Sellers E M, Naranjo C A, Cappell H, Sanchez-Craig M, Sykora K 1986
Withdrawal reaction after long-term therapeutic use of benzodiazepines. New England
Journal of Medicine 315: 854–859
Roncari G, Ziegler W H, Guentert T W 1986 Pharmacokinetics of the new benzodiazepine
antagonist Ro 15-1788 in man following intravenous and oral administration. British
Journal of Clinical Pharmacology 22: 421–428
Wolff J, Carl P, Calusen T G, Mikkelsen B O 1986 Ro 15-1788 for postoperative recovery.
A randomised clinical trial in patients undergoing minor surgical procedures under
midazolam anaesthesia. Anaesthesia 41: 1001–1006
Wyllie E, Wyllie R, Cruse R P, Rothner A D, Erenberg G 1986 The mechanisms of
nitrazepam induced drooling and aspiration. New England Journal of Medicine
314: 35–38

NITROUS OXIDE

Sweeney et al (1985) have shown that dentists who use nitrous oxide for
relative analgesia during prolonged dental treatment such as conservation
had reduced vitamin B_{12} activity with changes in bone marrow secondary
to impaired synthesis of DNA. The concentration of nitrous oxide in the
dental surgery may be as high as 7000 p.p.m. (parts per million). Midwives
and other staff working in the labour ward where nitrous oxide is used for
analgesia were exposed to not less than 100 p.p.m.: in one hospital the
average level was 360 p.p.m. but this was reduced to 2.5 with scavenging
(Munley et al 1986).

Nitrous oxide may precipitate a neurological complication of vitamin B_{12}
deficiency. Schilling (1986) described two patients who developed subacute
combined degeneration of the spinal cord within 8 weeks of being anaesthetized with nitrous oxide, investigations revealing the subclinical signs of
vitamin B_{12} deficiency.

Prolonged inhalation of nitrous oxide in experimental animals may result
in an increase in neutrophils and macrophages in lavage fluid. There is also
a loss of lung elastin which returns to normal when the nitrous oxide is
discontinued (see Starcher 1986).

It has been suggested that nitrous oxide is a partial agonist at mu, kappa
and sigma opioid receptors and hence may be addictive. An analysis of the
literature revealed 32 cases of myeloneuropathy associated with nitrous
oxide abuse as well as addiction (Gillman 1986). It is suggested that nitrous
oxide which is readily available commercially should be placed under
stricter control.

Greenberg et al (1985) have described the use of a computer-based system
to evaluate psychological performance following the inhalation of 20%
nitrous oxide and 80% oxygen. The results showed there was short term
impairment of CNS function. The tests involved the use of a COMPAQ
computer and the relevant software.

Lamas et al (1985) have described pacemaker malfunction following
nitrous oxide anaesthesia. A patient had a pacemaker inserted and the
following day was anaesthetized for total hip replacement with nitrous

oxide. Intermittent failure of the pacemaker took place and it was noticed that there was crepitus and distension of the pacemaker. It appears that the pacemaker may have contained some air into which the nitrous oxide diffused. On the day following operation crepitus had disappeared and this coincided with a return of full function of the pacemaker.

REFERENCES

Gillman M A 1986 Nitrous oxide, an opioid addictive agent. American Journal of Medicine 81: 97–102
Greenberg B D, Moore P A, Latz R, Baker E L 1985 Computerized assessment of human neurotoxicity: sensitivity to nitrous oxide exposure. Clinical Pharmacology and Therapeutics 38: 656–660
Lamas G A, Rebecca G S, Braunwald N S, Antman E M 1985 Pacemaker malfunction after nitrous oxide anesthesia. American Journal of Cardiology 56: 995
Munley A J, Reailton R, Gray W M, Carter K B 1986 Exposure of midwives to nitrous oxide in four hospitals. British Medical Journal 293: 1063–1064
Schilling R F 1986 Is nitrous oxide a dangerous anesthetic for vitamin B_{12} deficient subjects? Journal of the American Medical Association 255: 1605–1606
Starcher B C 1986 Elastin and the lung. Thorax 41: 577–585
Sweeney B, Bingham R M, Amos R J, Petty A C, Cole P V 1985 Toxicity of bond marrow in dentists exposed to nitrous oxide. British Medical Journal 291: 567–569

HALOTHANE

Hepatotoxicity has been reviewed in detail by Kaplowitz (1986) drawing attention to the fact that injury to the liver by drugs may mimic any form of acute or chronic liver disease. Hepatocellular necrosis may be caused by a variety of drugs resulting in a characteristic pattern. Centrilobular necrosis may be caused by acetaminophen or halothane, diffuse necrosis by isoniazid or alpha methyldopa — a pattern very similar to that of viral hepatitis, or infiltration of the liver with microvesicles of fat seen after tetracycline or valproic acid.

Cholestatic liver damage may be caused by steroids, estrogens, chlorpromazine or erythromycin. A mixed pattern may be seen following phenytoin, quinidine or allopurinol. The predictability of toxicity is also discussed by Kaplowitz (1986). Isoniazid toxicity often occurs in slow acetylators. Cytochrome P450 frequently breaks down drugs into electrophiles or free radicals. Halothane is reduced by cytochrome P450 to form free radicals leading to the formation of peroxy-fatty acid radicals which break down to form toxic alkanes and aldehydes. Glutathione and tocopherol may have a protective action.

Electrophiles formed by oxidation of cytochrome P450 drugs such as acetaminophen result in covalent binding to proteins. There is another method involving redox cycling and this affects drugs such as nitrofurantoin. The mechanism of cell death is also discussed by Kaplowitz (1986) as well as hepatotoxicity by drugs (Aw 1986), drug-induced cholestasis (Simon 1986) as well as drug-induced chronic liver disease (Stolz 1986).

Sherlock (1986) has also reviewed hepatotoxicity due to drugs and classi-fied the responses. Paracetamol liver damage is related to electrophilic metabolites. Cimetidine inhibits P450 but the dose required will be so large as to become impracticable.

In relation to the drugs outlined by Sherlock (1986) that can cause hepatotoxicity halothane appears to occupy only a small place. Farrell et al (1985) suggested that there was a familial susceptibility in patients who are predisposed to develop halothane hepatitis. In a study of HLA antigens Otsuka et al (1985) divided patients recovering from halothane hepatitis into two groups. In the non-jaundiced patients the HLA-Bw44 was high whereas the HLA-DR2 or Aw24-Bw52-DR2 were high in the jaundiced group. This study is of interest in that pyrexia was observed in all jaundiced patients but only in two-thirds of the non-jaundiced group. There were more females in the jaundiced group compared with the non-jaundiced and obes-ity, surprisingly, was more common in the non-jaundiced group. They sug-gested that the jaundiced patients were more likely to be sensitized to halothane whereas in the non-jaundiced group the mechanism may have been direct hepatic damage.

In a leading article (Lancet 1986) there is a discussion entitled 'Halo-thane-associated liver damage' in which the pathways of halothane metab-olism are summarized and it appears that under hypoxic conditions metabolites are formed which can cause liver damage. It is also a sad reflec-tion that patients who developed fulminating hepatic failure had fully docu-mented evidence of adverse response to halothane in a previous exposure. Children thought to be immune to halothane hepatotoxicity may also suffer liver damage (St Haxholdt et al 1986). On the other hand Wark et al (1986) while noting that some minor degrees of liver dysfunction did occur felt that, as a result of a prospective study of repeated halothane anaesthesia in children, there was no need to restrict its use according to the recommen-dations advocated for adults.

Blogg (1986) is of the opinion that the problem of 'halothane hepatitis' may only be solved by the use of alternative agents, especially if there is a family history or signs of possible hepatitis following a previous exposure. Unfortunately information of the drugs used at a previous operation are often not readily available especially if it took place at another hospital.

The Committee on Safety of Drugs (1986) analyzed 250 reports of cases of jaundice following halothane anaesthesia and have made the following recommendations.

1. A careful anaesthetic history should be taken to determine previous exposure and previous reactions to halothane.
2. Repeated exposure to halothane within a period of at least 3 months should be avoided unless there are over-riding clinical circumstances.
3. A history of unexplained jaundice or pyrexia in a patient following exposure to halothane is an absolute contra-indication to its future use in that patient.

Although there have been reports that enflurane may be hepatotoxic Eger et al (1986) have re-assessed the evidence (see also *Anaesthesia Review 3*). They evaluated 88 possible cases that might have occurred and were unable to find a convincing link between enflurane anaesthesia and subsequent liver damage. There was no characteristic liver damage such as centrilobular necrosis. Eger et al (1986) concluded that if enflurane could be implicated in causing hepatitis it was a very rare occurrence.

Anaesthesia and liver disease has been reviewed by McEvedy et al (1986) in which hepatic function was discussed in detail. Attention was also drawn to impairment of cardiovascular function, renal function, neurological function and problems of coagulation. The problems of the use of various anaesthetic agents are outline as well as the effect of reduced liver function on drug metabolism.

It is often forgotten that liver function may affect the metabolism of steroids. Oral prednisone can be given to patients with severe liver damage and although there is a reduction in conversion of prednisone to prednisolone there is also reduced metabolism of prednisolone. The amount of unbound prednisolone in patients with liver failure is higher than normal following oral prednisone or intravenous prednisolone and this may cause more pronounced effects (Renner et al 1986).

REFERENCES

Aw T K 1986 Drug-induced hepatotoxicity. Annals of Internal Medicine 104: 830–831
Blogg C E 1986 Halothane and the liver: the problem revisited and made obsolete. British Medical Journal 292: 1691–1692
Committee on Safety of Drugs 1986 No. 18
Eger E I, Smuckler E A, Ferrell L D, Choldsmith C H, Johnson B H 1986 Is enflurane hepatotoxic? Anesthesia and Analgesia 65: 21–30
Farrell G, Prendergast D, Murray M 1985 Halothane hepatitis. Detection of a constitutional susceptibility factor. New England Journal of Medicine 313: 1310–1314
Kaplowitz N 1986 Drug-induced hepatotoxicity. Annals of Internal Medicine 104: 826–839
Leading Article 1986 Halothane-associated liver damage. Lancet 1: 1251–1252
McEvedy B A, Shelly M P, Park G R 1986 Anaesthesia and liver disease. British Journal of Hospital Medicine 36: 26–34
Otsuka S, Yamamoto M, Kasuya S et al 1985 HLA antigens in patients with unexplained hepatitis following halothane anesthesia. Acta Anaesthesiologica Scandinavica 29: 497–501
Renner E, Horber F F, Jost G, Frey B M, Frey F J 1986 Effect of liver function on the metabolism of prednisone and prednisolone in humans. Gastroenterology 90: 819–828
St Haxholdt, O, Loft S, Clemmensen A, Hjortso E H 1986 Increased hepatic microsomal activity after halothane anaesthesia in children. Anaesthesia 41: 579–581
Sherlock S 1986 The spectrum of hepatotoxicity due to drugs. Lancet 2: 440–444
Simon F R 1986 Drug-induced hepatotoxicity. Annals of Internal Medicine 104: 831–834
Stolz A 1986 Drug-induced hepatotoxicity. Annals of Internal Medicine 104: 834–837
Wark H, O'Halloran M, Overton J 1986 Prospective study of liver function in children following multiple halothane anaesthetics at short intervals. British Journal of Anaesthesia 58: 1224–1228

ANALGESIC AGENTS

Fentanyl

The cardiovascular depressant effects of fentanyl including hypotension and bradycardia have been ascribed to its vagal effect. Anand et al (1987) reported favourably on the use of fentanyl (10 μg/kg) in reducing the stress response to ligation of patent ductus arteriosus leading to a possible improvement on the outcome of surgery.

In a recent study in animals Gautret & Schmitt (1985) demonstrated that there was not only a vagal action but in high doses it also appears to stimulate opioid receptors in the heart leading to bradycardia. There is also a direct central sympathomimetic stimulating action (alpha$_2$) which is masked by the vagal effect.

Alfentanil

In a reappraisal of alfentanil (Drug and Therapeutics Bulletin 1986) it was suggested that delayed respiratory arrest could occur in the postoperative period, not unlike that of the longer acting fentanyl. Bradycardia and asystole have been reported in patients who were not given atropine. Although alfentanil has attractive properties for day case surgery the possibility of adverse effects may limit its use.

Shafer et al (1986) demonstrated there was a wide range of clinical response to fixed doses of alfentanil and careful respiratory monitoring was recommended to minimize the possible hazards of postoperative respiratory depression.

In animal experiments Fone & Wilson (1986) showed that alfentanil prolonged inspiration by increasing the discharge duration of inspiratory neurones and expiration was delayed in onset. The effect can be prevented by pretreatment with naloxone. It is suggested that narcotic analgesics such as alfentanil and morphine, phenoperidine and fentanyl which also produce this effect do so by altering the mechanisms which determine the cessation of inspiration.

Hill et al (1986) conducted a study of subanaesthetic doses of alfentanil during painful dental stimulation assessing the response by reporting pain (PR) and by brain-evoked potentials (EP). The EP scores follow the distribution of alfentanil but the correlation was less during the elimination phase of the drug. The PR followed the elimination of alfentanil but not its distribution and the authors concluded that these two methods of assessment might identify different central effects with this analgesic.

Sufentanil

This is a potent synthetic agent related to fentanyl but is five to ten times more potent. It is 92% protein-bound and the volume distribution is smaller than that for fentanyl but larger than that for alfentanil.

Lofentanil

Lofentanil is 20 times more potent than fentanyl and has a much longer duration of action.

Morphine and prochlorperazine

Prochlorperazine, an anti-emetic drug, has no effect on resting ventilation or the respiratory response to hypercapnia. Morphine caused a significant fall in the ventilatory response to hypoxia. This was reversed by the administration of 12.5 mg of prochlorperazine but it did not affect the depression in the ventilatory response to hypercapnia caused by morphine (Olson et al 1986). Prochlorperazine may be acting as a dopamine antagonist at the site of carotid body. Somatostatin also has an inhibitory effect on the ventilatory response to hypoxia but has little effect on the hypercapniac response. Prochlorperazine increased the hypoxic response. This study suggested that the inhibitory action of somatostatin was on the carotid body (Maxwell et al 1986)

REFERENCES

Anand K J S, Sippell W G, Aynsley-Green A 1987 Randomised trial of fentanyl anaesthesia in preterm babies undergoing surgery: effects on the stress response. Lancet 1: 62–66
Drug and Therapeutics Bulletin 1986 Alfentanil in anaesthesia. Drug and Therapeutics Bulletin 24: 51–52
Fone K C F, Wilson H 1986 The effects of alfentanil and selected narcotic analgesics on the rate of action potential discharge of medullary respiratory neurones in anaesthetized rats. British Journal of Pharmacology 89: 67–76
Gautret B, Schmitt H 1985 Multiple sites for the cardiovascular actions of fentanyl in rats. Journal of Cardiovascular Pharmacology 7: 649–652
Hill H, Walter H, Saeger L, Sargur M, Sizemore W, Chapman C R 1986 Dose effects of alfentanil in human analgesia. Clinical Pharmacology and Therapeutics 40: 178–186
Maxwell D L, Nolop K B, Hughes J M B 1986 Effects of somatostatin, naloxone and prochlorperazine on the control of ventilation in man. Clinical Science 70: 547–554
Olson L G, Hensley M J, Saunders N A 1986 The effects of combined morphine and prochlorperazine on ventilatory control in humans. American Review of Respiratory Diseases 133: 558–561
Shafer A, Sung M-L, White P F 1986 Pharmacokinetics and pharmacodynamics of alfentanil infusions during general anesthesia. Anesthesia and Analgesia 65: 1021–1028

NALOXONE

Shock

In conscious rats following 20% haemorrhage of blood volume meptazinol led to a rapid and sustained increase in blood pressure to prehaemorrhage levels. Naloxone was equally effective. Meptazinol and naloxone increased blood pressure and total peripheral resistance but did not significantly alter heart rate or cardiac output. In 40% haemorrhage an infusion of meptazinol or naloxone partially restored blood pressure. In this study it was shown that meptazinol has a similar cardiovascular profile to naloxone but the former drug also had analgesic effects (Chance et al 1985).

Beta-endorphin

Beta-endorphin levels have been measured during the surgical removal of impacted wisdom teeth under local anaesthesia (Hargreaves et al 1986). Patients receiving naloxone had an increased level of beta-endorphin and pain compared with controls but the levels were reduced in patients given fentanyl and diazepam. Noradrenaline levels were increased in response to surgical stress except in patients receiving diazepam.

Phaeochromocytoma

Intravenous naloxone releases catecholamines in patients with phaeochromocytoma or paraganglioma. There was a marked rise in circulating noradrenaline despite the prior administration of phenoxybenzamine and propranolol. Two of the four patients investigated had marked rises in both systolic and diastolic blood pressure: these effects only occurred following 10 mg of naloxone but not after (2 mg). The mechanism for this effect may be due to the presence of naloxone-resistant opioid receptors in chromaffin tissue (Bouloux et al 1986).

Cushing's disease

In healthy subjects naloxone (0.2 mg/kg) increased plasma levels of ACTH, beta-endorphin and cortisol but in three patients out of nine with Cushing's disease (ACTH-dependent) levels were decreased (Baranowska et al 1985). It was suggested that there was some abnormality of the hypothalamic-pituitary-adrenal axis.

Insulin

Naloxone, 0.4 mg intravenously followed by an infusion at the rate of 0.066 mg/min for 2 hours, was shown to affect plasma insulin levels after oral glucose in obese subjects. These levels were reduced suggesting that opioids may affect the beta cell response to glucose (Vettor et al 1985). This response was similar to that previously reported in type 2 diabetics.

Captopril

Naloxone reverses the hypotension and bradycardia induced by captopril which appears to potentiate the effects of endogenous opioids. Oral captopril led to significant falls in blood pressure, but when it was administered after a bolus injection of 10 mg it was ineffectual. The heart rate was higher when the drugs were given together than during captopril alone. Neither captopril nor naloxone caused sedation when administered singly but in combination sedation resulted suggesting that captopril may have a central action as well (Ajayi et al 1985). In essential hypertensive patients naloxone does not appear to modify the antihypertensive action of captopril (Bernini et al 1985).

REFERENCES

Ajayi A A, Campbell B C, Rubin P C, Reid J L 1985 Effect of naloxone on the actions of captopril. Clinical Pharmacology and Therapeutics 38: 560–565
Baranowska B, Dorobek W, Misiorowski W, Jeske W, Abdel-Fattah M H 1985 The effect of naloxone on ACTH and beta-endorphin in patients with Cushing's disease. Acta Endocrinologica 110: 170–175
Bernini G, Taddei S, Graziadei L, Pedrinelli R, Salvetti A 1985 Naloxone does not modify the antihypertensive effect of captopril in essential hypertensive patients. Journal of Hypertension 3 (suppl 2): S117–S119
Bouloux P-M G, Grossman A, Besser G M 1986 Naloxone provokes catecholamine release in phaeochromocytomas and paragangliomas. Clinical Endocrinology 24: 319–325
Chance E, Paciorek P M, Todd M H, Waterfall J F 1985 Comparison of the cardiovascular effects of meptazinol and naloxone following haemorrhagic shock in rats. British Journal of Pharmacology 86: 43–53
Hargreaves K M, Dionne R A, Mueller G P, Goldstein D S, Dubner R 1986 Naloxone, fentanyl and diazepam modify plasma beta-endorphin levels during surgery. Clinical Pharmacology and Therapeutics 40: 165–171
Vettor R, Martini C, Manno M, Cestaro S, Federspil G, Sicolol N 1985 Effect of naloxone-induced opiate receptors blockade on insulin secretion in obesity. Hormone and Metabolic Research 17: 374–375

APPARATUS

Glass ampoules and needles

The hazards of injecting drugs from glass ampoules have been noted by Shaw & Lyall (1985) who found that glass particles could be aspirated into a syringe via a 19 but not a 21 gauge needle. They suggest that injections made through needles larger than 21 gauge should be made through a micropore filter. Waller & George (1986) reviewed many of the problems resulting from glass fragments and infusions and comment on the use of in-line filters. It may well be that glass will be replaced as a container for drugs in the future.

The dangers of needle-prick injuries has been restated by Nixon et al (1986) who describe the use of a device which would prevent injury during recapping of needles and which would make their disposal much safer. Accidents were five times less frequent when the protecting device was used.

Intravenous infusion

It is often assumed that drugs injected into the tubing of an intravenous administration set act perhaps almost instantaneously. Hutton & Thornberry (1986) have shown that when an extension piece (1250 mm in length) is attached to the set and the injection made at the end distal to the patient, it could take up to 3 minutes for 90% of a 1 ml or 3 ml injection to actually enter the patient's vein despite the fluid running as a continuous stream when observing the drip chamber. There was a hyperbolic relationship between the flow rate of the infusion and the time of delivery of a given percentage of the drug. A more effective way was flushing the drug in with a syringe of saline which produced a non-laminar flow.

Self-adhesive patches which release glyceryl trinitrate if applied to intravenous infusion sites led to a marked reduction of infusion failure whether it was due to extravasation or phlebitis (Wright et al 1985). The glyceryl trinitrate given transdermally acts by producing local venous dilatation. The only complication was headache which responded to simple analgesics.

Anaesthetic apparatus

Heneghan (1986) had drawn attention to the output of vaporizers and gas-driven ventilators such as the Blease-Manley. Although the concentration of vapour may be accurate on leaving the vaporizer outlet it was reduced when it reached the patient. Nunn (1986) confirmed that the Northwick Park anaesthetic apparatus delivered a vapour concentration 15% less than that indicated on the dial. Vaporizers based on the copper kettle principle and controlled by microprocessors may soon be available to deliver accurate and predictable concentrations of anaesthetic vapours (Hahn et al 1986).

Endotracheal tubes

Intracuff and 'leak-past' pressures of various types of tubes have been measured by Shah & Mapleson (1986) in which it was shown that air diffused out of the cuff irrespective of the material, whether it was red rubber, latex or PVC. The material of the cuff 'crept' under stress increasing cuff volume. The study showed that the 'leak-past' pressure decreased with red rubber and latex tubes but increased with PVC tubes for at least 75 minutes. Chandler (1986) has reviewed many of the factors affecting pressure changes in the cuff of endotracheal tubes including permeability coefficient, cuff thickness and volume and whether the cuff was filled with fluid or gas. The most important gas crossing the cuff membrane is oxygen and during oxygen therapy with 30% oxygen the pressure in the cuff could increase by 0.9 kPa (90 mm H_2O). Ideally the pressure in the cuff should be monitored.

Chandler & Crawley (1986) suggested that the size of endotracheal tube should be rationalized and they recommended a tube of 7.5 mm and 8.5 mm (internal diameter) for female and male patients respectively. As the trachea is capable of dilatation the diameter of low pressure high volume cuffs should be 20.5 mm for females and 27.5 mm for males.

The importance of these studies on tube size and cuff pressures is not only the possibility of mucosal damage to the larynx and trachea but also the dangers of vocal cord paralysis (Leading Article Lancet 1986) (see Complications).

Intubation aid

Although many aids to intubation have been described there have been few controlled studies on the success rate. Ellis et al (1986) have compared the use of a lighted stilette with the use of the laryngoscope. Intubation was performed under general anaesthesia with a non-depolarizing muscle relaxant and the patients monitored with non-invasive blood pressure recorders. More than one attempt had to be made using the stilette but there was no significant difference in the time required to intubate. There was also an increased incidence of cardiac arrhythmias of short duration when the stilette was used. The incidence of sore throat or hoarseness was comparable.

Patient monitoring

Mandatory standards

The Harvard Medical School have laid down mandatory standards for minimal patient monitoring during anaesthesia and these include the measurement of blood pressure and heart rate every 5 minutes and the continuous display of the ECG from induction of anaesthesia. During operation in addition to observation of respiratory and circulatory parameters they recommend the monitoring of end-tidal CO_2 and direct or indirect arterial blood pressure which where possible should be continuous. Automatic ventilator alarms indicating high pressure or disconnection are included as well as an oxygen analyzer to measure the concentration of oxygen in the circuit. The patient's temperature should also be measured at operation (Eichhorn et al 1986).

The indications for arterial blood gas analysis have been set out by Raffin (1986) and these include acute and chronic pulmonary disease, acute respiratory failure, cardiovascular disease with cardiac failure, pulmonary shunting and acid base disturbances. Excess amounts of heparin when obtaining the arterial sample may lead to spurious results (Bloom et al 1985).

Neuromuscular blockade

The desirability of monitoring the state of neuromuscular blockade was emphasized by Astley (see *Anaesthesia Review 4*). One of the problems has been to find suitable equipment for clinical use. Pollmaecher et al (1986) have described a pocket-sized battery-operated peripheral nerve stimulator with a calibrated constant current output. The Datex Relaxograph has been assessed by Carter et al (1986) and although only measuring the electrical response to nerve stimulation it appears to correlate satisfactorily with muscle output measured by a force transducer.

Blood pressure

A prototype finger sphygmomanometer has been developed as a screening device for patients with possible hypertension. Close et al (1986) found that the apparatus compared satisfactorily with the standard mercury column sphygmomanometer for systolic pressure.

There are occasions where access to an arm for measuring blood pressure is limited and blood pressure measurements are then taken from a cuff applied to the thigh. Goldthorp et al (1986) found there were significant differences in the thigh:arm systolic and diastolic pressures. The mean thigh pressure approximated to the calculated mean pressure for the arm.

Echocardiography

The theory, techniques and applications of Doppler echocardiography have been reviewed by Nishimura et al (1985) indicating the possibility of its use for measuring cardiac output, the magnitude of left to right shunts and possibility of assessing the patency of coronary bypass grafts.

Nuclear magnetic resonance spectroscopy

The use of a non-invasive technique involving nuclear magnetic resonance spectroscopy has been introduced to study the effects of tourniquet ischaemia in animals. During the period of ischaemia the pH within the muscle became acidic, phosphocreatine level decreased and inorganic phosphate rose. After 2 hours of tourniquet ischaemia phosphocreatine was absent and ATP was not detected after $3\frac{1}{2}$ hours. If ATP was present metabolic recovery occurred within 1 hour after tourniquet release but it took 3 hours or more if there was no ATP present. The ATP level could be maintained by releasing the tourniquet at hourly intervals for 10 minutes but if the intervals were only 5 minutes there was a lower protective effect and in fact the pH became more acidic. The use of heparin and steroids were without any beneficial effect (Newman 1984).

REFERENCES

Bloom S A, Canzanello V J, Strom J A, Madias N E 1985 Spurious assessment of acid-base status due to dilutional effect of heparin. American Journal of Medicine 79: 528–530
Carter J A, Arnold R, Yate P M, Flynn P J 1986 Assessment of the Datex Relaxograph during anaesthesia and atracurium-induced neuromuscular blockade. British Journal of Anaesthesia 58: 1447–1452
Chandler M 1986 Pressure changes in tracheal tube cuffs. Anaesthesia 41: 287–293
Chandler M, Crawley B E 1986 Rationalization of the selection tracheal tubes. British Journal of Anaesthesia 58: 111–116
Close A, Hamilton G, Muriss S 1986 Finger systolic pressure: its use in screening for hypertension and monitoring. British Medical Journal 293: 775–778

Eichhorn J H, Cooper J B, Cullen D J, Maier W R, Philip J H, Seeman R G 1986 Standards for patient monitoring during anesthesia at Harvard Medical School. Journal of the American Medical Association 256: 1017–1020

Ellis D G, Jakymec A, Kaplan R M et al 1986 Guided orotracheal intubation in the operating room using a lighted stylet: a comparison with direct laryngoscopic technique. Anesthesiology 64: 823–826

Goldthorp S L, Cameron A, Asbury A J 1986 Dinamap arm and thigh arterial pressure measurement. Anaesthesia 41: 1032–1038

Hahn C E W, Palayiwa E, Sugg B R, Lindsay-Scott 1986 A microprocessor-controlled anaesthetic vaporizer. British Journal of Anaesthesia 58: 1161–1166

Heneghan C P H 1986 Vaporizer output and gas driven ventilators. British Journal of Anaesthesia 58: 932

Hutton P, Thornberry E A 1986 Factors affecting delivery of drug through extension tubing. British Journal of Anaesthesia 58: 1141–1148

Leading Article 1986 Laryngeal paralysis after endotracheal intubation. Lancet 1: 536–537

Newman R J 1984 Metabolic effect of tourniquet ischaemia studied by nuclear magnetic resonance spectroscopy. Journal of Bone and Joint Surgery 66B: 434–440

Nishimura R A, Miller F A, Callahan M J, Benassi R C, Seward J B, Tajik A J 1985 Doppler echocardiography: theory, instrumentation, technique and application. Mayo Clinic Proceedings 60: 321–343

Nixon A D, Law R, Officer J A, Cleland J F, Goldwater P N 1986 Simple device to prevent accidental needle-prick injuries. Lancet 1: 888–889

Nunn J F 1986 British Journal of Anaesthesia 58: 932–933

Pollmaecher T, Steiert H, Buzello W 1986 A constant current peripheral nerve stimulator (Neurostim T4). Description and evaluation in volunteers. British Journal of Anaesthesia 58: 1443–1446

Raffin T A 1986 Indications for arterial blood gas analysis. Annals of Internal Medicine 105: 390–398

Shah M V, Mapleson W W 1986 Intracuff and 'leak-past' pressures of red rubber, latex and p.v.c. tubes. A laboratory and clinical study. British Journal of Anaesthesia 58: 103–110

Shaw N J, Lyall E G H 1985 Hazards of glass ampoules. British Medical Journal 291: 1390

Waller D G, George C F 1986 Ampoules, infusions and filters. British Medical Journal 292: 714–715

Wright A, Hecker J F, Lewis G B H 1985 Use of transdermal glyceryl trinitrate to reduce failure of intravenous infusion due to phlebitis and extravasation. Lancet 2: 1148–1150

Index